THE MAMMALIAN FETUS

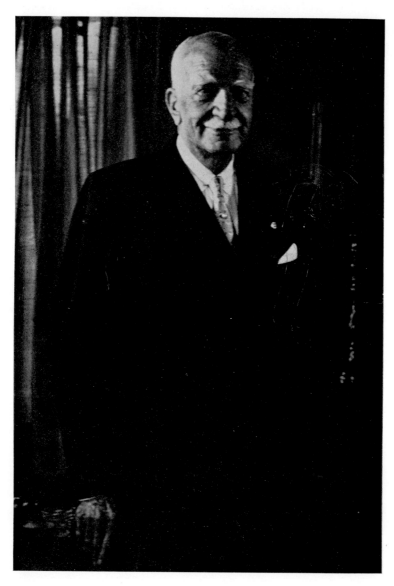

This volume is dedicated to Charles Stewart Mott (1875-1973) who contributed so richly to the improvement of the quality of life.

THE
MAMMALIAN
FETUS

COMPARATIVE BIOLOGY
AND METHODOLOGY

Edited by

E. S. E. HAFEZ

Reproductive Physiology Laboratories,
C. S. Mott Center
for Human Growth and Development
Wayne State University
School of Medicine
Detroit, Michigan

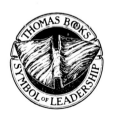

CHARLES C THOMAS · PUBLISHER
Springfield · Illinois · U.S.A.

Published and Distributed Throughout the World by
CHARLES C THOMAS • PUBLISHER
Bannerstone House
301-327 East Lawrence Avenue, Springfield, Illinois, U.S.A.

© 1975, by CHARLES C THOMAS • PUBLISHER
ISBN 0-398-03285-8
Library of Congress Catalog Card Number: 74-19867

Printed in the United States of America
W-2

Library of Congress Catalog Card Number: 74-19867

Hafez, E. S. E.
        Mammalian fetus.
Illinois   Charles C Thomas
Jan. 1975
                9-12-74

CONTRIBUTORS

H. W. BERENDES: *Fertility Regulating Methods Evaluation Branch, Center for Population Research, National Institute of Child Health and Human Development, Bethesda, Maryland.*

PAUL COSTILOE, Ph.D., *Department of Biostatistics and Epidemiology*

WARREN CROSBY, *Professor of Obstetrics and Gynecology, Department of Gynecology and Obstetrics*

T. N. EVANS: *Department of Gynecology-Obstetrics, Director, C. S. Mott Center for Human Growth and Development, Wayne State University School of Medicine, Detroit, Michigan.*

P. GRUENWALD: *Departments of Pathology and Pediatrics, Hahnemann Medical College and Hospital, Philadelphia, Pennsylvania.*

E. S. E. HAFEZ: *Departments of Gynecology-Obstetrics and Physiology, and C. S. Mott Center for Human Growth and Development, Wayne State University School of Medicine, Detroit, Michigan.*

V. HAMBURGER: *Department of Biology, Washington University, St. Louis, Missouri.*

P. G. HARDING: *Department of Obstetrics-Gynecology, St. Joseph's Hospital, London, Ontario.*

M. A. HEYMANN: *Departments of Pediatrics and Physiology, Cardiovascular Research Institute, University of California, San Francisco School of Medicine, San Francisco, California.*

H. S. HARNED, JR.: *The University of North Carolina at Chapel Hill, The School of Medicine, Senior Investigator of North*

Carolina Heart Association, Department of Pediatrics, Chapel Hill, North Carolina.

R. L. HENRY: *Department of Physiology, Wayne State University School of Medicine, Detroit, Michigan.*

GAIL JACOBSON, Ph.D., *Research Associate, Department of Pediatrics and Department of Biochemistry and Molecular Biology*

L. I. KLEINMAN: *Department of Environmental Health, University of Cincinnati Medical Center, Cincinnati, Ohio.*

G. KUPPE: *Department of Obstetrics-Gynecology, Medical School of University Essen, Essen, Germany.*

H. LUDWIG: *Department of Obstetrics and Gynecology, Medical School of University Essen, Essen, Germany.*

MOSTAFA MAMEESH, Ph.D., *Research Associate Professor, Department of Pediatrics and Department of Biochemistry and Molecular Biology*

JACK METCOFF, M.S., M.D., *Professor, Department of Pediatrics and Department of Biochemistry and Molecular Biology*

HILDEGARD METZGER: *Department of Obstetrics and Gynecology, Medical School of Essen, Essen, Germany.*

R. E. MYERS: *Laboratory of Perinatal Physiology, National Institute of Neurological Diseases and Stroke, Bethesda, Maryland.*

H. L. NADLER: *Department of Pediatrics, Northwestern University Medical School, Chicago, Illinois.*

R. M. NALBANDIAN: *Department of Pathology, Blodgett Memorial Hospital, Grand Rapids, Michigan.*

F. POSSMAYER: *Departments of Obstetrics and Biochemistry, University of Western Ontario Medical School, London, Ontario, Canada.*

A. M. RUDOLPH: *Professor of Pediatrics and Physiology, Cardiovascular Research Institute, University of California, San Francisco School of Medicine, San Francisco, California.*

E. RUOSLAHTI: *Department of Gynecology-Obstetrics and Department of Serology and Bacteriology, University of Helsinki, Helsinki, Finland.*

M. SEPPALA: *Department of Gynecology-Obstetrics and Department of Serology and Bacteriology, University of Helsinki, Helsinki, Finland.*

D. SECCOMBE: *Faculty of Graduate Studies, University of Western Ontario, London, Ontario, Canada.*

J. L. SEVER: *Collaborative and Field Research, Infectious Diseases Branch, National Institute of Neurological Diseases and Stroke, Bethesda, Maryland.*

J. SINCLAIR: *Department of Pediatrics, McMaster University, Hamilton, Ontario, Canada.*

P. I. TERASAKI: *Department of Surgery, School of Medicine, University of California, Los Angeles, California.*

J. B. WARSAW: *Department of Pediatrics and Obstetrics and Gynecology, Division of Perinatal Medicine, New Haven, Connecticut.*

FRANCINE WEHMER: *Departments of Psychology and Physiology and C. S. Mott Center for Human Growth and Development, Wayne State University School of Medicine, Detroit, Michigan.*

PREFACE

A SYMPOSIUM ON the comparative biology and methodology of "The Mammalian Fetus" was held on December 3 and 4, 1973, at the Purple Auditorium in Gordon Scott Basic Medical Sciences Building, to dedicate the foundation of C. S. Mott Center for Human Growth and Development. The elegant presentations and elaborate discussions dealt with modern concepts and recent advances in the control of fetal circulation, perinatal respiratory physiology, fetal behavior, lipid substrates and fetal development, perinatal energy metabolism, fetal water and electrolyte balance, fetal under-nutrition, biophysical techniques to study the fetus, feto-maternal incompatibility-HL-A antibody, intrauterine detection of biochemical disorders and fetal malnutrition, embryological basis of abnormal development, Müllerian defects, maternal health and fetal development, and fetal responses to asphyxia.

In the study of mammalian fetus one discovers the past and the future. The history of living organisms is written in the development of the embryo and fetus, revealing the patterns of anatomy, physiology, and behavior that may have characterized ancestral organisms. It is this past which may reveal answers to questions about the structure and function of contemporary man, just as archeology reveals the source of contemporary societies. The future of the individual, and of the social orders in which these individuals live, may also be determined by the strength of that foundation, which is manifested by fetal health. It is not yet known how much of the future of an individual is determined by conditions affecting his fetal life. When we have found the answers, we will have made a quantum leap to a new level of understanding, a level which will profoundly influence many biological and social disciplines.

It is apparent that important gaps in our knowledge still prevail; e.g. preventive mechanisms of intrauterine hypoxia, necessary nutrients for fetal growth, physiological and molecular mechanisms of intrauterine malnutrition and growth retardation, the effect and the extent of intrauterine malnutrition on postnatal physical and mental growth, the etiology of pregnancy toxemia, physiology of labor initiation, preventive mechanisms of premature labor, and genetic and embryonic manipulations to correct certain hereditary and congenital anomalies.

Thanks are due to Marlene Visconti and Kathy Perdonik for editorial skills, and to all the staff of Charles C Thomas.

E. S. E. HAFEZ

Detroit, Michigan

ACKNOWLEDGMENTS

THE MANUSCRIPT OF Doctor A. Rudolph and Michael A. Heymann was supported by Program Project Grant HE-06285 from the National Heart and Lung Institute.

The chapter authored by Doctor Francine Wehmer and Doctor E. S. E. Hafez was supported in part by Ford Foundation Grant No. 710-0287A and the National Institute of Child Health and Human Development Grant No. HD 06234.

The manuscript of Doctor Leonard I. Kleiman was supported by NIH Grants HD-06337 ES00159.

Doctor John L. Sever and Doctor Paul I. Terasaki, wish to acknowledge the assistance of Mrs. Mary Ruth Gilkeson, Doctor Shiela C. Mitchell and Mrs. Dianne Edwards of the National Institute of Health.

The manuscript of Doctor Jack Metcoff, Doctor Mostafa Mameesh, Doctor Gail Jacobson, Doctor Paul Costiloe and Doctor Warren Crosby was supported by grant POIHD-06915 from the National Institute of Child Health and Development, NIH, USPHS.

The manuscript of Doctor Markku Seppala, and Doctor Erkki Ruoslahti was supported by grants from the Sigrid Juselius Foundation and the Finnish Medical Research Council. Doctor Markku Seppala, and Doctor Erkki Ruoslahti extend thanks to Professor P. Vara, M.D. and Professor S. Timmonen, M.D. for the clinical material, and Miss Lea Salo, Miss Sirpa Ristimaki, and Miss Sirkka Soikkeli for technical assistance. Statistical advice was provided by Mr. Timo Partanen, M.Sc.

The Mammalian Fetus Symposium was sponsored by Hoffmann-LaRoche, Ortho Pharmaceutical, Parke-Davis, Samuel Higby Camp Foundation, Upjohn and C. S. Mott Center for Human Growth and Development.

E.S.E.H.

CONTENTS

THE MAMMALIAN FETUS

SECTION I

PERINATAL PHYSIOLOGY

Chapter 1

CONTROL OF THE
FETAL CIRCULATION

A. M. RUDOLPH AND M. A. HEYMANN

INTRODUCTION

C IRCULATORY ADJUSTMENTS IN the adult animal result from an integration of homeometric responses of the cardiac ventricles, and the numerous autonomic and hormonal factors influencing myocardial performance and vasomotor activity in the peripheral circulation. There is considerable evidence indicating that although the general patterns of circulatory regulation are similar in newborn animals, there are differences in the degree of response. Little information is available, however, regarding the maturation of the various factors which regulate circulation in the fetus, knowledge of which is most important in understanding how the fetal circulation responds to stress at various stages of gestation. In this chapter we will discuss some of our studies measuring cardiac output in the mammalian fetus and observations on the control of cardiac output and its distribution.

Until quite recently, studies of fetal cardiovascular function have been conducted in ovine fetuses which were delivered from the uterus, with placental circulation continuing for several hours. It was assumed that as long as the fetus was not permitted to breathe, normal fetal circulation was maintained. We know now, however, that not only is the fetal circulation influenced by the anesthesia given to the mother and by the surgical procedures employed, but that exteriorization of the fetus from the uterus results in a progressive decrease in umbilical blood flow.[1] Since, as we have shown recently, the placental circulation receives about 40 percent of the total cardiac output in the fetus, an interference in the circulation may modify the total output and blood flow to other fetal organs. Exteriorization of the fetus may also interfere with many other physiological functions. Thus sympathetic nervous stimulation and release of catecholamines from the adrenal may affect the circulation for a considerable period of time; it has also been shown that adrenal cortical activity is increased for several days.[2]

Recently attempts have been made to study the fetus *in utero* to avoid the influences of anesthesia, surgery and exteriorization. Meschia, *et al.*[3] placed catheters in the umbilical artery and vein in fetal lambs and studied the fetus for several days. We developed techniques for chronic maintenance of catheters in hindlimb and forelimb arteries and veins of fetal lambs for several weeks. Although these developments permitted us to monitor fetal blood gases, arterial and venous pressures and umbilical-placental blood flow, it was not possible to measure fetal cardiac output.

The usual methods of measuring cardiac output, as used in adult animals, are not readily applicable to the fetus. In adult circulation the right and left ventricular outputs are in series, and it has become customary to refer to the output of either ventricle as "Cardiac Output." In the fetus, where there is admixture of oxygenated and systemic venous bloods and in which the two ventricles function somewhat in parallel because of the large communications between the atria, and the aorta and pulmonary artery, it is more convenient to consider the output of the two ventricles as "Combined Ventricular Output." The Fick method, as applied in the adult, entails measurement of oxygen content of arterial and mixed venous blood and oxygen consumption. In the fetus, oxygen consumption is difficult to measure. Also, the course of superior and inferior vena caval return is different in the fetal circulation; superior vena caval blood passes almost exclusively into the right ventricle and is then directed across the ductus arteriosus to the descending aorta; part of the inferior vena caval blood enters the left atrium and left ventricle and is distributed to the coronary vessels, head, neck and forelimbs. It is therefore, not possible to obtain a representative mixed arterial or mixed venous sample. Dawes, *et al.*[4] attempted to calculate the proportions of cardiac output flowing through various fetal vessels and intracardiac shunts by measuring oxygen content of blood in many sites in the heart and great vessels. This required exteriorization of the lamb fetus and rather extensive surgical procedures; also, since many of the sites of sampling were very close to each other, questions of adequacy of mixing arose. Indicator dilution techniques as used in adult animals to measure cardiac output cannot be applied to the fetal circulation in view of the number of shunts present. Mahon, *et al.*[5] used the dye dilution method to measure right and left ventricular outputs separately in exteriorized fetal lambs. They injected indocyanine green dye through the left and right ventricle and sampled blood from the carotid artery and pulmonary trunk or ductus arteriosus respectively. This technique may be criticized since the dye may not mix adequately, and the distance between the injection and sampling sites is very small, and the errors in measurement may be considerable. Mahon, *et al.*[5] found that in late gestation lambs the outputs of the left and right ventricles were similar, although there was suggestive predominance of right ventricular output; the combined output of the two ventricles was about 360/ml/kg/min.[5] Assali, *et al.*[6] used a more direct method of measuring cardiac output; they applied electromagnetic flow transducers around the ascending aorta, pulmonary trunk and ductus arteriosus in various combinations. All these studies were done acutely in exteriorized lamb fetuses in which extensive surgery was performed. They recorded combined ventricular outputs of 240 ml/kg/min in late gestation lambs and noted that right ventricular output exceeded that of the left ventricle by 30 to 40 percent.

We have measured fetal cardiac output in fetal lambs *in utero,* after allowing several days for recovery from the surgical procedure necessary to place catheters and other recording devices for chronic observation. We have used two main approaches for measuring cardiac output. The first method comprises the injection of radionuclide-labelled microspheres into tributaries of the inferior and superior vena cavae while blood is withdrawn at a continuous rate from a fetal femoral and carotid or subclavian artery; the second approach consists of chronic implantation of precalibrated electromagnetic flow transducers around the pulmonary trunk or ascending aorta to measure right and left ventricular outputs respectively.

Radionuclide-labelled Microsphere Technique

The principle of this technique is that when microspheres are injected into the circulation and are mixed evenly, they will be distributed in relation to blood flow to various parts of the body.[7] They lodge in the precapillary vessels and by counting the number of microspheres in each organ the flow to that organ can be estimated. If the microspheres are of uniform size and evenly labelled with radionuclides, the amount of radioactivity is proportional to the number of microspheres and thus to the flow to the organ. If a blood sample is withdrawn at a constant continuous rate from an artery in the same distribution pattern as the organs of interest, it can be used as a reference to calculate actual flows to each organ. In the adult animal, if microspheres are injected into the left atrium or ventricle, they are distributed to the whole body. By relating the amount of radioactivity in the arterial reference sample to that in any body organ or tissue, the flow can be calculated. Thus, if the reference sample is withdrawn at 10/ml/min. and has 10,000 counts/min., an organ with 50,000 counts/min. would have a blood flow of 50/ml/min. In our first studies we used microspheres with a diameter of 50μ, but then changed to 15 or 25μ diameter spheres. This was done since it was appreciated that the accuracy of flow measurement could be improved by increasing the number of microspheres to each organ or organ segment being studied. Statistically it has been shown that flow can be measured accurately to within about 10 percent if at least 400 microspheres are present in the reference sample and the individual organ or part of the organ. The total cardiac output can be calculated by measuring the total amount of radioactivity injected and relating it to that in the reference sample. If a total of 10^7 counts/min. are injected and the reference sample withdrawn at eight ml/min. contains 10^4 counts/min., the cardiac output is $8 \times 10^7/10^4$ or 8,000 ml/min.

In the fetus the method is somewhat more difficult to apply because the superior and inferior vena caval bloods are distributed differently, and because the blood distributed from the ascending aorta has a different composition than that in the descending aorta. We have, however, taken advantage of the presence of shunts in the fetal circulation to avoid having to place and maintain catheters in the cardiac ventricles. Two sets of microspheres with different gamma radionuclide labels are injected simultaneously into a hindlimb and either a forelimb or jugular vein, and reference blood samples are withdrawn from a femoral and a carotid or axillary artery during the injections. This permits calculation of the proportions of superior and inferior vena caval blood distributed to each organ, and actual flows to each organ can be determined. To determine cardiac output, the superior and inferior vena caval flows, coronary flow and pulmonary flow are all added. This provides a measure of the total output of the two ventricles or combined ventricular output rather than, as in the adult, the output of each ventricle.

Although it is possible to calculate the flow patterns across the foramen ovale and ductus arteriosus and the output of each ventricle from the data, a much more reliable measure of these flows can be derived if a third reference blood sample is withdrawn simultaneously from the main or branch pulmonary artery. Using this approach, we measured the patterns of flow in chronically instrumented fetal lambs *in utero* at various gestational ages. The proportions of combined ventricular output ejected by each ventricle and passing through various fetal channels and to individual organs are shown in Figure 1-1 and Table 1-1. The right ventricle is responsible for ejecting 67 percent of combined ventricular output (CVO), while the left ventricle ejects only half that of the right. Only about 8 percent of CVO passes to the lungs; the remaining 59 percent of CVO ejected by the right ventricle crosses the ductus arteriosus to the descending aorta. Of the 33 percent of CVO ejected by the left ventricle, most is distributed to the coronary circulation,

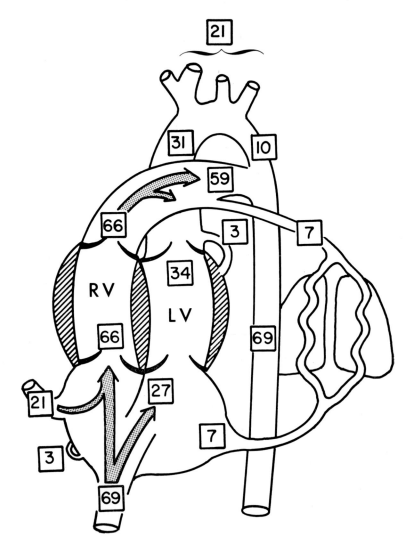

FETAL CIRCULATION-DISTRIBUTION OF C. V. O.

Figure 1-1. The proportions of combined ventricular output which are ejected by each ventricle and which flow through the major vessels and shunts in the fetal heart are shown in the square within each chamber or vessel. RV—right ventricle. LV—left ventricle. For detailed description refer to text.

TABLE 1-I

PERCENTAGE OF COMBINED VENTRICULAR OUTPUT
DISTRIBUTED TO FETAL ORGANS

Placenta	39.7
Heart	3.0
Brain	3.0
Kidneys	2.2
Gut	5.5
Lungs	7.5
Spleen	0.8
Lower trunk	18.0
Upper trunk	18.0

brain and upper trunk including the head and forelimbs, and only 8 to 10 percent of CVO crosses the aortic isthmus to the descending aorta. The umbilical-placental circulation received about 40 percent of the CVO. Negligible quantities of superior vena caval blood cross the foramen ovale to the left atrium, but about one third of inferior vena caval blood returning to the heart crosses the foramen; this represents about 25 percent of the CVO.

The levels of combined ventricular output were considerably higher in our studies than in those previously reported. Combined ventricular outputs of 450 to 500 ml/kg/min were measured in fetal lambs *in utero* as compared with levels of 360 ml/kg/min reported by Mahon, *et al.*[5] and about 240 ml/kg/min presented by Assali, *et al.*[6] The lower values reported previously are probably due to the acute effects of anesthesia and surgery as well as to exteriorization of the fetus. Exteriorization is probably also responsible for the lower proportion of CVO ejected by the right ventricle. Since most of the right ventricular blood is ejected through the ductus arteriosus to the descending aorta, and since 40 percent of CVO is distributed to the placenta, an increase of umbilical-placental vascular resistance could markedly influence the right ventricular ejection. We have shown that exteriorization of the fetus produces a progressive fall in umbilical blood flow,[1] and since fetal arterial pressure did not change, umbilical-placental vascular resistance must have increased.

We have developed techniques for separating the gamma peaks from five different radionuclides, ^{125}I, [141]Ce, ^{51}Cr, [85]Sr and [95]Nb. This permits us to measure cardiac output and distribution both during a control period and after an experimental change in the same fetus. We have used the labelled microsphere technique for studying the effects of fetal hypoxia and of reduction of fetal blood volume on cardiac output and its distribution in lambs *in utero*. Fetal femoral arterial pO_2 was reduced from control levels of about 20 torr to levels of about 13 torr by administering low oxygen gas mixtures to conscious ewes through a hood placed over their heads. This degree of fetal hypoxemia produced a decrease in fetal heart rate and in combined ventricular output, while arterial pressure increased. The proportion of the combined ventricular output distributed to the myocardium, brain, adrenal and placenta increased, so that while combined ventricular output fell, blood flow to the heart, brain and adrenal were maintained or actually increased, and umbilical-placental flow was also maintained. Flow to the kidneys, lungs and particularly to the peripheral circulation dropped markedly.[8] When fetal blood volume was reduced by 15 percent of its control values, fetal heart rate, arterial blood pressure and combined ventricular output fell. Myocardial and cerebral blood flows were maintained, but in contrast with hypoxic stress, umbilical-placental flow was significantly reduced.[9]

The radionuclide-labelled microsphere technique has been most valuable in studying the fetal circulation *in utero*.[7, 10] Among the advantages of the method are the relatively minor surgical procedures necessary, with minimal interference to the fetus, and the opportunity to measure blood flow to each organ of the body. The main disadvantage of the method is the limitation to the number of observations that can be made, and cardiac output can only be measured at specific moments; it is not possible to make numerous sequential or continuous measurements.

Electromagnetic Flowmeter Studies

We elected to use the electromagnetic flowmeter for measuring flow continuously in fetal lambs *in utero*. The flow transducers are placed around the vessels through which flow is to be measured. The main disadvantages of the method are that the transducer is heavy and bulky and the diameter of the vessel is fixed. The transducer may occlude the aorta when placed on the pulmonary trunk or vice versa; it may also rotate and kink the vessel and occlude it. For these reasons, the flow transducers currently available to measure ventricular output cannot be used in lamb fetuses of less than 100 days gestation. The great advantages of the electromagnetic flow transducer are that it can be precalibrated to measure flow directly and instantaneous changes of stroke volume and flow can be recorded. We have used the Statham SP 2202 flowmeter with an electrical zero and with precalibrated flow transducers. Since the right ventricle contributes 66 percent of combined ventricular output, we have studied mainly the normal output of the right ventricle and factors influencing it. We have done fewer studies on left ventricular output, and in a few fetuses have been able to examine left and right ventricular output in the same animal.

The ewe was anesthetized with low spinal anesthesia and the uterus exposed through a midline incision. The fetal hind-limb was exposed through a small uterine incision and catheters passed through a hindlimb vein to the inferior vena cava and through a femoral artery into the descending aorta. In some animals a small balloon catheter was passed through a femoral artery to the descending aorta; by inflating the balloon, the aorta is occluded and ventricular outflow resistance increased. Through a second uterine incision the fetal head and neck were exposed and catheters placed in a carotid artery and jugular vein. A catheter was also passed through a pursestring suture in the trachea and advanced into the thorax to monitor respiratory movements. In some fetuses electrodes were placed in the parietal region of the skull to record electrocortical activity. A thoracotomy was then performed in the third left intercostal space. An electromagnetic flow transducer was placed around the pulmonary trunk just beyond the valve to measure right ventricular output. To record left ventricular output, the trans-ducer was placed around the ascending aorta just above the coronary arteries so that coronary flow was not included in the measurement. As measured by the radionuclide labelled microsphere technique, coronary flow represents about 3 percent of combined ventricular output, and since left ventricular output is about 33 percent of CVO, the flowmeter measurement represents an underestimate of about 10 percent. A catheter or catheter tip transducer was also inserted into the right ventricular cavity and in some instances platinum electrodes were placed on the left atrium for pacing, and on the vagus in the neck to stimulate the nerve electrically.

The chest was sutured, all the catheters and electrodes exteriorized to the maternal flank, and the uterine and abdominal incisions closed. Measurements were made immediately, and also for several days to three weeks after the ewe and lamb had recovered from the surgical procedures. Studies were conducted with the ewe standing quietly in a specially constructed pen.

Right ventricular output (RVO) was reduced to variable degrees on the day of the operation, but it gradually increased over the next two to three days to reach levels of about 300-350 ml/kg/min. This flow corresponded well with the measurements made with the radionuclide-labelled microsphere method. The fetal heart rate varied considerably; spontaneous increases and decreases in heart rate occurred without apparent relation to fetal movement or disturbance of the sheep. In those fetuses in which electrocortical activity was being monitored the onset of electrocortical activity which has been interpreted by Dawes, *et al.*[11] as being characteristic of rapid eye movement sleep, was often associated with rapid respiratory movements and tachycardia. However episodes of tachycardia and bradycardia occurred without relation to changes in electrocortical activity or respiratory pattern. We noted that mean right ventricular output changed in relation to heart rate; a rise in heart rate was accompanied by an increase in RVO; whereas RVO fell when heart rate was decreased; we, therefore, systematically examined the effects of changing heart rates on RVO. The heart rate was increased above its resting rate of 160-180/min by pacing the left atrium by means of the chronically implanted platinum electrodes. Heart rate was decreased by stimulating the vagus nerve through the electrodes implanted on the nerve in the neck. Since the nerve was not severed, violent respiratory movements occurred during stimulation; in order to study the effects of changes in heart rate alone, the fetus was paralyzed with succinylcholine chloride. The heart rate could be reduced to 112-120/min. by vagal stimulation. Using a combination of these two procedures, we examined the effects of changing heart rate over the range of 115 to 330/min. on RVO. Increasing heart rate always produced an increase in RVO (Fig. 1-2), while decrease in rate caused a dramatic fall in RVO (Fig. 1-3). The magnitude and pattern of changes in RVO are shown in Figure 1-4. RVO increased by 15 to 20 percent when heart rate was raised from the resting level of 160-180/min. to rates of 240-270/min. Above this level, it reached a plateau and only at rates above 315-330/min. did it again fall. Reduction of heart rate to about 120/min. caused a fall of RVO of almost 50 percent. In Figure 1-5, right ventricular stroke volume was plotted against heart rate; it is noted that when heart rate was reduced below the resting level of 160-180/min., very little increase in stroke volume occurred, hence the marked fall in RVO.

We observed the effect of increasing afterload or outflow resistance of the right ventricle by inflating a balloon catheter

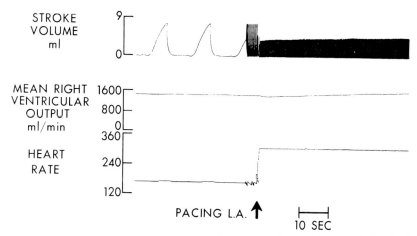

Figure 1-2. The effects of increasing heart rate from the control level of about 160/min. to about 285/min. by electrically pacing the left atrium are shown in a fetal lamb. Note the decrease in right ventricular stroke volume, but mean right ventricular output increases.

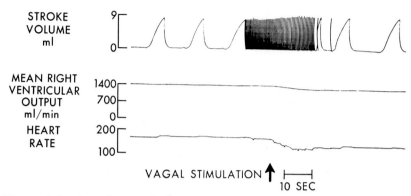

STROKE VOLUME ml

MEAN RIGHT VENTRICULAR OUTPUT ml/min

HEART RATE

VAGAL STIMULATION   10 SEC

Figure 1-3. Stimulation of the vagus nerve in the neck resulted in a decrease in heart rate, and this was associated with a fall in mean right ventricular output and only a minimal increase in stroke volume of the right ventricle.

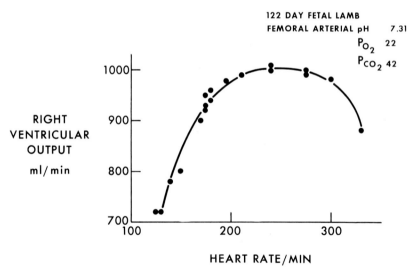

122 DAY FETAL LAMB
FEMORAL ARTERIAL pH   7.31
P_{O_2} 22
P_{CO_2} 42

RIGHT VENTRICULAR OUTPUT ml/min

HEART RATE/MIN

Figure 1-4. The effects of changing heart rates on mean right ventricular output are shown in a fetal lamb of 122 days gestation, studied *in utero*. The data were obtained by cervical vagus stimulation to decrease heart rate, and by left atrial pacing to increase heart rate. Note the slight increase in output when heart rate is increased above resting rate of 160-180/min.. reaching a peak at a rate of 250-270/min. Output drops precipitously when heart rate is decreased.

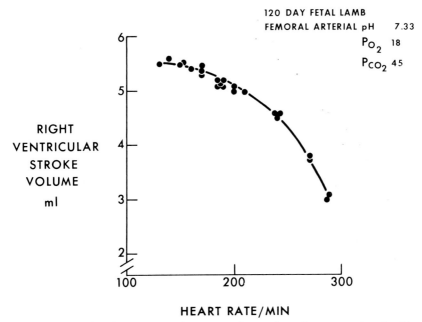

Figure 1-5. The changes in right ventricular stroke volume associated with changes in heart rate are shown in a fetal lamb studied *in utero*. Note that a decrease in heart rate below the resting level of 160-180/min. is associated with only a minimal increase in right ventricular stroke volume.

in the descending aorta. The procedure increases pressure in both the pulmonary trunk and ascending aorta and causes a slowing of heart rate through the baroreflex mechanism. We obviated the bradycardia either by administering atropine before the balloon inflation, or by pacing the left atrium. Whereas in the adult animal an increase in afterload causes a fall of stroke volume with recovery within a few beats, in the fetal lambs stroke volume fell and was reduced as long as the balloon was inflated. We also studied the effects of increasing preload on the right ventricle by infusing warm saline rapidly into a large catheter in the fetal jugular vein at rates of 20 to 30 ml/kg/min. This procedure results in a marked increase in cardiac output in adult animals.[12] In the fetal lambs RVO increased only slightly even though right ventricular endiastolic pressure was raised by 15 to 20 mm Hg.[13]

These findings all indicate that the fetal heart has limited ability to increase stroke volume, either when heart rate is reduced, when afterload is increased or when preload is increased. At present we are not sure whether this is due to inability of the fetal myocardium to increase its performance in response to an increased demand as compared with the adult, or whether the fetal heart is less compliant than the adult heart. Thus an increase in endiastolic pressure may not increase the endiastolic volume to invoke the same magnitude of Frank-Starling response as in the adult. Both a decrease in myocardial compliance and a decrease in myocardial contractility may explain the poor functional performance of the fetal heart. The fetal cardiac output is thus largely regulated by changes in heart rate; an increase in heart rate produces a modest increase in RVO, but a fall in heart rate causes a marked decrease in right ventricular output.

REFERENCES

1. Heymann, M. A., and Rudolph, A. M.: Effect of exteriorization of the sheep fetus on its cardiovascular function. *Circ Res, 21*:741, 1967.
2. Bassett, J. M., and Thorburn, G. D.: Foetal plasma corticosteroids and the initiation of parturition in sheep. *J Endocrinol, 44*:285, 1969.
3. Meschia, G.; Cotter, J. R.; Makowski, E. L., and Barron, D. H.: Simultaneous measurement of uterine and umbilical blood flows and oxygen uptakes. *Q J Exp Physiol, 52*:1, 1967.
4. Dawes, G. S.; Mott, J. C., and Widdicombe. J. G.: The foetal circulation in the lamb. *J Physiol,* London, *126*:563, 1954.
5. Mahon, W. A.; Goodwin, J. W., and Paul, W. M.: Measurement of individual ventricular outputs in the fetal lamb by a dye dilution technique. *Circ Res, 19*:191, 1966.
6. Assali, N. S.; Morris, J. A., and Beck, R.: Cardiovascular haemodynamics in the fetal lamb before and after lung expansion. *Am J Physiol, 208*:122, 1965.
7. Rudolph, A. M., and Heymann, M. A.: The circulation of the fetus *in utero*: methods for studying distribution of blood flow, cardiac output and organ blood flow. *Circ Res, 21*:163, 1967.
8. Cohn, H. E.; Sacks, E. J.; Heymann, M. A., and Rudolph, A. M.: Cardiovascular responses to hypoxemia and acidemia in unanesthetized fetal lambs. *Pediatr Res, 6*:342, 1972.

9. Toubas, P. L.; Silverman, N. H.; Heymann, M. A., and Rudolph, A. M.: Cardiovascular responses to acute hemorrhage in the fetal lamb. *Circulation, 48*:IV-38, 1973.

10. Rudolph, A. M., and Heymann, M. A.: Circulatory changes during growth in the fetal lamb. *Circ Res, 26*:289, 1970.

11. Dawes, G. S.; Fox, H. E.; Leduc, B. M.; Liggins, G. C., and Richards, R. T.: Respiratory movements and rapid eye movement sleep in the foetal lamb. *J Physiol,* London, *220*:119, 1971.

12. Bishop, V. S.; Stone, H. L., and Guyton, A. C.: Cardiac function curves in conscious dogs. *Am J Physiol, 207*:677, 1964.

13. Heymann, M. A., and Rudolph, A. M.: Effects of increasing preload on right ventricular output in fetal lambs *in utero. Circulation, 48*:IV-37, 1973.

Chapter 2

EARLY FETAL DEATH, MECHANISMS OF INTRAUTERINE HEMOGLOBIN SYNTHESIS, AND VARIANT HEMOGLOBIN MOLECULES

R. L. Henry, T. N. Evans, and R. M. Nalbandian

THEORETICAL CONSIDERATIONS OF genetic control mechanisms for embryonic, fetal, and neonatal hemoglobin synthesis with sites of erythrocytogenesis provide a basis to explain occurrences of a variety of abnormal hemoglobins as well as peak fetal death near the end of the first trimester of pregnancy.

Several molecular species of hemoglobin found in intrauterine and neonatal life are shown in Figure 2-1. Each globin chain possesses specific and constant amino acid sequences under structural control of genetic mechanisms.[1, 2] The genetic mechanisms control production of specific chains and, therefore, indirectly control the composition of hemoglobin molecules or tetramers. The four specific hemoglobin chains associated to form molecules are those chains available at the time of erythrocytogenesis. More than 160 hemoglobin types have been recognized from various combinations of different hemoglobin chains.[3] Only a few are referred to here because of their possible importance during intrauterine and neonatal life.

Structural genes control amino acid sequences of hemoglobin chains, activator genes control initiation of production of hemoglobin chains, and repressor genes inhibit or shut off production of hemoglobin chains. Alpha, beta, gamma, delta, and epsilon

20

HEMOGLOBIN TYPE	DESIGNATION	MOLECULAR ORIENTATION
GOWER-1	ξ_4	ξ ξ / ξ ξ
GOWER-2	$\alpha_2 \xi_2$	α α / ξ ξ
A$_2$	$\alpha_2 \delta_2$	α α / δ δ
F	$\alpha_2 \gamma_2$	α α / γ γ
A	$\alpha_2 \beta_2$	α α / β β
S	$\alpha_2 \beta_2^{S}$	α α / β^S β^S
BART'S	γ_4	γ γ / γ γ
H	β_4	β β / β β

Figure 2-1. Molecular globin chain structures of hemoglobin commonly found in embryonic, fetal, and neonatal life. The name of each hemoglobin species is given in the left column, with its conventional notation of globin composition in the middle column, and its tetrameric hemoglobin structure represented in the right column.

chains are normally produced during specific periods of intrauterine and neonatal life. Each may have abnormal variations
as determined genetically by each specific operon. Relative
abundance and production of five globin chain types are shown
in Figure 2-2 and are plotted against specific time spans of
intrauterine and neonatal life according to data published.[4, 5, 6, 7, 8]
Note that alpha chains appear early in the first trimester of
pregnancy and normally remain in high abundance throughout
the life of an individual. Although a heme group is associated
with each globin chain, hemoglobin molecules associated without
alpha chains do not have the capacity to carry oxygen for normal
cellular respiration. Epsilon globin chains appear for a brief
period only during the first trimester. The gamma chain increases

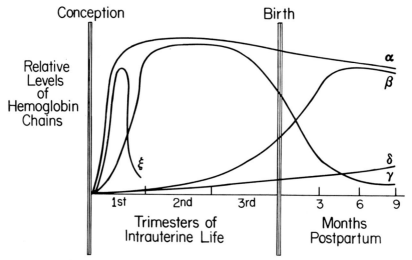

Figure 2-2. Production and abundance of globin chains are represented
in relation to intrauterine and neonatal life. Onset, levels, and duration
of each globin chain is under independent control by activator, repressor,
and structural genes. Hemoglobin types can easily be visualized at any
point along the time scale by associating dyads of globin chains. For
instance, at birth, alpha and gamma chains associate to form fetal hemoglobin as the predominant type. Rising levels of beta chains indicate that
hemoglobin A will also be present at birth by association of alpha and
beta chains. Hemoglobin A_2 may also be present at birth by alpha and
delta chain association.

in abundance as the epsilon chain disappears in the first trimester. It remains high until late in the third trimester where it seems to disappear in a reciprocal relationship with beta chains. Beta chains rise to meet alpha chain levels in the late third trimester and neonatal periods. Delta chains normally remain low throughout the time span indicated.

Comparison of Figures 2-1 and 2-2 will allow determination of hemoglobin molecular type expected from dyad associations at any given time during intrauterine, neonatal, and adult life. Red cells containing Gower-1 and Gower-2 hemoglobin will appear early in the first trimester. Both types normally disappear toward the end of the first trimester as gamma chains increase. Dyads of gamma chains associate with alpha globin dyads to form hemoglobin F as the predominant type during the second and most of the third trimester. During the third trimester activator genes initiate beta chain production and repressor genes inhibit gamma chain production progressively. These events result in a mixture of hemoglobins A and F at birth and a gradual replacement of F with A within six months after birth.

Before considering clinical applications of observations surrounding the genetic control of globin chain synthesis, attention should be given to embryonic and fetal erythrocytogenesis. Custer correlated erythrocytogenesis with organ site of production during intrauterine and neonatal life.[9] His work indicates that red cell production occurs predominently in the yolk sac during most of the first trimester. The liver and spleen take over erythrocytogenesis during the second trimester, with the liver continuing significantly throughout the third trimester. However, bone marrow production of red blood cells begins in the second trimester and becomes increasingly more prominent during the third trimester, becoming the primary site of erythrocytogenesis after birth. Turning once again to Figure 2-2, alpha globin chains must be generated by all organ sites of red cell production. Epsilon globin chains must be produced in the yolk sac while the gamma chains are produced primarily in the liver. Beta globin chains appear coincident with the increase in erythrocytogenesis by bone marrow. The capability of production of any globin chain may be inherent in each of the organ sites, but specific chain types are initiated or inhibited by activator or repressor genes respectively. However, the work of Bloom and Bartelmez[10] and Gilmour[11] would indicate that there exists a complicated but distinct sequence of overlapping erythropoietic cell populations within the various organ sites. Summary of their elegant work with known appearances, abundance, and disappearances of specific globin chains; with identification of molecular hemoglobin species; and with organ sites of erythrocytogenesis results in the following conclusions.[12] Primitive megaloblastic erythroblasts in the yolk sac and body stalk synthesize alpha and epsilon globin chains during most of the first trimester, accounting for the identification of Gower-1 and Gower-2 molecular hemoglobin during this period (see Figs. 2-1 and 2-2). These primitive megaloblastic erythroblasts first appear in blood islands at about nineteen days after conception and disappear by eleven weeks. About six weeks after conception definitive megaloblastic erythroblasts begin to appear primarily in the liver and to a lesser extent in the yolk sac, spleen and bone marrow. These blast cells gradually disappear from these sites of erythrocytogenesis five to fifteen days after birth. They synthesize alpha and gamma globin chains and so produce hemoglobin F. Peak levels of alpha and gamma chains as well as hemoglobin F occur in the second and third trimester and rapidly disappear late in the third trimester and within a few months after birth, corresponding well with the appearance and disappearance of definitive megaloblastic erythroblasts.

Definitive normoblastic erythroblasts appear in bone marrow beginning in the second trimester and become prominent during the third trimester. These cells presumbaly synthesize alpha, beta, and delta globin chains and thus induce, by dyad formation and association, A and A_2 type hemoglobin molecules. Production of gamma globin chains by definitive megaloblastic erythroblasts of the liver becomes inhibited by repressor genes, while beta globin chains predominently initiated by activator genes on definitive normoblastic erythroblasts of bone marrow are increased.

Theoretical considerations of genetic control of globin chains, and thus molecular hemoglobin types, can now be extended to clinical applications. Hemoglobin F, although predominant at birth, declines in concentration while hemoglobin A gains in prominence. Ingram,[1, 2] Gerald,[13] Weatherall,[14] and Baglioni[4] have discussed in detail the complicated mechanisms resulting in initiation and inhibition of globin chain synthesis. Such inter-actions account for the rise and decline of specific globin chain dyads which form hemoglobin molecules by specific cell types in specific sites of erythrocytogenesis. Concentrations of hemo-globin F can be correlated with gestational age and hence infant maturity.[2]

Sickle cell hemoglobin is a quantitatively delayed genetic abnormality.[15, 16, 17] Structural genes misdirect the synthesis of beta globin chains with valine instead of glutamic acid in the sixth position from the amino end.[18] Homozygous, red blood cells containing sickle hemoglobin can have devastating effects by deforming when relatively deoxygenated, and thus block vascular flow to tissues.[19] The onset of such events has been observed to be delayed for several months after birth. Sickling by deoxygenat-ing blood samples at birth may be as low as 3 percent and as high as 97 percent in the same individual some five or six months after birth.[12] Since sickle cell hemoglobin is a tetramer of alpha and beta-S globin chains ($\alpha_2\beta_2{}^s$) it stands to reason that significant degrees of sickling will be delayed until the bone marrow produces enough cells containing the newly initiated β^s globin chains and production of γ chains to form fetal hemo-globin ($\alpha_2\gamma_2$) which has been repressed (see Figs. 2-1 and 2-2).

Hemoglobin Bart's (Bartholomew) is a homogeneous tetra-mer of gamma globin chains (γ_4). This hemoglobin does not contain alpha chains and is most frequently seen in alpha thalassemia where there is a reduction or absence of alpha chains. The synthesis of alpha chains has been repressed while dyads of gamma chains become associated to form hemoglobin Bart's. Complete suppression of α chain synthesis in homozygous α thalassemia results in death *in utero* from failure of hemoglobin Bart's to release its oxygen.[3] It can be predicted from Figure 2-2 that hemoglobin Bart's will be replaced near birth and during the neonatal period by hemoglobin H formed from dyads of beta chains (β_4). Such an event has been well documented.[7, 16] In beta thalassemia the production of beta chains would be markedly depressed and one would expect a persistance of fetal hemoglobin or an appearance of hemoglobin A_2. Failure of genetic mechanisms to initiate or repress synthesis of specific globin chains may result in the formation of other abnormal hemoglobins. Tetramers of alpha chains (α_4) and delta chains (δ_4) have also been reported.[17, 20] Coupled with structural abnormalities a tremendous number of hemoglobinopathies can be expected and have been reported.[21]

Finally, abortions occurring near the end of the first trimester may be primarily due to failure of activator and repressor genes to function properly.[12] Modern investigative techniques should be utilized to study this possibility. It is important to recognize the age of embryonic development rather than time of abortion to correlate with erythropoietic cell populations and relative concentrations of specific globin chains. Near the end of the first trimester the molecular hemoglobin type prevalent normally changes from Gower to F. If failure to initiate gamma chains occurs, resulting in insufficient quantities of F hemoglobin, while production of epsilon chains and Gower hemoglobin is inhibited, the embryo would be left with no hemoglobin production and thus death would ensue. Peak incidence of abortions at the end of the first trimester has been recognized for years.[22] These abortions can only partially be explained by hormonal insufficiency. Failure of activator genes, as early as six to eight weeks of gestation, to induce gamma chain production while repressor genes normally inhibit epsilon chain production results in a relentless and devastating fall in Gower hemoglobin. Identification and measurement of these events is within the realm of investigative possibility.

REFERENCES

1. Ingram, V. M.: Control mechanisms in hemoglobin synthesis. *Medicine,* 43:759, 1964.
2. Ingram, V. M.: Biochemical genetics at the molecular level. *Am J Med,* 34:674, 1963.

3. Lorkin, P. A.: Fetal and embryonic haemoglobins. *J Med Genet,* *10*:50, 1973.
4. Baglioni, C.: Correlation between genetics and chemistry of human hemoglobins. In J. Herbert Taylor (Ed.): *Molecular Genetics.* New York, Acad Pr, 1963, p. 405.
5. Hecht, F.; Motulsky, A. G.; Lemire, R. J., and Shepard, T. E.: Predominance of hemoglobin Gower 1 in early human embryonic development. *Science, 152*:91, 1966.
6. Huehns, E. R.; Dance, N.; Beaven, G. H.; Hecht, F., and Motulsky, A. G.: Human embryonic hemoglobins. *Cold Springs, Harbor Symp Quant Biol, 19*:327, 1964.
7. Huehns, E. R., and Shooter, E. M.: Human haemoglobins. *J Med Genet, 2*:48, 1965.
8. Zuckerkandl, E.: The evolution of hemoglobin. *Sci Am, 212*:110, 1965.
9. Custer, P. R.: *An Atlas of the Blood and Bone Marrow.* Philadelphia, Saunders, 1949, p. 16.
10. Bloom, W., and Bartelmez, G. W.: Hematopoiesis in young human embryos. *Am J Anat, 67*:21, 1940.
11. Gilmour, J. R.: Normal haemopoiesis in intrauterine and neonatal life. *J Pathol, 52*:25, 1941.
12. Nalbandian, R. M.; Henry, R. L.; Camp, F. R.; Wolf, P. L., and Evans, T. N.: Embryonic, fetal and neonatal hemoglobin synthesis: Relationship to abortion and thalassemia. *Obstet Gynecol Survey, 26*:185, 1971.
13. Gerald, P. S.: Genetic determination of hemoglobin structure. *Medicine, 43*:747, 1964.
14. Weatherall, D. J.: *The Thalassaemia Syndromes.* Philadelphia, Davis Co., 1965.
15. Diggs, L. W.; Ahmann, C. P., and Bibb, J.: The incidence and significance of the sickle cell trait. *Ann Intern Med, 7*:769, 1933.
16. Porter, F. S., and Thurman, W. G.: Studies of sickle cell disease. *Am J Dis Child, 106*:35, 1963.
17. Schneider, R. G., and Haggard, M. D.: Sickling, a quantitatively delayed genetic character. *Proc Soc Exp Biol Med, 89*:196, 1955.
18. Hunt, J. A., and Ingram, V. M.: A terminal peptide sequence of human hemoglobin. *Nature, 184*:640, 1959.
19. Murayama, M., and Nalbandian, R. M.: *Sickle Cell Hemoglobin: Molecule to Man.* Boston, Little, 1973.
20. Dance, N., and Huehns, E. R.: A haemoglobin containing only δ chains. *Biochem Biophys Res Commun, 7*:444, 1962.
21. Stamatoyannopoulos, G.: The molecular basis of hemoglobin disease. *Annu Rev Genet, 47*:47, 1972.
22. Bateman, D. E. R.: *J Obstet Gynaec Br Commonw, 75*:1169, 1968.

Chapter 3

PERINATAL RESPIRATORY PHYSIOLOGY; THE INITIATION OF BREATHING

Herbert S. Harned, Jr.

DESPITE THEIR DRAMATIC nature and vital importance, the physiological events occurring during birth of the infant are not completely understood. The infant must survive the transition from a state in which it is entirely dependent on its mother for its respiratory function to an entirely independent state in which its own respiration is promptly initiated and maintained. This transition, sufficiently important that it provides a legal definition of life itself, represents a focus of interest involving the obstetrician, the pediatrician and the physiologist. Some of the facts relating to the onset of breathing have been established through astute clinical observations, but many have been established through physiological observations in acute and chronic preparations of fetal sheep and primates. The classic work of Barcroft[1] has been supplemented by recent productive experiments by a variety of investigators. In this article, the present state of knowledge of respiratory physiology pertaining to the onset of breathing will be reviewed and related to the findings of experiments performed in our laboratory.

Fetal Respiration

The fetal ambient environment is a comfortable one where stimuli from the outside are minimal. The fetus lives in a warm amniotic fluid pool, maintained at maternal core temperature where heat loss is minimal. There is very little stimulation from

the sensory modalities which will be present during and immediately after birth, such as cold, pain, touch, light, sound and
proprioceptive stimuli. A relatively inactive and obtunded state
is maintained, but various motor activities are performed which
will prepare the fetus for the major exertions needed for survival
at birth. Respiratory activity appears to take the form of rapid
irregular respiratory movements occurring three to four times
per second. This type of respiratory activity, documented initially
by Merlet, *et al,*[2] has been described in detail by Dawes.[3] The
respiratory patterns, not observed readily in acute fetal sheep
preparations, perhaps because of inhibitory effects from operative
procedures and restraint of the animal, have been noted in chronic
fetal lamb preparations where pressure catheters have been
inserted into the fetal trachea and flowmeter recordings taken
from the trachea slightly below the larynx. The characteristics
of this type of respiratory activity are listed in Table 3-I.

In addition to this type of respiratory activity, periodic gasping and sighing efforts have been documented which occur at
one to four per minute for about 5 percent of the time and
generate pressures as high as 20 mm Hg. These are not associated
with fetal blood gas changes or the electrocorticographic changes
of rapid eye movement sleep. In addition, asphyxial gasps have
also been documented. Finally, the fetal sheep appears to be
capable of panting at a rate of approximately 4 Hz and protrudes
the tongue, if the amniotic temperature is raised one degree.[4]

The documentation of these fetal respiratory movements in

TABLE 3-I

FETAL RESPIRATORY ACTIVITY IN SHEEP

Irregular rate (3 to 4 Hz) and depth (usually shallow, can reach 30 mm Hg.
    pressure).
Increase in rate and depth from eighty days' gestation to term. May occur at
    forty days.
Back and forth flow of fluid in trachea usually 1 ml. (insufficient to clear 8 to 10
    ml tracheal dead space).
Movement noted in chest wall and respiratory muscles—not detectable on
    maternal abdomen.
Occur in episodes, lasting for 1 min. to 1 hr., which are present about 40 percent
    of time.
Circadian rhythm with greatest flow (rate and depth increase) at 2100 hours.
Related to rapid eye movement sleep (REM) as documented by electrocorticogram.

lambs has been supplemented by observations in humans. Ahlfeld[5] observed rhythmic fetal movements through the maternal abdominal wall as early as 1888, which he attributed to fetal respiratory efforts. Boddy and Mantell[6] recently have taken simultaneous tracings of movements noted on the maternal abdominal surface below the level of the umbilicus and of fetal respiratory movements as recorded by ultrasound. The rates of these motions were the same and differed from the maternal cardiac rate. Although these abdominal wall movements may be difficult to see and may be transmitted above the umbilicus if a fetal limb lies in position between the fetal chest and lower abdominal wall, Boddy and Mantell[6] state that the mother often can locate them. Thus, astute observations by nineteenth century clinicians and modern mothers again have substantiated the findings of the lamb physiologists.

Under normal conditions, the fetal internal milieu consists of acid-base conditions similar to the adult animal in its arterial pH and pCO_2 as well as electrolyte modalities, but with much lower pO_2 level. The pH and pCO_2 levels are determined by the state of maternal hyperventilation associated with pregnancy, the pO_2 by the necessary oxygen pressure gradient across the placenta. The degree of placental inefficiency which results in this pressure drop to carotid arterial pO_2 levels of approximately 25 mm Hg. does not reflect a state of fetal hypoxia, but it does set a condition wherein strong stimulation of peripheral chemoreceptors would be occurring if the glomera were operating as they are destined to function after birth.

Interestingly, the rapid respiratory movements described above appear to be diminished by mild fetal hypoxia; lowering of fetal PaO_2 from 25 to 16 mm Hg decreased these movements.[3] These particular respiratory movements do not appear to be influenced by hypoxic stimulation of peripheral chemoreceptors. However, high pCO_2 induced in the fetus by altering the maternal inspired gases did increase these rapid respiratory movements.[3]

It is probable that these rapid, irregular respiratory movements are highly important in the preparation of the fetal muscles of respiration and other mechanical features of the respiratory apparatus for the intense efforts of establishing breathing. They may also be important in establishing respiratory rhythmicity and in developing the asynchrony of respiratory activity and deglutition. In relation to the latter function, there appears to be a periodic movement of fluid during this respiratory activity from the lower respiratory tract to the supralaryngeal region. Swallowing of such fluid probably occurs.[7]

Fetal Chemosensor Function

Certain observations about fetal chemoreceptor function will be reviewed, but conclusions relating to this complex subject must be minimal. The peripheral carotid glomera do not function in the fetus as in the independently breathing animal or the fetus would show more readily identifiable chemoreceptive carotid sinus nerve potentials and would probably have gasping respiratory efforts with normal fetal pO_2 levels. Baroreceptor potentials, readily recorded in the fetal lamb's carotid sinus nerve at blood pressures as low as 25 mm Hg,[8] interfere with recordings of chemoreceptor potentials. However, Biscoe and associates,[9] as ourselves[10, 11] have been unable to record chemo-potentials from the fetal lamb's carotid sinus nerve, nor were such potentials recorded after NaCN was injected into the ipsilateral carotid artery. Also, we were unable to initiate respiratory activity in the fetal lamb when various gas mixtures were administered to the ewe which were designed to produce a degree of fetal hypoxia or hypercarbia similar to that observed in the lamb at the time of the first breath.[12] A review of these particular experiments proves interesting in view of new information now available.

After the ewe was given spinal anesthesia, the lamb's head, thorax and left forelimb were delivered and the lamb was capped with an air-tight unit attached to an anesthesic bag filled with nitrogen. Brachial arterial blood gases were continuously monitored by a cuvette electrode assembly. When gas mixtures were administered to the ewe to lower pO_2 or raise pCO_2, a degree of maternal hyperventilation occurred. Thus, when a gas mixture of 10% O_2–90% N_2 was given to the ewe, fetal PaO_2 dropped to 6.6 mm Hg, but the ewe's hyperventilation changed fetal $PaCO_2$

from 39.4 mm Hg. to as low as 31.5 mm Hg. Also, when the gas mixture contained 6.5% CO_2, 21% O_2 and 72.50 N_2 and fetal $PaCO_2$ was raised to as high as 63 mm Hg, the PaO_2 was also raised by maternal hyperventilation.

These observations may be related to certain clinical conditions. During pregnancy, presence of decreased maternal PaO_2 caused by low FiO_2 as in high altitude) or by such other factors as right to left vascular shunts could induce hyperventilation which would result in a decrease in fetal $PaCO_2$. This might blunt the effect of hypoxic stimulation in inducing fetal intrauterine gasping efforts. It is important to realize that no such mechanism is available to protect the fetus from such intrauterine respiratory efforts in response to interruption of placental-fetal gas exchange. Interference with placental function or cord blood flow, for example, would result in the combined effect of decreased pO_2 and increased pCO_2 which, as will be shown later, appears to have a greater tendency to provoke fetal respirations.

In the foregoing discussion, we have stressed the fetal respiratory patterns which appear to be unique and the observation that low fetal PaO_2, which would produce strong stimulation of active breathing in the adult, simply does not invoke fetal respiratory activity. We must keep in mind that other factors are present during gestation which would blunt fetal respiratory responses and which should be evaluated when exteriorized fetal animal preparations are interpreted. Several of these factors have been mentioned, in particular the lack of sensory stimulation, especially from cold, and the immersed state, especially involving presence of fluid in the supralaryngeal region. The importance of these conditions in relation to initiation of breathing will become apparent in the subsequent discussion.

Initiation of Respiration

From the preceding discussion, one can see that the fetus is in a state of readiness for initiating the vigorous breathing needed to sustain life, but various triggering mechanisms will be needed to set this process in action. Burns[13] has proposed that rhythmic activity of the respiratory centers is enhanced by sensory input from a variety of modalities which reaches a degree such that the motor respiratory apparatus is activated and breathing starts. This hypothesis, substantiated by excellent experiments in adult animals, does not indicate priorities for the sensory inputs. Also, in view of the demonstration that various fetal rhythmic respiratory movements are occurring *in utero*, along with "practice" gasps and panting, it would seem that the fetal respiratory centers are more active than was formerly believed.

Effects of Occlusion of the Umbilical Cord

In assigning priorities to the neural inputs which might initiate breathing, one must evaluate the results of additional experiments. One becomes impressed with the utter consistency of initiating respiration of the fetal lamb by occlusion of the umbilical cord and this occurs, despite various experimental conditions. The respiratory efforts, which do not occur immediately, but always begin within three minutes after cord occlusion, are strong and gasping in nature and are almost always associated with violent movement of the fetus[14] and are associated with a marked secretion of catecholamines presumably from hypoxic stimulation of the fetal adrenal gland.[15] The circulatory changes occurring at this time are similar to those of the hypoxic adult animal—including decrease in peripheral blood flow, with preservation of cerebral and myocardial blood flow[16] renal blood flow and descending aortic flow decrease, possibly resulting in diminished perfusion by mesenteric arteries as well as adrenal arterial vessels. The delay in initiation of respiration after cord occlusion suggests that threshold levels of arterial blood gases need to be reached or that humoral factors such as norepinephrine and epinephrine release and mobilization of the sympathetic nervous system may be involved to potentiate the blood gas effects. We would suggest that both mechanisms are operative; that there does appear to be a critical relationship of fetal arterial blood gases to onset of breathing and that fetal arousal into the "fight or flight" state may potentiate sensory inputs from the variety of modalities mentioned previously.

In addition to this, mobilization of the sympathetic nervous system may have important implications in the response of chemoreceptors to blood gas changes. Biscoe and Purves[9, 17, 18] have suggested that peripheral chemoreceptor activity, as indicated by the potentials recorded from individual nerve fibers in the carotid sinus nerve, is potentiated by stimulation of sympathetic nerves. They have demonstrated that this phenomenon occurs in the fetal sheep by recording carotid sinus nerve potentials induced by asphyxia or injection of NaCN before and after stimulation of sympathetic nerves affecting the blood flow to the carotid glomus. They proposed initially that vasoconstriction of the arteries supplying the glomus could potentiate its responses to hypoxic, hypercarbic and acidic stimulation, resulting in strong peripheral chemoreceptive activity at the time of the first breath but this mechanism has not been proved. Also, we have noted a great increase in potentials recorded from a nerve slip of the carotid sinus nerve after cord occlusion, which shows no relationship to the blood pressure.[11]

Effects of Blood Gas Alterations at Birth

Effects of fetal blood gas changes (hypoxemia, hypercarbia and hyperhydermia) in initiating respiration have been studied with interesting findings. Several of these experiments have involved carotid arterial perfusions. Avery et al.[20] performed a study on a fetal lamb in which they injected blood with low pO_2 and later with high pCO_2 into the carotid artery. The hypercarbic blood invoked an immediate gasp, the hypoxic blood did not. We also perfused a carotid artery of an exteriorized fetal lamb with blood low in oxygen, but with normal pCO_2 and pH and elicited inconsistent respiratory activity in two of four animals.[10] Since we were interested at that time in carotid chemoreceptor responses, we altered the blood perfused so that the pO_2 and pH were low but pCO_2 was unchanged, changes that should affect peripheral chemoreceptors rather than the central chemosensors known at that time. This latter perfusion resulted in far more persistent respiratory effort which started too soon after the challenge to be related to pH change in the spinal fluid bathing the ventrolateral medullary chemosensors described by Loeschcke[21] in the adult animal. We interpreted this to mean that there was potentiation of the stimulus for initiating respiratory activity from combined hypoxemia and hyperhydremia. We did not rule out central chemosensor stimulation nor did we test for potentiation by combined hypoxemia and hypercarbia.

Experiments by Woodrum, *et al.*[22] indicate that a step decrease in pO_2 or increase in pCO_2 produced by perfusion of the fetal sheep's carotid artery can cause ventilatory activity, although not all their animals showed this. Interestingly, these investigators showed a difference in the time required for initiation of respiration after perfusions of blood low in oxygen and those of blood high in CO_2. The mean time before the first gasp was nine seconds for the hypoxic challenge and twenty-nine seconds for the hypercarbic challenge. The delay in response to the step changes in PaO_2 in Woodrum's experiments, also noted in ours where the mean time from onset of perfusion to first gasp was eighteen seconds, is considerably greater than that found in the adult animal. This again reflects a degree of refractoriness in the fetal chemosensor responses. Woodrum, *et al.*[22] speculated that the slower pCO_2 effect may indicate that the central chemosensing mechanisms are involved primarily in the response to CO_2 whereas peripheral chemoreceptors may be responsible for the pO_2 effect. Even so, the lag time between increased pCO_2 challenge and respiratory gasp is much longer than that of seven to fifteen seconds found by Biscoe and Purves[19] in the newborn lamb after alteration of pCO_2. One must also be aware that these carotid perfusion experiments are testing carotid glomic effects and perhaps central chemosensing mechanisms rather than aortic chemoreceptor effects. There is evidence that the aortic chemoreceptors may play an important part in altering the fetal circulation, but their role in initiating respiration has not been defined.

The interesting experiments by Pagtakhan, *et al.*[23] and by Chernick and Jansen[24] add other nuances. Using a newborn lamb to control fetal blood gases by a complex cross transfusion preparation, these authors have been able to maintain fetal circulation. They have also found relative inactivity of the peripheral chemoreceptors, but have induced breathing by hypoxia alone (pO_2 5 mm Hg.) or by predictable alterations of

pCO_2 and pO_2. Breathing was initiated by an approximate pO_2 of 5 mm Hg. and pCO_2 of 40 mm Hg., a pO_2 of 6 to 14 mm Hg. and pCO_2 of 40 to 100 mm Hg. or by a pO_2 of 17 to 20 mm Hg. and pCO_2 of 100 mm Hg. Interestingly, when carotid sinus and vagus nerves were cut to eliminate peripheral chemoreceptor activity, breathing was initiated with a PaO_2 of 10 to 12 mm Hg. at various levels of pCO_2 from 40 to 110 mm Hg. They believe this suggested that the peripheral chemosensors are sensitive to $PaCO_2$, not to PaO_2. In addition, by injecting NaCN peripherally and into the ventral brain stem region, these authors have concluded that a central chemosensor is present which is sensitive to oxygen and is capable of initiating fetal respiratory movements. These experiments, while raising many provocative questions, do suggest answers to others. They confirm a reciprocal relationship between PaO_2 and pCO_2 suggested by our experiments and the levels of fetal PaO_2 and $PaCO_2$ which they found capable of invoking respirations are very similar to those we have observed under differing experimental conditions. As a corrollary observation, they also substantiated the contention that blood gas changes, unaccompanied by blood pressure and flow changes are a sufficient stimulus for onset of respiration. Finally, by inducing respiratory activity using slow change in blood gas tensions, they showed that such change (analogous to that at normal birth) is capable of initiating respiration.

The degrees of importance of peripheral and central chemosensing mechanisms in the initiation of respiration need additional elaboration. We believe that both of these units are involved in the initial respiratory activity. Peripheral chemoreceptor activity has been shown to be important in the initiation of effective breathing by an experiment in which the carotid sinus nerves were divided before respiration was initiated by cord occlusion. Fetal sheep, in which the nerves were divided, initiated breathing, but did not survive as did mock-operated animals.[25] Also, breathing newborn lambs, in which the sinus nerves were divided, showed depression of ventilation which was of several minutes duration.[26] Equally important, it was apparent from these experiments that central chemosensing mechanisms were also active during the perinatal period. This has been substantiated by experiments in which fetal lambs with bilaterally divided carotid sinus and vagus nerves (presumably eliminating the known peripheral chemosensor activity) were still able to initiate a degree of effective respiratory activity.[27] However, we were unable to show sensitivity of the ventrolateral regions of the medulla to increasing acidity of perfused mock spinal fluid in the fetal sheep. This proved to be an extremely difficult technique in the fetal lamb because of the degree of vascularity of the bony structures and meninges overlying the region and is even a more difficult area to expose than in the cat.

We believe these experiments indicate that the central chemosensing mechanisms are effectively active in the term fetal lamb as it is exposed to other birth processes and these mechanisms are capable of responding appropriately to changes in pCO_2 and pH.

Effects of Temperature Change

In addition to the consistent initiation of respiration by occlusion of the umbilical cord and blood gas change, alteration in the ambient temperature of the fetal lamb can invariably result in initiation of forceful breathing. This has been demonstrated under different conditions. Dawes[28] trained an electric fan on the moistened fleece of a lamb, with an intact umbilical circulation, lying at its mother's side. The cooling from this initiated breathing even though the fetus was probably affected by the ewe's urethane-chloralose anesthesia. Merlet, *et al.*[29] introduced cool water into a plastic bag surrounding the fetal head and induced breathing. Recently, we have been delivering lambs into a warm water bath (40° C) which has permitted maintenance of a more basal fetal state than an air environment. The umbilical venous flows of 210 to 230 ml/min/Kg compare reasonably well with those obtained in chronic fetal preparations. By altering the water temperature slowly over a period of five to six minutes to 27° C, we have been able to induce breathing in over thirty consecutive experiments.[30] When the temperature was returned to 39° to 40° C, breathing has invariably stopped. Figure 3-1 reveals the rhythmic, rapid strong breathing induced by this method. This type of breathing, which is not character-

The Mammalian Fetus

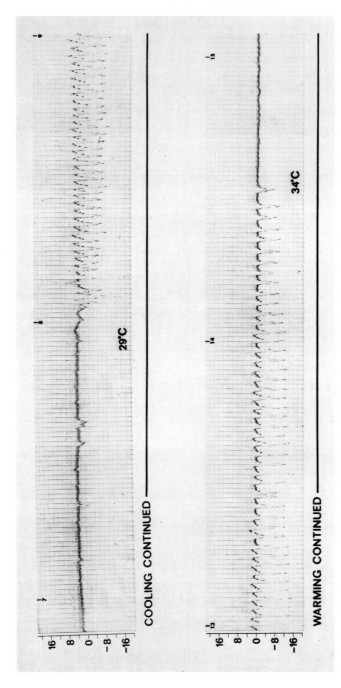

Figure 3-1. Respiratory activity recorded by pressure change in the right atrium of a term fetal lamb. Some respiratory activity was observed beginning 2½ minutes after cooling of water surrounding the immersed animal. Occasional minimal efforts are shown in the upper tracing between seven and eight minutes after cooling was started and consistent, rhythmic respirations began shortly after eight minutes. Note also the decrease in strength and rate of respirations with rewarming with cessation of respiratory activity when ambient temperature of 34° reached.

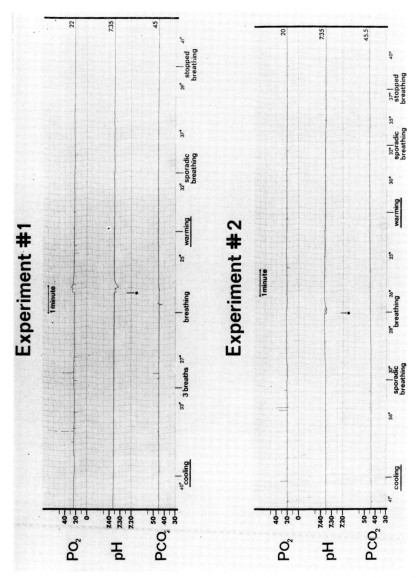

Figure 3-2. Two experiments are shown with continuous recording of pO_2, pH and pCO_2 by a cuvette electrode assembly. The lack of variation in these parameters during the sequences of cooling and rewarming is shown. Comments are entered of the breathing patterns observed. The system was flushed with saline shortly after sustained breathing occurred in both experiments causing the transient alterations in readings. (H. S. Harned and J. Ferreiro, Initiation of breathing by cold stimulation: Effect of change in ambient temperature on respiratory activity of the full-term lamb. *J Pediatr*, 83:663, 1973).

ized by gasps, is generally slower than normal breathing after birth of the lamb, but is much more vigorous than the type of respiratory activity of lambs *in utero* described by Merlet, *et al.* and Dawes.[3] The strong negative pressures developed would be expected to move air well, but we did not permit this to occur in animals in which a fluid column was maintained in the upper respiratory passages. Use of a flow-through cuvette assembly to monitor pO_2, pCO_2 and pH concurrently with monitoring of respiratory activity revealed no change in the blood gases to correspond with the onset or cessation of breathing (Fig. 3-2). This is a sure demonstration that this type of rhythmic breathing was related to the effects of ambient temperature change and not alteration of blood gases. Interestingly, no detectable change was noted in rectal temperature during these alterations of environmental temperature. This also provides a useful model for study of other parameters related to initiation of breathing as will be mentioned later.

Alteration of environmental temperature by releasing the lamb from an immersed state (at 40° C) into room air (at 25° C) did not invoke respiratory activity under these conditions, nor did change from warm air (40° C) to room air. We concluded that this meant that the change in water temperature was associated with considerably more cold stimulation, since immersion in water eliminates the boundary layer of air in the lamb's wool coat which protects him during exposure to a cold air environment.

In addition, studies have been performed under these circumstances in which patterns of blood flow have been measured by electromagnetic flowmeters. In these experiments, the expected decrease in femoral artery flow was noted as peripheral vasoconstriction occurred. There appeared to be less fall in flow through the internal maxillary artery than in the carotid artery, indicating a degree of preservation of blood flow to the brain. There was a minimal increase in adrenal norepinephrine and epinephrine excretion which was quite transient. The changes in blood flow patterns did not differ substantially in the group of lambs which invariably initiated respiratory activity from those noted in the group of lambs subjected to change from a warm water to warm air environment which did not initiate breathing. Thus, we obtained no evidence that circulatory effects influenced the onset of breathing under these circumstances. The conclusion was that cold stimulation *per se* was a sufficient stimulus to initiate breathing under certain conditions, even when the lamb's trachea remained filled with fluid and the lamb was totally submerged.

Effects of Immersion and of Fluid in the Upper Respiratory Passages

Previously, we had shown that total immersion of a lamb in water inhibits breathing markedly.[31]. This was especially apparent in experiments where lambs, tracheotomized to provide a lifeline to room air, were delivered and immersed in water at 40° C and then induced to breathe by clamping of the umbilical cord (Fig. 3-3). Other experiments indicated that the presence of water in the supralaryngeal region was the prime deterrent to breathing. When water at 40° C was introduced into the trachea via a rostrally directed catheter, there was marked decrease in ventilation of newborn lambs (Fig. 3-4). We observed these animals to swallow very vigorously and questioned whether we were not observing reflex inhibition of respiration resulting from this active swallowing. The depression of respiration resulting from fluid in the laryngeal region was observed concurrently by Tchobroutsky, *et al.*[32] who proposed that the afferent limb of this reflex was mediated by the superior laryngeal nerve, but they also suggested afferent trigeminal stimulation as an alternate mechanism.

The former reflex has been studied by Johnson, *et al.*[33] with very interesting findings. They submerged lambs delivered in a warm saline bath at the mother's side and maintained the placental circulation intact. The lambs were then induced to breathe by occlusion of the umbilical cord and they established rhythmic ventilation which appeared to be far more effective than that which we had observed in lambs immersed in water. They also noted that introduction of water into the upper airway resulted in apnea, which was not associated with swallowing. A variety of fluids have been tested as shown in Table 3-II. We

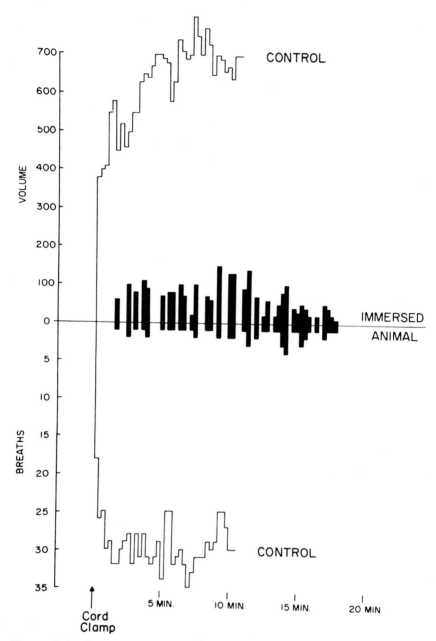

Figure 3-3. Representative experiment showing the suppression of respiration during complete immersion of a lamb in warm water. After initiation of breathing by occlusion of the umbilical cord, both the volume and number of breaths are markedly decreased over that observed in a control animal.

TABLE 3-II

Perfusing Fluid	Apnea	Swallowing
Saline (0.077 M to 0.616M)	—	—
Water	+	+
HCl (0.01 N)	+	+
Sucrose (1 M)	+	+
Glucose (0.11 M to 2.22 M)	+	+
Amniotic fluid	—	—
Tracheal fluid	—	—
Sheep's milk	—	—
Cow's milk	+	+
Allantoic fluid	+	+

also have introduced small quantities of water into the supra-laryngeal region of the fetal lamb induced to breathe by cooling the environment as described above and have noted rapid appearance of apnea, but swallowing has been noted consistently. Also, warm saline has a markedly different effect in that usually no swallowing occurs and no hyponea develops. On some occasions, however, there was a decrease in the respiratory rate.

These authors believe the discrimination of these different fluids means that taste sensors must be involved. They, like Tchobroutsky, have shown the superior laryngeal nerve is the afferent pathway for the reflex since division of this nerve abolishes the apnea caused by introducing water into the laryngeal region. They propose that this reflex may have important implications in drowning and possibly in the sudden death syndrome of infancy.

Effects of Other Sensory Stimuli

We have not been particularly impressed with the importance of other sensory modalities which might provide stimuli for initiation of breathing. Tactile and pain stimuli[10] appear to invoke single breaths and may increase the activity of the lamb, but they do not appear to cause rhythmic respiratory activity. Pro-

---

Each animal was tracheotomized and ventilation was measured by a Fleisch pneumotachometer. Respiratory activity of the control animal was not measured after about ten minutes, respiratory activity of the immersed animal ceased as shown. (H. S. Harned, Jr.; R. T. Herrington, and J. Ferreiro, The effects of immersion and temperature on respiration in newborn lambs, *Pediatrics*, 45:598, 1970).

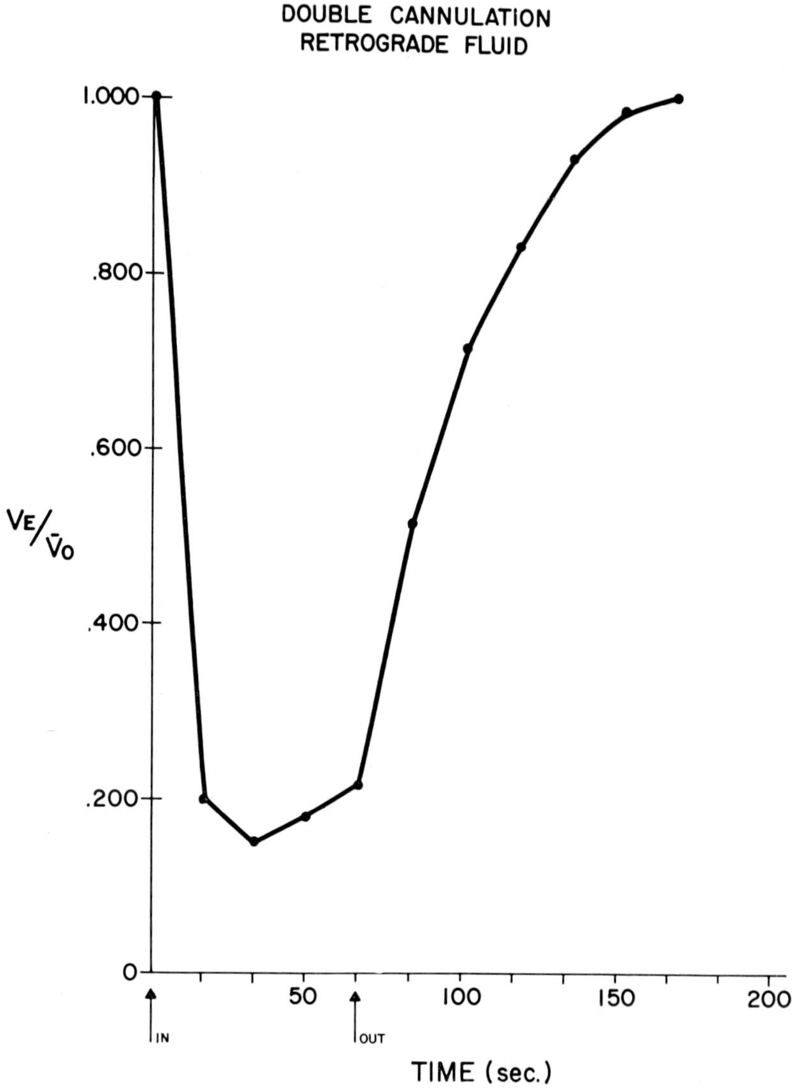

DOUBLE CANNULATION
RETROGRADE FLUID

$V_E/\bar{V}_O$

TIME (sec.)

Figure 3-4. Representative experiment of the effect on ventilation of introduction of warm water into a rostrally directed cannula in the trachea of an actively breathing term lamb. The ordinate expresses the ratio of ventilation measured to ventilation before the challenge, as measured by a pneumotachometer attached to a cannula directed candad in the trachea below the other cannula. Note the precipitous decline in ventilation during the perfusion of fluid and rapid recovery afterwards. (H. S. Harned, Jr.; R. T. Herrington, and J. Ferreiro, The effects of immersion and temperature on respiration in newborn lambs, *Pediatrics, 45*:598, 1970).

prioceptive stimuli seem to have the same transient effects. The stimuli of light and sound may arouse the animal to a degree, but are not strong stimuli. Despite this, tactile stimulation of the newborn infant may initiate the first cry and gasp at a time which is desirable during the delivery. From these animal experiments, it would appear that repeated tactile and proprioceptive stimulation would not be particularly effective in sustaining respiratory activity.

Summary and Speculation

The most important triggering mechanism for the onset of breathing appears to be the changes in blood gases; the hypoxemic, hypercarbic and hyperhydric effects of diminished maternal fetal gas exchange exert strong stimulation on peripheral and central chemosensors. The activation of the sympathetic-adrenal systems arouses the newborn into a state of "fight or flight" in which the major effects are alterations in the capability of the central nervous system to receive sensory stimuli and change in the peripheral chemoreceptors' ability to respond to the blood gas changes occurring concurrently.

Cold stimulation would appear to be the most important sensory modality, especially in producing persistent respiratory stimulation. Again, this may result in arousal of the newborn but apparently through mechanisms other than adrenal stimulation.

Finally, the role of immersion in inhibiting respiratory activity is important, especially the local effects of fluid in the supralaryngeal regon. The reciprocal functions of respiration and deglutition are revealed in reflexes where the newborn can differentiate between fluids located in the supralaryngeal region, some of which induce swallowing. In swallowing, the infant may inhibit respiration to a degree which can delay or compromise the initiation of effective breathing.

All of these mechanisms demand further elaboration for they provide important insights into the medical procedures needed to assist the infant in the initiation of breathing. Most studies have been performed in the lamb and some projections of these findings to primates are indicated. A more complete understanding of these mechanisms should result in alterations of some of the methods used in neonatal resuscitation and in respiratory care of the newborn.

REFERENCES

1. Barcroft, J.: *Researches on Prenatal Life.* Oxford, England, Blackwell Scientific Publications, 1946.
2. Merlet, C.; Hoerter, J.; Devilleneuve, C., and Tchobroutsky, C.: Mise en evidence de mouvements respiratoires chez le foetus d'agneau *in utero* au cours du demier mois de la gestation. *CR Acad Sci* [D] (Paris) *270*:2462, 1970.
3. Dawes, G. S.: Breathing and rapid-eye-movement sleep before birth, in Foetal and Neonatal Physiology. Proceedings of the Sir Joseph Barcroft Centenary Symposium. Cambridge, England, Cambridge University Press, 1973, pp. 49-62.
4. Robinson, J. S.: (Unpublished) cited in Dawes, G. S.: Breathing and rapid-eye-movement sleep before birth, in Foetal and Neonatal Physiology. Proceedings of the Sir Joseph Barcroft Centenary Symposium, Cambridge, England, Cambridge University Press, 1973, p. 55.
5. Ahlfeld, F.: Die intrauterine tägtigkeit der thorax und zwerchfell muskulatur, intrauterine atmung. Mschr. Geburtsh. *Gynack, 21*: 143. 1905.
6. Boddy, K., and Mantell, C. D.: Observations of fetal breathing movements transmitted through maternal abdominal wall. *Lancet, 2*: 1219, Dec. 9, 1972.
7. Adams, F. H.; Desilets, D. T., and Towers, B.: Control of flow of fetal lung fluid at the laryngeal outlet. *Respir Physiol, 2*:302, 1967.
8. Harned, H. S., Jr.: Respiration and the respiratory system. In Stave, U.:*Physiology of the Perinatal Period.* New York, Appleton, 1970, p. 73.
9. Biscoe, T. J.; Purves, M. J., and Sampson, S. R.: Types of nervous activity which may be recorded from the carotid sinus nerve in the sheep foetus. *J Physiol* (London), *202*:1, 1969.
10. Harned. H. S., Jr.; MacKinney,. L. G.; Berryhill, W. S., Jr., and Holmes, C. K.: Effects of hypoxia and acidity on the initiation of breathing in the fetal lamb at term. *Am J Dis Child, 112*:334, 1966.
11. Harned, H. S., Jr.; Griffin, C. A.; Berryhill, W. S., Jr.; MacKinney, L. G., and Sugioka, K.: Role of hypoxia and pH decrease in initiation of respiration, in Exerpta Medica Monograph 1967. Intra-uterine dangers to the Foetus. Proceedings of a Symposium, Prague, Czechoslovakia, October 11-14, 1966.

12. Harned, H. S., Jr.; Rowshan, G.; MacKinney, L. G., and Sugioka, K.: Relationships of pO_2, pCO_2 and pH to onset of breathing of the term lamb as studied by a flow-through cuvette electrode assembly. *Pediatrics, 33*:672, 1964.

13. Burns, B. D.: The central control of respiratory movements. *Br Med Bull, 19*:7, 1963.

14. Dawes, G. S.: In *Foetal and Neonatal Physiology.* A comparative study of the changes at birth. Chicago, Yearbook Medical Publishers, 1968, p. 131.

15. Comline, R. S., and Silver, M.: Development of activity in the adrenal medulla of the foetus and new-born animal. *Br Med Bull, 22*:16, 1966.

16. Campbell, A. G. M.; Dawes, G. S.; Fishman, A. P., and Hyman, A. I.: Regional redistribution of blood flow in the mature fetal lamb. *Circ Res, 21*:229, 1967.

17. Biscoe, T. J., and Purves, M. J.: Cervical sympathetic and chemoreceptor activity before and after the first breath of the newborn lamb. *J Physiol* (London), *181*:70, 1965.

18. Biscoe, T. J., and Purves, M. J.: Observations on carotid body chemoreceptor activity and cervical sympathetic discharge in the cat. *J Physiol* (London), *190*:413, 1967.

19. Biscoe, T., and Purves, M.: Carotid body chemoreceptor activity in the newborn lamb. *J Physiol, 190*:443, 1967.

20. Avery, M. E.; Chernick, V., and Young, M.: Fetal respiratory movements in response to rapid changes of CO_2 in carotid artery. *J Applied Physiol, 20*:225, 1965.

21. Loeschcke, H. H.: Intracranielle chemorezeptoren mit wirkung aut die atmung. *Helv Physiol Pharmacol Acta, 15*:25, 1957.

22. Woodrum, D. E.; Parer, J. T.; Wennberg, R. P., and Hodson, W. A.: Chemoreceptor response in initiation of breathing in the fetal lamb. *J Applied Physiol, 33*:120, 1972.

23. Paglakhan, R. D.; Faridy, E. E., and Chernick, V.: Interaction between arterial pO_2 and pCO_2 in the initiation of respiration of fetal sheep. *J Applied Physol, 30*:382, 1971.

24. Chernick, V., and Jansen, A. H.: Initiation of respiratory movements in foetal sheep by hypoxic stimulation of foetal central chemoreceptor, in *Foetal and Neonatal Physiology.* Proceedings of the Sir Joseph Barcroft Centenary Symposium, Cambridge, England, Cambridge University Press, 1973, p. 213.

25. Harned, H. S., Jr.; Griffin, C. A.; Berryhill, W. S., Jr.; MacKinney, L. G., and Sugioka, K.: Role of carotid chemoreceptors in the initiation of effective breathing of the lamb at term. *Pediatrics, 39*:329, 1967.

26. Harned, H. S., Jr.; Herrington, R. T.; Griffin, S. A.; Berryhill, W. S., Jr., and MacKinney, L. G.: Respiratory effects of division of the carotid sinus nerve in the lamb soon after initiation of breathing. *Pediat Res,* 2:264, 1968.

27. Herrington, R. T.; Harned, H. S., Jr.; Ferreiro, J. I., and Griffin, C. A.: The role of the central nervous system in perinatal respiration: Studies of chemoregulatory mechanisms in the term lamb. *Pediatrics,* 47:857, 1971.

28. Dawes, G. S.: In *Foetal and Neonatal Physiology.* A comparative study of the changes at birth. Chicago, Yearbook Medical Publishers, 1968, p. 132.

29. Merlet, C.; Leandri, J.; Rey, P., and Tchobroutsky, C.: Action du refroidissement localise dans le declenchement de la respiration chez L'agneau a la Naissance. *J Physiol* (Paris), 59:457, 1967.

30. Harned, H. S., Jr., and Ferreiro, J.: Initiation of breathing by cold stimulation: Effect of change in ambient temperature on respiratory activity of the full-term lamb. *J Pediatr,* 83:663, 1973.

31. Harned, H. S., Jr.; Herrington, R. T., and Ferreiro, J.: The effects of immersion and temperature on respiration in newborn lambs. *Pediatrics,* 45:598, 1970.

32. Tchobroutsky, C.; Merlet, C., and Rey, P.: The diving reflex in rabbit, sheep and newborn lamb and its afferent pathways. *Resp Physiol,* 8:108, 1969.

33. Johnson, P.; Robinson, J. S., and Salisbury, D.: The onset and control of breathing after birth, in *Foetal and Neonatal Physiology,* Proceedings of the Sir Joseph Barcroft Centenary Symposium, Cambridge, England, Cambridge University Press, 1973, p. 217.

Chapter 4

ULTRASTRUCTURAL CHANGES OF THE HUMAN PLACENTA AS SEEN BY SCANNING ELECTRON MICROSCOPY

G. Kuppe, Hildegard Metzger, and H. Ludwig

Fetal development depends to a great extent on undisturbed placental function, i.e. rapid exchange of nutrients and waste products over the surface membrane of the placenta to and from the maternal blood in the intervillous space. Morphological changes of the placenta surface, then must lead to a severe impairment of fetal nutrition.

Pathological surface changes of the placenta include the following:

a) an increased number of placenta infarcts on gross inspection.

b) an increase of syncytiotrophoblastic sprouts, looked upon as a trial of the organ to compensate for the loss of no longer functioning villi.

c) a thickening of the subtrophoblastic basement layer of the villi, most prominent in the area of intervillous fibrin deposition.[1]

d) areas of villous mesenchyme not covered by a syncytiotrophoblast layer.[24]

e) Fibrin deposition in the intervillous space with subsequent thrombotic occlusion and degeneration of neighboring villi.

f) Thickening of the wall of the fetal vessels within the villi; fibrin deposition in these blood vessels and occasionally thrombotic occlusions. In addition to these findings that were principally obtained by light and transmission electron microscopy, the SEM reveals:

g) Relatively more villi with a swollen appearance.

h) Areas of rarefication of villi.

i) A higher degree of microvillous arborization similar to that seen in early placentas.

j) Fibrin fibers, identified under SEM by their typical "cross-linkage," inserting on the villous surface with inclusions of maternal erythrocytes and platelet aggregates.

It is generally accepted that a spasm of uterine arterioles of a still unknown origin precedes the above mentioned surface changes of the human placenta in primary pre-eclampsia.

Ludwig[24] has developed the concept of primary and secondary infarction of the placenta instead of the purely descriptive terms of "white and red" infarction.

Primary infarction means the sequence of events due to reduced uterine arteriole blood flow following spasm or occlusion of these vessels with subsequent impairment of blood flow in the intervillous space and hypoxic degeneration of the adjacent microvilli. Secondary infarction means the changes of the utero-placental unit that have become independent and self-supporting, i.e. fibrin apposition leading to further slowing of the blood stream in the intervillous space, hence to hypercoagulability and further degeneration of microvilli.

The purpose of this chapter is to describe the morphological changes in normal and abnormal human placentae as observed by scanning electron microscopy.

METHODOLOGY

Twenty-eight human placentae were examined. Eighteen placentae were obtained from pregnancies complicated by primary pre-eclampsia as defined by an elevation of blood pressure above 140/90, proteinuria and edema and ten placentas from normal pregnancies and deliveries. All patients included in this study were delivered vaginally within the thirty-eighth week and term. More than one half of the preeclamptic patients were primiparas.

A 2 x 2 cm specimen was excised from the maternal side of the placenta immediately after birth both from normal appearing and infarcted areas. The specimens were washed in saline and fixed in buffered (pH 7.2) glutaraldehyde. Dehydration in ascending alcohol series and drying by the critical point method with partial vacuum was done. The dried specimens were glued to steel object carriers and vaporized with atomic carbon and gold in the high vacuum chamber.[19, 31, 32]

Detached edges were covered with conductive silver. Observation under SEM (Cambridge S4-10) allowed for magnifications between 200 x and 20,000 x. Suitable areas were photographed with a Praktica L- Camera. The original size on the screen corresponds to a picture 10 x 10 cm. Maternal erythrocytes did not lose their normal biconcave shape by the fixation procedure, which indicates that gross artifacts are unlikely. Comparing the size of erythrocytes it can be concluded that the fixation process leads to shrinkage of about 16 percent.

OBSERVATIONS

Normal Placentas

Noninfarcted Area
The syncytiotrophoblastic surface is covered by a dense uninterrupted turf of microvilli (Fig. 4-1a). During maturation the villous tree of the normal placenta diminishes in diameter. Multiple subdivisions into tertiary and occasionally quarternary villi can be identified. Quarternary villi are often bulged by knots and syncytio-sprouts. The differences between knots and sprouts as seen by SEM are: 1) Knots are slightly hilly variations of the round villous top. 2) A sprout is a ramification of a villous top. Most tops are divided into two sprouts. It is uncommon to find only one sprout of tertiary villus in a mature placenta.

During maturation the microvilli undergo significant changes: their average length in the midplacenta varies in the first trimenon from 0.75 to 1.25 μ and thickness from 0.12 to 0.17 μ; whereas, at term these values are 0.50 to 0.70 for length and 0.08 to 0.14 μ

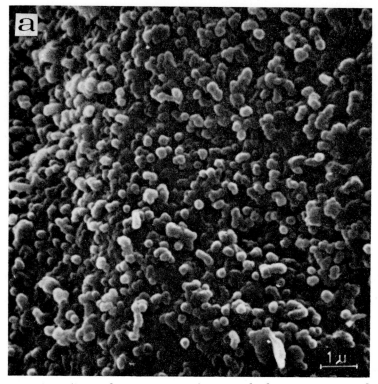

Figure 4-1a.   (Magnification 9,000 x.)   Normal placenta at term: dense uninterrupted microvillous turf.

for thickness.[27] The microvilli become smaller and more slender, thus providing better conditions for diffusion. Another feature is the approximate twofold increased density of microvilli near term as compared with early placentas. Figure 4-1a clearly reveals all the features of mature microvilli: slender, short structures with frequently seen bulgings of their tops. There is no area without microvilli; clumping of microvilli is insignificant. In the mature placenta there are some luxury forms of microvilli with an extreme length up to fourfold of the normal. See Figure 4-1b. These were never seen in immature placentas.

Area of Infarction

Infarction also occurs in undisturbed pregnancies and is often referred to as a sign of physiologic degeneration. It is not the

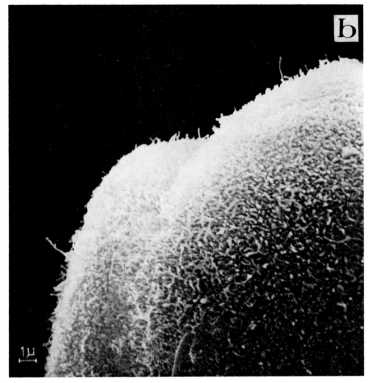

Figure 4-1b. (Magnification 4,500 x.) Normal placenta at term: two microvilli with extreme length are shown.

existence of placenta infarction as such, but rather the amount of trophoblastic surface involved that makes the difference between normal and pathological placenta-function (Figs. 4-1c & 4-1d). In infarction the density, the length and thickness of the microvillous protrusions are different from the normal. High power magnification (Fig. 4-1d) shows several microvilli with a shadow-like appearance, probably indicating degenerating villi. Clumping of the microvilli is not markedly increased.[25]

Pre-eclampsia

Figures 4-1e & 4-1f show a case of mild pre-eclampsia. The survey and low-power magnification shows a slight variation of the microvilli in length and thickness, suggesting the microvillous turf is composed of villi of different ages, i.e. older and younger

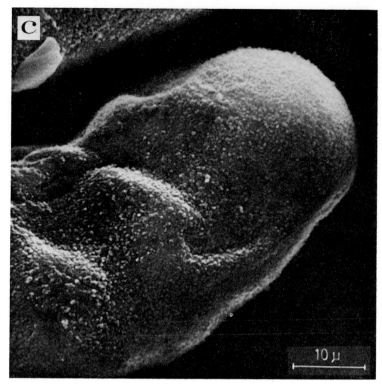

Figure 4-1c. (Magnification 2,000 x.) Same placenta as in Figures 1 and 2: Area of infarction: Density, length and thickness of microvillous protrusions vary.

ones. This finding is consistent with light-microscopy findings showing syncytiosprouts.[21]

In summary this case must be looked upon as borderline to normal as it indicates either an early stage of pre-eclampsia or the specimen has been taken from a relatively undisturbed area.

The changes of pre-eclampsia are similar to those seen in infarction, although they are diffuse rather than localized, subacute rather than acute in nature. Figures 4-1g and 4-1h represent a case of severe pre-eclampsia. The survey and low-power magnification shows areas of rarefication of the microvillous turf. Some of the microvilli have a shadow-like appearance resembling placenta infarction. The high-power magnifica-

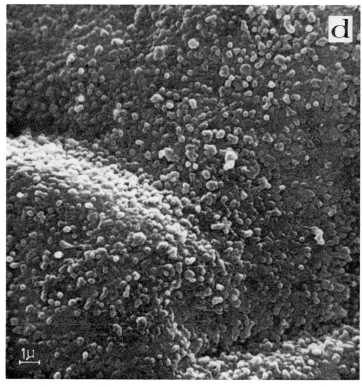

Figure 4-1d. (Magnification 5,000 x.) Same as Figure 3. Variation of microvilli is shown in detail. Degenerating and newly outgrowing micro-villi compose the area.

tion shows two maternal erythrocytes with an almost normal biconcave appearance, thus excluding severe artifacts (Figure 4 1g). The microvilli show a marked difference in length and thickness. There is swelling and clumping of microvilli. These changes must be interpreted as degeneration and growing of new villi. Concurrently, there is an indication of contrast in that the normal turnover of villi was increased or that the causative mechanism for pre-eclampsia does not always act with the same strength but allows for periods of regeneration. Again in contrast to infarction the changes are rather diffuse and subacute in nature.

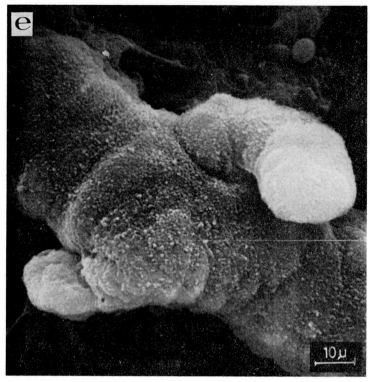

Figure 4-1e.   (Magnification 1,250 x.)   Mild pre-eclampsia.   Microvilli of different ages, length and thickness are present.

Figures 4-1i and 4-1j show a specimen from severe pre-eclampsia representing all the features of pre-eclampsia: infarction and fibrin deposition, and thrombus formation in the inter-villous space. Fibrin deposition starts with small bridges between the flanks or tops of terminal villi. These fibrin bridges show a typical cross-linkage which is the identifying sign for fibrin or SEM visualization. Fibers of other composition do not show this phenomenon. While scanning the amnion, it was found that the elastic fibers present have a typical curly appearance similar to light microscopy visualization. Besides, there is no cross linkage between fibers, although bundles of fibers do not always take a parallel course but in fact do cross each other. In transmission electron microscopy the identifying sign of fibrin

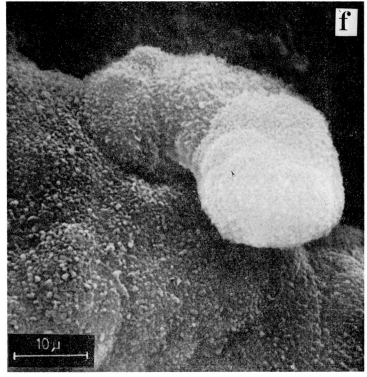

Figure 4-1f. (Magnification 2,000 x.) Mild pre-eclapsia. Microvilli of different ages and size. SEM equivalent of syncytiosprouts.

is a 250 Å period that obviously cannot be seen by SEM. Whenever fibrin is formed in the intervillous space it is proof of thrombus formation, i.e. platelet aggregation including erythrocytes. The slender fibrin fibers form a network which is transformed to a dense layer by apposition of erythrocytes and involving platelet aggregation. Thrombus formation in the intervillous space follows the same rules inside the blood vessels i.e. stasis, hypercoagulability, endothelial defects.[23, 26]

Erythrocytes fixed by fibrin fibers lose their normal biconcave shapes, and as a consequence of the contraction of the fibrin fibers, they become bizarre structures. The thrombus grows by continuous thrombin formation within the deposition Ultimately, the intervillous thrombus extends to villi with a normal surface

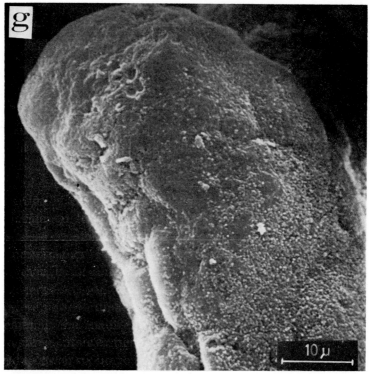

Figure 4-1g. (Magnification 1,800 x.) Severe pre-eclampsia. Areas of rarefication of the microvillous turf are present. Microvilli vary in age, length and thickness.

and causes secondary immobilization of these villi. Thrombus formation means several villi are cut off from circulation and subsequently undergo degeneration. The thrombus formation finally becomes self-supporting and leads to secondary infarction.[24]

COMMENTS

Normal Development of Chorionic Villi

Since the chorionic villi have been identified as the essential structures for placental function, many investigators have concentrated on them and have tried to reveal their function by light microscopy, transmission electron microscopy and scanning

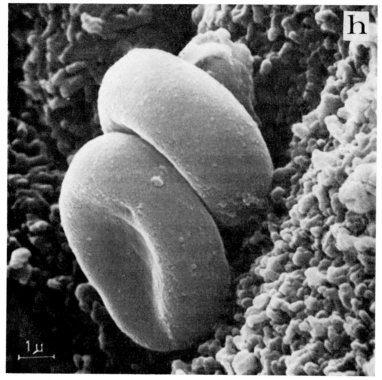

Figure 4-1h. (Magnification 10,000 x.) Severe pre-eclampsia. Platelet deposition on maternal erythrocytes. Swelling and clumping of microvilli.

electron microscopy. Efforts have been made to delineate the normal and correlate the seemingly abnormal to the various groups of placenta insufficiency. The term "placenta insufficiency" has aroused much controversy, due to the fact that the placenta is a rapidly growing organ with a short span of life. Thus growth and degeneration, the two morphologial essentials of life, must occur simultaneously under normal circumstances. It is reasonable to evaluate and categorize the normal and abnormal according to the quantitative degree and amount of degeneration.[22, 34]

The primary villi arise from the syncytium of the intervillous space. These primary villi are histological aggregations of cytotrophoblastic cells,[9, 21] that still show no tendency to bud into the intervillous space formed by the confluence of the lacunae

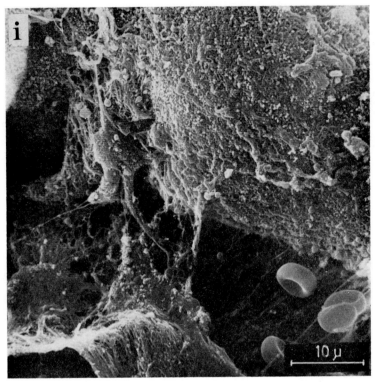

Figure 4-1i. (Magnification 2,000 x.) Severe pre-eclampsia. Fibrin deposition in intervillous space. Fibrin fibers show typical cross-linkage. Included in the network are maternal erythrocytes and platelet aggregates.

in the very early trophoblastic syncytium.[13] It should be noted that primary villi have neither mesenchyme nor blood vessels. The majority of primary villi are transient structures. As soon as mesenchyme assembles below and invades the primary villi, the features of secondary villi are present, i.e. a longitudinal shape with an outer trophoblastic and an inner mesenchymal layer on section. The identifying sign of tertiary villi is the presence of fetal vessels in the villous stroma. Quarternary villi are divisions of tertiary villi at later stages of pregnancy when the cytotrophoblastic layer has disappeared.

Tertiary and quarternary villi are sometimes referred to as resorptive villi, because not before that stage does placental

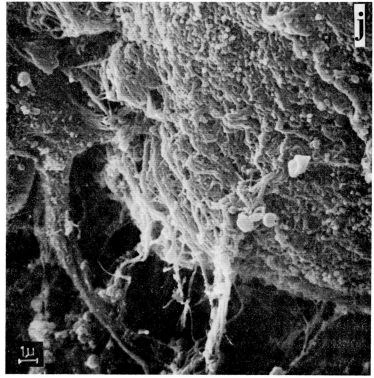

Figure 4-1j. (Magnification 5,000 x.) Severe pre-eclampsia. Fibrin network including degenerating maternal erythrocytes and platelet aggregates. The microvillous turf shows some variation in length, density and thickness.

function take place. Even in mature and postmature placentas primary and secondary villi can be found, which may be a regenerative effort to compensate for the loss of villi.[40, 42]

Maturation and Aging of Villi

Terminal villi in different stages of pregnancy have the same basic architecture, but some important variations are due to maturation. These include a decrease in length and thickness,[27] disappearance of the cytotrophoblastic layer, attenuation of the basement membrane, increased stromal fibrosis, fibrin deposition, infarction and degenerative changes of fetal vessels.[13]. These changes are sometimes looked upon as signs of premature aging[6] with the clinical syndrome of placenta insufficiency related to it.

Since the above mentioned alterations are difficult to quantify, conclusions drawn from them must remain debatable. Several investigators[7, 11, 15, 16, 36] ascribe the cited phenomena to normal maturation rather than to a pathological mechanism. This point is further substantiated by noting that in almost every placenta there are striking differences between villi of a comparable stage as found in specimens taken from different areas of the same placenta.

Pathological changes such as infarcts and fibrin deposition do increase in number and amount during pregnancy. However, they are so variable that no firm conclusions as to placental age can be drawn from them.[4, 6]

The following criteria are frequently considered to be signs of maturity of the placenta[3, 5, 6]: a) decrease in the villous diameter with increase in the surface of the individual villi; b) increase in the fetal vascular spaces in the villi; c) diminuition of the peripheral intravillous connective tissue with increase in the number of syncytial bridges; and d) marked increase in the connective tissue sheaths of the vessels in the trunci chorii.

Features of Villi at Light; Transmission and Scanning Electron Microscopy

Light Microscopy

Chorionic villi composing the brush border of the syncytium vary in structure and distribution.[37] This is thought to be a sign of continuous growth and degeneration of the trophoblast. On light microscopy a brush border can be readily identified on almost any free villus-trunk in all stages of gestation.

Transmission Electron Microscopy

In addition to the ordinary features of a human cell such as mitochondria Golgi apparatus, centrioles, ribosomes, polysomes, lysosomes, microfilaments and microtubules the syncytiotrophoblastic cell has vesicles and vacuoles indicating resorptive function.[13] The microvilli being slender protrusions of the syncytium are the basis of the brush border seen on light microscopy.[1, 2, 10, 12, 38, 39] Near term the microvilli vary much less in thickness than in length, which is the basis of the luxury length observed. The syncytioplasma is continuous as had been suspected from light microscopy findings. Transmission electron microscopy reveals that the microvilli are not evenly distributed and that in fact there are some smooth areas.[13]

Since microvilli and the vesicles and vacuoles which are the morphological equivalent of resorptive function, it is tempting to assume that their presence or absence is indicative of placental function. Again, it must be stated that it is not the existence of microvilli and vesicles as such, but their presence in quantity which leads to insufficiency of placental function. A certain amount of turnover of microvilli must be considered normal.

Scanning Electron Microscopy

On scanning electron microscopy the microvilli have a hairlike and sometimes cone-shaped appearance with bulbous tops.[8, 14, 23] In the course of pregnancy there is a marked decrease in length and thickness of microvilli, except for some luxury forms with an extreme length. On the other hand the density of microvilli rises sharply, about twofold, in comparison to early pregnancy.[27] As previously outlined, the tops of quarternary villi may show knots and syncytiosprouts.

Pathology of Microvilli and Intervillous Space

Fibrin Deposition

Fibrin in the intervillous space and between microvilli increases during pregnancy. In fact it has been stated[35] that the area of syncytium covered by fibrin is seven times greater at term than at the end of the first trimester. In the placenta fibrin occurs in other locations, for instance in Rohr's and Nitabuch's layer but apparently in SEM it can be seen only in the intervillous space. Fibrin deposition in the intervillous space takes place in much the same way as it does inside blood vessels, impaired blood flow, hypercoagulability and defects of the endothelial layer, this latter being degenerating syncytiotrophoblast. Some authors[11, 17, 18] feel that stasis might be the predominant factor, whereas others[33, 36, 41] think that ischemic necrosis is the precipitating factor. Nilsen[30] concluded from his SEM studies that fibrin deposition was due to a hyper-coagulability due to lack of fibrinolytic activity in the intervillous space near term.

In early placentas fibrin in the intervillous space can be demonstrated.[20] It is thought to be a protective mechanism for the decidua against syncytial cytolytic activity.[28] In advanced stages of pregnancy fibrin deposition does not seem to offer any advantage, and may possibly be a sign of aging[29] or a clearcut pathological feature, depending upon the amount of deposition.

Identification of Fibrin

Histologically the presence of fibrin is proven by special stains. On TEM there is a typical 250 Å period identifying a fiber as fibrin. On SEM cross-linkage of fibers has only been observed with fibrin fibers.

Placenta Infarction

On gross inspection infarctions of the placenta appear either white or red, indicating they are either of ischemic or hemorrhagic origin. In addition to these purely descriptive terms it has been suggested[24] that primary infarction can be defined as ischemic degeneration of villi due to impaired blood flow in the maternal uterine arterioles. In secondary infarction, the consequences of this degeneration are hemorrhagic infiltration and fibrin deposition in the infarcted area. Secondary infarction might become self-supporting and thus involve larger areas of the syncytiotrophoblastic surface.

Light microscopic changes of infarction include degeneration of the syncytiotrophoblast with fibrin deposition on the villous surface, degeneration of the villous stroma and the fetal vessels in the villi. Transmission electron microscopy reveals the degeneration of subcellular structures and the deposition of fibrin on the surface. SEM reveals swelling, or even absence of micro-villi in addition to fibrin deposition. One notes that next to the area of degeneration there frequently appear regenerative structures such as syncytiosprouts forming new villi.

REFERENCES

1. Anderson, W. R., and McKay, D. G.: Electron microscope study of the trophoblast in normal and toxemic placentas. *Am J Obstet Gynecol, 95*:1134, 1966.
2. Bargmann, F., and Knoop, A.: Elektronenmikroskopische Untersuchungen an Plazentarzotten des Menschen. Bemerkungen zum Synzytiumproblem. *Z Zellf, 50*:472, 1959.
3. Becker, V.: Über die Reifung der plazentaren Zotten. *Klin Wochenschr, 37*:1204, 1959.
4. Becker, V.: Über maturitas praecox placentae. *Verh Dtsch Path Ges, 44*:256, 1960.
5. Becker, V., and Bleyl, U.: Plazentarzotte bei Schwangerschaftstoxikose und fetaler Erythroblastose im fluoreszenzmikroskopischen Bilde. *Virchow's Arch Path Anat, 334*:516, 1961.
6. Becker, V.: Mechanismus der Reifung fetaler Organe. *Verh Dtsch Path Ges, 46*:309, 1962.
7. Benirschke, K., and Driscoll, S. G.: The Pathology of the human placenta. Berlin, Springer Verlag, 1967.
8. Bergström, S.: Surface ultrastructure of human amnion and chorion in early pregnancy. A scanning and electron microscope study. *Obstet Gynecol, 38*:513, 1971.
9. Boving, B. G., and Laren, J. F.: In Hafez, E. S. E., and Evans, T. N. (Eds.): *Human Reproduction.* Hagerstown, 1973.
10. Boyd, J. D., and Hughes, A. F. W.: Observations on human chorionic villi using the electron microscope. *J Anat Lond, 88*:356, 1959.
11. Boyd, J. D., and Hamilton, W. J.: Development and structure of the human placenta from the end of the 3rd month of gestation. *J Obstet Gynaec Br Commw, 74*:161, 1967.
12. Boyd, J. D.; Hamilton, W. J., and Boyd, C. A. R.: The surface of the syncytium of the human chorionic villus. *J Anat Lond, 102*:553, 1968.
13. Boyd, J. D., and Hamilton, W. J.: *The Human Placenta.* Cambridge, Heffer, 1970.
14. Ferenczy, A., and Richart, R. M.: Scanning electron microscopic study of normal and molar Trophoblast. *Gyn Oncol, 1*:95, 1972.
15. Fox, H.: The pattern of villous variability in the normal placenta. *J Obstet Gynaec Br Commw, 71*:749, 1964.
16. Fox, H.: The villous cytotrophoblast as an index of placental ischemia. *J Obstet Gynaec Br Commw, 71*:885, 1964.
17. Fox, H.: Perivillous fibrin deposition in the human placenta. *Am J Obstet Gynecol, 98*:245, 1967.

18. Fox, H.: Fibrinoid necrosis of placental villi. *J Obstet Gynaec Br Commw*, 75:448, 1968.
19. Frost, H.; Hess, H., and Richter, J.: Untersuchungen zur Pathogenese der arteriellen Verschluβkrankheiten. *Klin Wochenschr*, 46:1099, 1967.
20. Hamilton, W. J., and Boyd, J. D.: Development of the human placenta in the first three months of gestation. *J Anat Lond*, 94:297, 1960.
21. Janovski, N. A., and Dubrauszki, V.: *Atlas of Gynecologic and Obstetric Diagnostic Histopathology*. New York, 1967.
22. Kubli, F., and Budliger, H.: Beitrag zur Morphologie der insuffizienten Plazenta. *Geburtsh. Frauenh*, 23:37, 1963.
23. Ludwig, H.; Junkermann, H., and Klingele, H.: Oberflächenstrukturen der menschlichen Plazenta im Rasterelektronenmikroskop. *Arch Gynaek*, 210:1, 1971.
24. Ludwig, H.: In Rippmann E. T. (Ed.): *Die Spätgestose. Pathologische Fibrinierung bei der Spätgestose*. Basel, 1970.
25. Ludwig, H.: Surface structure of the human term placenta and of the uterine wall post partum in the screen scan electron microscope. *Am J Obstet Gynecol*, 111:328, 1971.
26. Ludwig, H., and Metzger, H.: Das uterine Plazentarbett post partum im Rasterelektronenmikroskop, zugleich ein Beitrag zur Frage der extravasalen Fibrinbildung. *Arch Gynaek*, 210:251, 1971.
27. Ludwig, H.: Surface structure of the human placenta. *The Placenta*. In K. S. Moghissi and E. S. E. Hafez (Eds.), Springfield, 1974.
28. Ludwig, K. S.: Die Rolle des Fibrins bei der Bildung der menschlichen Plazenta. *Acta Anat*, 38:323, 1959.
29. Martin, C. B.: The Anatomy and Circulation of the Placenta. In Barnes, Allan C. (Ed.): *Intra-uterine Development*. Philadelphia, Lea & Febiger, 1968.
30. Nilsen, P. A.: The mechanism of hypofibrinogenemia in premature separation of the normally implanted placenta. *Acta Obstet Gynecol Scand*, 42:Suppl. 2, 1963.
31. Reumuth, H.: Die Rasterelektronenmikroskopie. *Dtsch Med Wochenschr*, 94:1832, 1967.
32. Reumuth, H., and Becker, V.: Stereoscan, ein neues Elektronenmikroskop. Erste anatomische Bilder: Zugleich ein Beitrag zur Blut-Gefäβwand-Beziehung. *Klin Wochenschr*, 46:81, 1968.
33. Tighe, J. R.; Garvod, P. R., and Curran, R. C.: The trophoblast of the human chorionic villus. *J Path Bact*, 93:559, 1967.
34. Villée, C. A.: *The Placenta and Fetal Membranes*. Baltimore, Williams & Wilkins, 1960.
35. Wilkin, P., and Bursztein, M.: Etude quantitative de l'èvolution au cours de la grosesse, de la superficie de la membrane d'échange du

placenta humain. In Snoeck (Ed.): *Le Placenta Humain.* Paris, 1958.

36. Wilkin, P.: *Pathologie du Placenta.* Paris, Masson, 1965.
37. Wislocki, G. B., and Benett, H. S.: Histology and cytology of the human and monkey placenta with special reference to the trophoblast. *Am J Anat, 73*:335, 1943.
38. Wislocki, G. B., and Dempsey, E. W.: Electron microscopy of the human placenta. *Anat Rev, 123*:133, 1955.
39. Wislocki, G. B., and Padykula, H. A.: Histochemistry and electron microscopy of the placenta. In Young (Ed.): *Sex and Internal Secretions.* Baltimore, Williams & Wilkins, 1961.
40. Wynn, R. M.: Morphology of the placenta. In Assali (Ed.): *Biology of Gestation.* New York, Acad Pr, 1968, Vol. 1, p. 93.
41. Zacks, S. J., and Blazar, A. S.: Chorionic villi in normal pregnancy, pre-eclamptic toxemia, erythroblastosis and diabetes mellitus. *Obstet Gynecol, 22*:149, 1963.
42. Zhemkova, Z. P., and Topchieva, O. J.: Compensatory growth of villi in postmature human placentae. *Nature, 204*:703, 1964.

The Mammalian Fetus
ed. E. S. E. Hafez
1975
Publisher: Charles C. Thomas, Springfield, Ill.

Chapter 5————————————————————————

FETAL BEHAVIOR

V. Hamburger

INTRODUCTION

THE STUDY OF fetal behavior is an elusive venture. The mammalian fetus is well hidden from the inquisitive eye of the investigator, and once exposed, its performance is usually short-lived and not necessarily normal, unless great precaution is taken to provide for adequate environmental conditions. Nevertheless, a considerable body of information on fetal behavior has accumulated, mainly during the thirties and forties, through efforts of neuroembryologists like Coghill, Windle, Hooker, Humphrey, and developmental psychologists like Kuo and Carmichael.[3] For the neuroembryologist, one of the basic issues was, and still is, the relationship of the structural differentiation of the nervous system to the development of motility and behavior. In contrast, psychologists are particularly interested in the role which sensory input and prenatal "experiences" play in the molding of behavior patterns. More recently, an entirely different approach has been taken. The great interest in human and mammalian sleep-patterns has been extended to neonatal and prenatal stages and prematures, with the intent of elucidating the origins of these patterns. These rather divergent concepts will be amalgamated at the conclusion of this chapter.

SOME BROAD GENERALIZATIONS

Before dealing with the more intricate and controversial issues, a few basic points should be made. Most investigators will agree, as to what applies to Vertebrate embryos in general.

1. Motility begins at remarkably *early developmental stages.* In lower forms, behavior starts earlier than in higher forms (in relation to overall body development). In the human embryo, the first turning of the head occurs at seven and one-half to eight weeks menstrual age (20 to 23 mm CR length). The head bending to the side is universally the first expression of motility in Vertebrate embryos. From there motility extends to trunk and tail, usually in the form of sinusoid waves. In lower aquatic forms, that is fishes and amphibian larvae, these rostro-caudal waves, when performed with more force, lead to swimming. In higher forms, this pattern breaks up soon after its inception into more localized movements.

2. Movements are *neurogenic* from the beginning, that is, they result from nervous activity. An early myogenic phase, based on autonomous muscle contraction, has been demonstrated experimentally only for dogfish embryos.[18]

3. These two points imply that both neural and muscular structures are capable of functional activity in *very immature stages* of differentiation, before typical neuromuscular junctions are formed, and before myelination begins. Likewise, responses to stimulation are obtained before specialized sensory receptors are differentiated.

4. *Tactile sensitivity* is the first of the sensory modalities that becomes functional. Two generalizations concerning tactile stimulation in embryos can be stated. The area that becomes sensitive first is the skin of the face, innervated by the trigeminal nerve; in some mammals, including primates and man, the palmar surface of the hand becomes sensitive at the same time. The originally narrow reflexogenic zone or zones gradually expands to other parts of the body skin. Furthermore, in higher forms there is an early phase of considerable length during which tactile stimulation elicits a generalized, total body activity of a seemingly uncoordinated nature. In the human, this phase of generalized response (F) is the prevailing activity

between eight and thirteen weeks. Local reflexes emerge from the generalized response, gradually combining to become organized into more complex functional sequences. Some of these become the antecedents of postnatal behavioral acts such as suckling or grasping.[20]

EVOKED VERSUS SPONTANEOUS MOTILITY

It is essential to realize that in practically all studies done in the thirties and forties, tactile stimulation experiments were the universal procedure in dealing with fetal activity; almost no attention was paid to unevoked, spontaneous motility. This was understandable for two reasons. Spontaneously generated electrical activity of nervous tissue had just been discovered, and a decade or more passed until it was accepted as an important phenomenon in its own right.[1] Furthermore, the predominant contemporary theory of behavior was based on the Stimulus-Response concept. Since the generalized total response, mentioned above, was difficult to interpret, the local reflexes moved to the center of the stage, and the theory emerged that local reflexes were the building blocks of behavior development.[32] A representative statement of that time is one by D. Hooker who had done extensive investigations of the human fetus: ". . . the behavior of vertebrate animals, including man, has its genesis in the early exteroceptive responses exhibited during embryonic, larval or fetal life."[19] This general theory had the virtue of conforming to the then prevailing bias in psychology toward the all-powerful role of sensory input and "experiences," broadly defined, in shaping behavior. The theory was strongly endorsed by prominent psychobiologists like Schneirla, Lehrman, and Kuo and still has its followers. It should be mentioned that other viewpoints were promulgated; for instance Coghill[4] envisaged behavior as being integrated, from its inception through adult activities such as swimming, walking, and food getting. These holistic theoretical and philosophical ideas had a considerable impact on contemporary thinking.

It turns out that all these earlier theories of embryonic motility are untenable, at least as broad generalizations, and definitely not applicable to the origins or the major part of embryonic and fetal motility of higher forms. The general theory which emerged from our observations and experiments is based on that element which had been overlooked or ignored by previous investigators, that is, *spontaneous motility* (defined tentatively as not evoked by obvious stimulation). This had been observed and mentioned casually, but did not fit in any acceptable paradigm at that time. Actually, spontaneous embryonic motility had been recognized as a significant phenomenon during the 1880's by an exceptionally perspicacious German psychologist, F. W. Preyer[26] the founder of behavioral embryology, but it remained in oblivion for almost eight decades.[11]

SPONTANEOUS MOTILITY IN THE CHICK EMBRYO

In order to probe more deeply into the roots of behavior, it is necessary to proceed from simple, direct observation, which is always the first step of inquiry to *analysis,* which uses the powerful tool of the analytical experiment. Since the mammalian embryo and fetus resists penetration into its privacy, the chick embryo became the victim of this approach, partly due to its early accessibility through a window in the shell, and partly to my long familiarity with microsurgical experimentation on its nervous system, which the embryo tolerates with remarkable forbearance. Of course, there was hope from the beginning that whatever the chick embryo revealed would be relevant to the mammalian fetus.

As was mentioned, *spontaneous motility* begins at three and one-half to four days with a slight bending of the head, and extends from there to other parts. At six and one-half to seven days, the neuromuscular system of wings and legs becomes sufficiently mature to initiate their movements. Other parts, like beak, eyelid and tongue become motile at later stages. The motility up to seventeen days is characterized by several features: overall motility, measured either in terms of percent activity during a standard observation period (usually 15 minutes) or the number of movements per minute, increases up to thirteen days and then declines to hatching. The movements are mostly jerky twitches of the limbs, wriggling of the body, slow opening and closing or clapping of the beak, and others. A prominent feature is the apparent *absence of coordination* of parts. Any combination of parts can move simultaneously, but the combinations are unpredictable. Coordinated wing flapping or alternating leg movements are rarely seen, even at late stages. A *periodicity,* that is, an alternation of activity and inactivity phases, is pronounced up to thirteen days and then resumes later. But during peak activity the motility appears almost continuous, since the inactivity phases are reduced to seconds. We have designated the spontaneous activity characterized by these features as *type I.* Type II are startles, that is, tremors shaking the whole body. At day seventeen a new type of highly coordinated activity is initiated (type III). It involves the embryo in the preparation for hatching and in the hatching act.[16]

Direct observations yielded many more details that cannot be elaborated. We proceeded from there to the *experimental analysis* by means of microsurgery on early embryos. Two points of fundamental importance for the understanding of behavior origin were established. It was demonstrated first that embryonic motility (type I) is essentially a spinal phenomenon, triggered and sustained by spinal neural mechanisms; and second, that the type I embryonic motility does not require sensory input. Chronic isolation of the spinal cord was achieved by early embryonic extirpation of segments of the cervical spinal cord. The isolated cord generates activity which is quantitatively below normal from the eighth day on, but qualitatively normal with respect to behavioral criteria.[14] Brain influences on type I behavior cannot be detected by our methods until day seventeen,[6] but different parts of the brain are indispensable for different facets of later prehatching and hatching (type III) behavior.[23] The spinal orgin of head, body, and limb motility cannot be disputed, though more refined electrophysiological investigations may well reveal subtle supraspinal influences on the performance of the spinal cord which are not detectable by behavioral observation. Of course, eye and beak movements are controlled by brain stem motor nuclei; likewise, they are spontaneous and not coordinated with movements of other parts.

Concerning the role of *sensory input*, Preyer[26] made the important discovery of a prereflexogenic period in the chick embryo. No response to tactile or other stimulation was attainable before seven or seven and one-half days of incubation. Hence, activity during the first four days was definitely nonreflexogenic. Neurological data supported this finding.[31, 33] How about the subsequent period? A complete chronic deafferentation of the leg level was achieved by a double operation performed on very early (2-day) embryos. Peripheral input was eliminated completely by extirpation of the dorsal half of the lumbosacral spinal cord, which includes the neural crest precursor of spinal ganglia. The latter contained both extero- and proprioceptive sensory neurons. All supraspinal input was eliminated by additional extirpation of a segment of the thoracic spinal cord immediately in front of the limb-innervating level. The intact motor and adjacent internuncial system was capable of maintaining leg motility, quantitatively within the normal range, up to fifteen to seventeen days. Of course, the legs were completely insensitive. Controls were embryos with a thoracic spinal gap only.[17]. Similarly, it was possible to deafferent the entire face and beak by early embryonic bilateral extirpation of the precursors of the trigeminal ganglia. Again, motility of the head, limbs and body was quantitatively and qualitatively normal.[15] Obviously, type I motility does not require sensory input. The experiments also refute the earlier-held view that self-stimulation, for instance the brushing of legs against the head, or proprioceptive stimuli, plays a role in the molding of embryonic behavior. Since none of the deafferented embryos hatched, the question of whether prehatching and hatching activity are controlled by sensory cues remains unanswered.

The data thus far have led to the view that the overt uncoordinated spontaneous behavior of the chick embryo is generated in the spinal cord and is entirely nonreflexogenic. At this point, it was desirable to obtain direct *electrophysiological evidence of spinal cord activity*. The technique of recording from chick embryos *in situ* was worked out by Provine, *et al.*[28] The results of subsequent investigations along this line are briefly stated here.[27] Recordings from lumbosacral cords of curarized embryos showed a very close correlation of polyneuronal burst activity patterns in the ventral cord with overt motility patterns, and a rise in burst activity up to day thirteen, when both the bursts and the activity phases attained their peak. Using floating tungsten electrodes, it was possible to record from freely moving legs. Motility could then be recorded simultaneously with burst activity, and the synchrony of the two events was confirmed. Finally, burst activity was recorded for fifteen minutes each, before, during, and after curarization. The burst activity pattern was maintained throughout the period of leg immobilization. Hence, burst activity is the primary, autonomous event and not a movement artifact, or due to sensory feedback from the leg. These and other recordings leave no doubt that the polyneuronal burst discharges are the electrophysiological correlate of behavior. "Spontaneous" activity can now be defined more rigorously, resulting from self-generated discontinuous discharges of the ventral spinal cord, not requiring sensory input. The simultaneous activation of several body parts in an uncoordinated fashion during behavioral activity phases presupposes near-simultaneous discharges in different parts of the spinal cord. Indeed, Provine,[27] recording concurrently electrophysiological activity with two electrodes placed at two different sites along the main axis of the spinal cord, found "almost identical discharges . . . at different loci within spinal cords of 6- and 20-day embryos." Hence, generalized behavioral activity, designated as type I, is paralleled by the spreading of electrical activity in a seemingly diffuse neuronal network. However, caution is in order in interpreting the behavioral and related electrophysiological data. While they are perfectly consistent, permitting the conclusions that were drawn, both the recording of burst patterns and direct observations of overt motility have their limitations. It is certain that while both burst and motility patterns show little basic changes in their general appearance between five and twenty days, the neural organization of the spinal cord can be expected to undergo progressive differentiation, specific pathways are elaborated and intricate control by higher centers is gradually established. None of this seems to be reflected in the burst patterns or the behavior patterns.[13] Studies are now underway to detect the more subtle organizational changes that go on under the surface, by monitoring the motor outflow from the cord, through EMG recordings from synergistic and antagonistic leg muscles, *in situ,* during undisturbed spontaneous activity.[2]

SPONTANEOUS ACTIVITY IN THE MAMMALIAN FETUS

Can the concept that self-generated spontaneous discharges of the spinal cord are the basis of overt motility in the chick embryo, be extended to mammals? There are numerous references to spontaneous motility in older literature, referring to a variety of fetuses, but, as previously stated, little attention was paid to them. These were incidental to studies of evoked behavior. Nevertheless, there is clear recognition in all these investigations that spontaneous performance is usually a generalized, total, or mass activity, though local movements did occur. Designations such as "generalized" or "mass" actions imply that the body movements were not coordinated, but were more of a convulsive type, resembling the main characteristic of type I motility in the chick embryo. Reinvestigation of the behavior of rat fetuses, with special focus on spontaneous motility, also included evoked responses.[22] Pregnant females were immobilized by spinal transection at the lumbar level, thus avoiding anesthesia, and were fixed on Plexiglas® board. The body, except for the head, was submerged in warm saline and the fetuses carefully released into the bath, with placenta intact. Such preparations, after acclimatization, showed the same type of performance for several hours. Spontaneous movements were recorded both *in utero* and *ex utero.* Rat fetuses displayed as much spontaneous activity as chick embryos. Distinction was made between total, regional, and local movements. An example of regional movements is represented by a combination of head and forelimb movements, while other parts are at rest. Motility in rat fetuses begins at fifteen and one-half days. Our studies extended through days sixteen to twenty.

The gist of our observations is that spontaneous motility in the rat fetus shares major characteristics with that of the chick

embryo. Lack of coordination is indeed the most outstanding
feature. This is particularly striking in forelimbs which are the
most vigorously active parts; rarely does one observe coordinated
or alternating movements of left and right forelimbs. Resemblance was found in other features that had not been observed
before: movements are discontinuous bursts of activity of variable
duration alternating with quiescence. Furthermore, activity rises
to a peak, attained at day eighteen when the fetus or parts are in
motion 38 percent of the time *in utero,* and 48 percent *ex utero.*
Motility then declines, as it does in the chick embryo.

On the basis of these similarities in overt behavior, one is
inclined to draw a close parallel to type I behavior in the chick
embryo. At this time, however, the comparison cannot be carried
further. We have neither deafferentation experiments nor
electrical recordings *in vivo* to prove rigorously that motility of
the mammalian fetus is nonreflexogenic and self-generated in the
neurons of the spinal cord. Nor is there a prereflexogenic period
in mammals that would give some clues. Responses to tactile
stimulation can be elicited from the onset of motility. We have
excluded only one possible source of stimulation: uterine contrac-
tions are in no way related to fetal movements. Nevertheless,
the lack of coordination of parts and periodicity are strong
arguments in favor of the thesis that spontaneous embryonic
motility in higher Vertebrates, generally results from autonomous self-generated, non-reflexogenic discharges of the spinal
cord. This implies that environmental stimuli play a minor role
in the molding of behavior and in the underlying structural and
functional differentiation during the major part of embryonic and
fetal life. The situation changes in the perinatal and postnatal
period, when the major sensory systems, particularly visual and
acoustic systems become functional. There is increasing evidence
that environmental influences are instrumental in the final steps
of structural and behavioral maturation.[10]

RELATION OF FETAL MOTILITY AND SLEEP PATTERNS

The question arises whether the spontaneous motility with
which we have dealt can be linked in any way to sleep-wakeful-

ness patterns. One might entertain the notion, for instance, that type I motility may be related to the phasic movements which are observed during active (REM) sleep, or occasionally during quiet sleep. There is some resemblance inasmuch as both are spontaneous, and often manifested in uncoordinated jerks and twitches. However, it would be inadvisable to consider type I as an atypical, primitive state of active (REM) sleep. In the adult, two states of sleep, active and quiet, can be identified by a number of characteristics. In quiet sleep, one finds an association of spindles and slow-wave, high voltage EEG, usually a diminution of muscle tone, and a regular heart beat and respiratory rate. Active sleep is characterized by low voltage, fast wave EEG, disappearance of tone in antigravity, particularly in neck muscles, irregular twitches and rapid eye movements, irregular heart and respiratory rate, and high threshold for skin reflexes and behavioral arousal. Such identification becomes increasingly difficult when the states are traced back to the newborn or to prenatal stages. One criterion after another becomes atypical or gets lost altogether, and, eventually, the designation of states becomes arbitrary or impossible. The different components such as EEG, or hypotonia, or rapid eye movements, mature independently of each other until they are gradually assembled and coupled according to an intrinsic schedule, which is different for different species, eventually constituting the equivalents of the adult states. The gradual organization of sleep patterns has been studied in the human before and after birth.[7, 8]

A fairly clear picture of the emergence of the sleep-waking pattern has been outlined.[24, 25] In the human, this process extends over several months. Episodes identified as reasonably typical active (REM) sleep are not found until thirty-five weeks, and quiet sleep episodes at thirty-seven weeks. But, all components of quiet sleep are not fully stabilized until several months after birth. A similar situation holds for mammals.[9, 21, 30] For instance, in the kitten, during the first week after birth, sleep-waking states can be identified by behavioral criteria, but EEG patterns are indistinguishable.

Preceding the first appearance of episodes which might be considered as incipient active or quiet sleep, there exists a condition which bears no resemblance to typical active sleep. To be specific: in previable twenty-four to twenty-seven-week human premature infants, the EEG is atypial, eye movements are rare, hypotonia is not yet present, the EKG is regular. Dreyfus-Brisac[7] states: "We must admit that the state of sleep in such babies is unclassifiable, for it is too atypical, with a dissociation of the criteria characteristic of quiet or active sleep." In the rat and rabbit which are born in a very immature state, a similar condition prevails for several days after birth. It would seem advisable, in designating this particular state, to avoid any reference to sleep. Sterman[29] has expressed a similar view. I shall refer to this state tentatively as the *"pre-sleep"* state.

What are the characteristics of this state? One can characterize it only by behavioral criteria. The outstanding feature of human prematures of twenty-four to twenty-seven weeks, and of corresponding mammalian fetuses or newborns, is their high activity rate which ranges from almost continuous motility to intermittent activity with rest phases of several seconds duration. The activity is spontaneous; none of the observers suggest that it might be reflexogenic. The movements are seemingly uncoordinated, consisting of irregular rapid jerks and twitches, and slower movements of the body. Dreyfus-Brisac[7] lists for the previable human infant six different types: partly rapid and jerky, partly slow, partly generalized, and partly local. This repertory is more diversified than that observed by us in the chick and rat embryos. However, this point should not obscure the remarkable behavioral similarity between type I motility and what has been referred to as *pre-sleep* state. In both, the motility is spontaneous, nearly continuous (at least during peak activity in the chick and rat) and seemingly uncoordinated. On this basis, it is tempting to suggest that the *pre-sleep* state, like type I motility, is basically the expression of *autonomous electrophysiological activity* of the spinal cord and brain stem motor nuclei, with minimal or no control by higher centers.

Beginning with this primitive state, the sleep and wakefulness states would become gradually organized when the different brain centers which control their different components mature, according to their built-in time table. The unorganized embryonic type I movements would then be the primitive, elementary building blocks which later are incorporated in *active sleep,* as its phasic motility component, similar movements reappear as the occasional phasic movements of *quiet sleep.* If this notion could be validated by electrophysiological data on spinal cord activity in the pre-sleep state then the *continuity of the spontaneous activity in the embryo through infancy to the adult* would be established. Corner, *et al.,*[5] have a different interpretation of the relation of embryonic and hatching motility in the chick to sleep patterns.

The interesting question of the possible biological *adaptive significance* of spontaneous uncoordinated activity of embryos and fetuses has been raised. This type of motility may be necessary to guarantee the normal development and maintenance of joints and musculature.[12] Furthermore, electrical discharges may play a role in the functional or structural maturation of neurons. Future findings may place the peculiar acrobatics of embryos and fetuses into an as yet unforeseen perspective.

REFERENCES

1. Adrian, E. D.: Potential changes in the isolated nervous system of *Dytiscus marginalis. J Physiol, 72*:132, 1931.
2. Bekoff, A.: Development of motor coordination in seventeen- to twenty-one-day chick embryos. *Soc f Neurosci,* Third Annual Meeting, abstracts: 1973, p. 368.
3. Carmichael, L.: The onset and early development of behavior. In Mussen (Ed.): *Carmichael's Manual of Child Psychology.* New York, Wiley, 1970.
4. Coghill, G. E.: *Anatomy and the Problem of Behaviour.* Cambridge U Pr, 1929.
5. Corner, M. A.; Bakhuis, W. L., and van Wingerden, C.: Sleep and wakefulness in the domestic chicken, and their relationship to hatching and embryonic motility. In Gottlieb (Ed.): *Behavioral Embryology.* New York and London, Acad Pr, 1973.
6. Decker, J. D., and Hamburger, V.: The influence of different brain regions on periodic motility in the chick embryo. *J Exp Zool, 165*:371, 1967.
7. Dreyfus-Brisac, C.: Sleep ontogenesis in early human prematurity from twenty-four to twenty-seven weeks of conceptual age. *Dev Psychobiol, 1*:162, 1968.

8. Dreyfus-Brisac, C.: Ontogenesis of sleep in human prematures after thirty-two weeks of conceptional age. *Dev Psychobiol, 3*:91, 1970.

9. Garma, L., and Verley, R.: Ontogénèse des états de veille et de sommeil chez les mammiferès. *Rev Neuropsychiat Inf, 17*:487, 1969.

10. Gottlieb, G.: Introduction to behavioral embryology. In Gottlieb (Ed.): *Behavioral Embryology.* New York and London, Acad Pr, 1973.

11. Hamburger, V.: Some aspects of the embryology of behavior. *Quart Rev of Biol, 38*:342, 1963.

12. Hamburger, V.: Emergence of nervous coordination. Origins of integrated behavior. *Develop Biol Suppl, 2*:251, 1968.

13. Hamburger, V.: Anatomical and physiological basis of embryonic motility in birds and mammals. In Gottlieb (Ed.): *Behavioral Embryology.* New York and London, Acad Pr, 1973.

14. Hamburger, V.; Balaban, M.; Oppenheim, R., and Wenger E.: Periodic motility of normal and spinal chick embryos between eight and seventeen days of incubation. *J Exp Zool, 159*:1, 1965.

15. Hamburger, V., and Narayanan, C. H.: Effects of the deafferentation of the trigeminal area on the motility of the chick embryo. *J Exp Zool, 170*:411, 1969.

16. Hamburger, V., and Oppenheim, R.: Prehatching motility and hatching behavior in the chick. *J Exp Zool, 166*:171, 1967.

17. Hamburger, V.; Wenger, E., and Oppenheim, R.: Motility in the chick embryo in the absence of sensory input. *J Exp Zool, 162*:133, 1966.

18. Harris, J. E., and Whiting, H. P.: Structure and function in the locomotory system of the dogfish embryo. The myogenic state of movement. *J Exp Biol, 31*:501, 1954.

19. Hooker, D.: *The Prenatal Origin of Behavior.* Lawrence, U of Kansas Pr, 1952.

20. Humphrey, T.: Postnatal repetition of human prenatal activity sequences with some suggestions of their neuroanatomical basis. In Robinson (Ed.): *Brain and Early Behavior.* London, Acad Pr, 1969.

21. Jouvet-Mounier, D.; Astic, D., and Lacote, D.: Ontogenesis of the states of sleep in rat, cat and guinea pig during the first postnatal month. *Devel Psychobiol, 2*:216, 1969.

22. Narayanan, C. H.; Fox, M. W., and Hamburger, V.: Prenatal development of spontaneous and evoked activity in the rat (*Rattus norvegicus albinus*). *Behaviour, 40*:100, 1971.

23. Oppenheim, R.: Experimental studies on hatching behavior in the chick. III The role of the midbrain and forebrain. *J Comp Neur, 146*:479, 1972.

24. Parmelee, A. H.; Wenner, W. H.; Akayama, Y.; Schultz, M., and Stern, E.: Sleep states in premature infants. *Developm Med Child Neurol,* 9:70, 1967.

25. Parmelee, A. H., and Stern, E.: Development of states in infants. In Clemente, Purpura and Mayer (Eds.): *Sleep and the Maturing Nervous System.* New York and London, Acad Pr, 1972.

26. Preyer, W.: *Specielle Physiologie des Embryo.* Leipzig, Grieben. 1885.

27. Provine, R.: Neurophysiological aspects of behavior development in the chick embryo. In Gottlieb (Ed.): *Behavioral Embryology.* New York and London, Acad Pr, 1973.

28. Provine, R.; Sharma, S. C.; Sandel, T. T., and Hamburger, V.: Electrical activity in the spinal cord of the chick embryo *in situ. Proc Natl Acad Sci,* 65:508, 1970.

29. Sterman, M. B.: The basic rest-activity cycle and sleep: Developmental considerations in man and cats. In Clemente, Purpura and Mayer (Eds.): *Sleep and the Maturing Nervous System.* New York and London, Acad Pr, 1972.

30. Valatx, J. L.; Jouvet, D., and Jouvet, M.: Évolution électroencéphalographique des differents états de sommeil chez le chaton. *Electroenceph, Clin Neurophysiol,* 17:218, 1964.

31. Visintini, F., and Levi-Montalcini, R.: Relazione tra differenziazione strutturale e funzionale dei centri e delle vie nervose nell' embrione di pollo. *Arch Suisses Neurol Psychiat,* 43:1, 1939.

32. Windle, W. F.: *Physiology of the Fetus.* Philadelphia, Saunders, 1940.

33. Windle, F. W., and Orr, D. W.: The development of behavior in chick embryos; spinal cord structure correlated with early somatic motility. *J Comp Neur,* 60:287, 1934.

SECTION II

NUTRITION AND FETAL GROWTH AND DEVELOPMENT

Chapter 6

LIPID SUBSTRATES AND FETAL DEVELOPMENT

P. Harding, F. Possmayer, and D. Seccombe

$\mathbf{T}$HE EXTENT TO which carbohydrate, as opposed to other nutritional substrates, provides oxidative energy and biochemical precursors for the fetus has until recently seemed a somewhat academic question. The discovery of hormonal mechanisms that regulate the availability of nutrients to the fetus and our increasing awareness of the fetal compromise represented by a disturbance in this nutritional flow from mother to fetus, has prompted renewed interest in this area of fetal metabolism. Although glucose constitutes the major fetal substrate under normal circumstances, lipids, synthesized either by the fetus or acquired transplacentally from the mother, play important roles during fetal development as well. These include:

1. Adipose tissue lipids that are accumulated by the fetus in late pregnancy and constitute an important source of nutritional reserves during the immediate neonatal period when carbohydrate stores rapidly become exhausted.

2. The contribution of lipids during fetal development to the various phospholipids that are involved in the synthesis of such widely diversified and essential compounds as myeline and lung surfactant as well as cell membranes.

The mechanism by which the fetus conserves and protects these lipid reserves during late pregnancy is vital to its future well being and a study of such mechanisms must concern itself initially with the biochemical pathways and the fetal organs involved in fat synthesis and its deposition. In addition the question of whether the fetus utilizes his own lipid reserves under normal or abnormal circumstances, and if so by which tissues, is also of great practical interest. Whether certain organs such as the brain can and do oxidize other than carbohydrate substrates including the lipids and their water soluble analogues, the ketone bodies, particularly during glucose deficient periods is unresolved. This chapter is concerned with the role of fetal insulin as a regulator of lipid metabolism and secondly with the fetal metabolism of ketones, specifically β-hydroxybutyrate. The data has been obtained from our studies in the rat, rabbit and human.

INSULIN AND FETAL LIPID METABOLISM

In the postnatal animal, insulin coordinates metabolic events that occur during periods of nutritional abundance. Under these circumstances the anabolic process of energy storage involves the conservation of carbohydrate as glycogen and nutritional fat as triglyceride. In addition, insulin facilitates the accumulation of amino acids within the cell and thereby enhances protein synthesis.[1] In its own right therefore, insulin functions as a growth stimulating hormone as originally proposed by Salter and Best.[2]

The role of insulin in the fetus however is less well understood. In general the fetus is not exposed to fluctuations in the availability of nutritional energy as is the meal eating or foraging adult. A relatively constant supply of glucose and other substrates is available to the fetus under normal circumstances *in utero*. This steady flow of nutrients is determined by the mechanism that achieves homeostasis of plasma nutrients in the mother. Furthermore the intrauterine environment ensures that energy consumption is uniform since there is little need for bursts of muscle activity, or heat production by the fetus. The major metabolic concern of the fetus therefore is not homeostasis but constant anabolism that will ultimately result in the promotion of rapid growth and differentiation. As parturition nears[7] this anabolism is directed towards the conservation of energy reserves in the form of glycogen and triglyceride. This nutritional preparation by the fetus in anticipation of the expensive energy support required in the early neonatal period for thermogenesis, respiration and muscle activity is vital to the survival of the newborn.

Whether insulin is essential to this anabolic process is undetermined. It is widely accepted that the secretion and release of fetal insulin is in part controlled by the mean concentration of maternal blood glucose.[3] Chez, *et al.*[4] have demonstrated that the fetus exposed to a hyperglycemic environment responds to an acute glucose challenge in a more sensitive way than the fetus who has previously been euglycemic. In the offspring of the human diabetic, the concentration of insulin in cord blood correlates well with the mean level of maternal blood glucose during late gestation.[5] Therefore the presence of adequate amounts of insulin coinciding with that of abundant glucose as is present in the normal fetus, represents a circumstance that in general physiologic terms promotes a strongly anabolic and lipogenic state. It was with this hypothesis in mind that we embarked on our studies concerned with the effects of insulin on fetal fat metabolism.

The Effects of Insulin on Fetal Brown Adipose Tissue

To determine the physiologic importance of insulin in promoting glucose uptake in brown adipose tissue, Yeomans and O'Hea[16] to whom we are indebted for permission to present this current data, incubated this organ *in vitro* with glucose-C[14]. The experimental brown adipose tissue homogenates were incubated with glucagon-free insulin in concentrations of 100, and 1000 microunits per ml. Controls were incubated in the absence of insulin. The concentrations of both insulin and glucose were calculated to be within the physiologic range of the *in vivo* circumstance.

The presence of insulin in the incubating medium significantly enhanced the incorporation of glucose-C[14] into the fatty acid and glyceride-glycerol fraction of brown adipose tissue lipid (Fig. 6-1). It also increased the conversion of glucose to CO_2 (Fig. 6-2). Insulin exerted no significant effect on glucose utilization by fetal liver or diaphragm under similar circumstances.

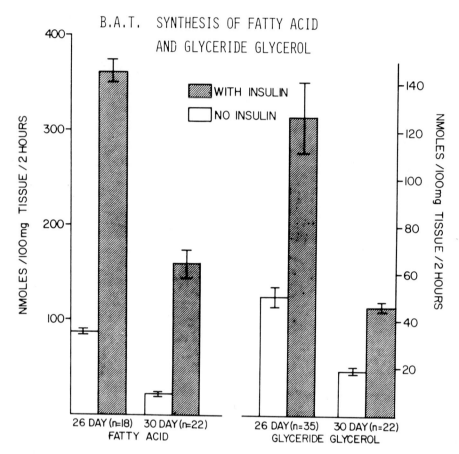

Figure 6-1.   The effect of insulin on the incorporation of glucose-C^{14} into the fatty acid and glyceride-glycerol fraction of brown adipose tissue lipid *in vitro* (26 and 30 day rabbit fetuses).

A comparable experiment conducted *in vivo* in which glucose-C^{14} with or without insulin (4 units) was injected intraperitoneally into the rabbit fetus *in utero*, revealed a threefold increase in the incorporation of glucose into the total lipid component of brown adipose tissue under the influence of the injected insulin (Fig. 6-3).

In spite of evidence from this study as well as others that glucose represents a relatively ineffective challenge to the release

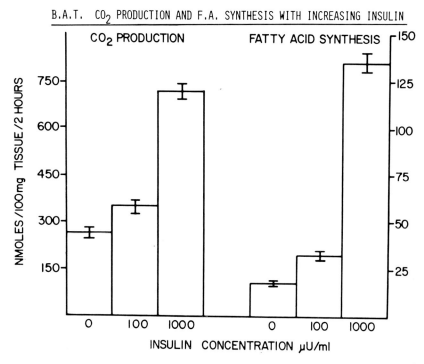

Figure 6-2. The effect of insulin concentration on the conversion of glucose-C^{14} to CO$_2$ and fatty acid in brown adipose tissue lipid *in vitro* (term rabbit fetuses).

of fetal insulin, certain fetal tissues, possibly those most concerned with the conservation of nutrients, such as adipose tissue, have acquired a sensitivity to insulin during the latter part of pregnancy. It is postulated that fetal insulin under these circumstances primarily exerts an anabolic function rather than performing a homeostatic role at least during the latter part of intrauterine life.

The neuroendocrine influence of the central nervous system on fetal lipid metabolism has been emphasized by Jack & Milner[6] who have observed that decapitation of the rabbit fetus on day twenty-four results in an increase in fetal plasm insulin on day twenty-nine (term 31 days). In addition, under *in vitro* conditions the pancreas of the decapitated fetus secretes more insulin

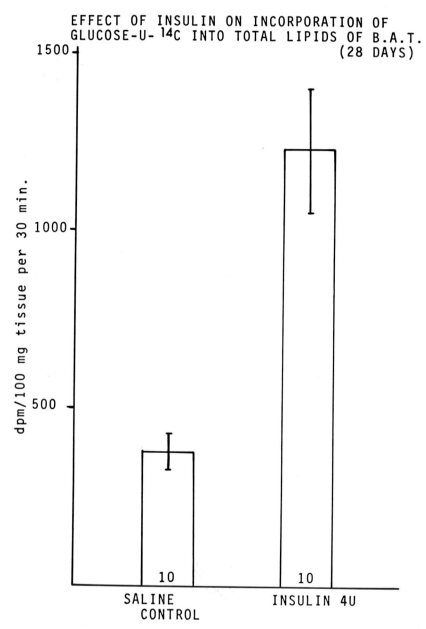

Figure 6-3. The effect of insulin on the incorporation of glucose-C[14] into lipid of fetal brown adipose tissue *in vivo*. Rabbit fetuses injected in utero on day 28 of gestation.

than do those of intact fetuses. Glucagon does not influence this secretion. It was suggested by Milner that the lipogenesis observed in decapitated fetuses may represent an important effect of this increased insulin secretion. The anencephalic human fetus without significant pituitary function also demonstrates an accentuated rate of fat deposition. This cephalic concept implies that the integrated regulation of lipid metabolism in the fetus involves glucose, insulin and lipogenesis and the latter can be suppressed through some form of central control.

The other end of the nutritional spectrum in the fetus, i.e. the effect of deficient fetal glucose and insulin and its possible role in inducing intrauterine fetal growth retardation is of interest as well. Does this common syndrome merely result from a deficiency of glucose and/or other substrates and thus secondary hypoinsulinemia; or is the pathophysiologic deficiency a more complex one involving such possibilities as a failure of response of the insulin-secreting mechanism that normally releases insulin following a substrate challenge? It may well be asked whether the therapeutic provision of glucose to the fetus by nonplacental routes will improve the anabolic state if, perchance, the release of insulin in response to the substrate is deficient. Experiments presently under way in our laboratory have resulted in the induction of fetal hypoinsulinemia during the latter part of pregnancy in the rabbit. The effects of this hypoinsulinemic state on fetal lipid metabolism are being studied.

Ketone Metabolism in the Fetus

Recent interest in the role and effect of ketones in the fetus has been generated by concern regarding the human fetus in two areas:

1. That acute maternal starvation may prove detrimental to the fetus through a mechanism involving a transfer of maternal ketone bodies across the placenta.

2. That the undernourished fetus may be capable of utilizing previously accumulated fat reserves to meet his energy requirements if and when the availability of glucose declines. It is a well established biochemical principle that when lipolysis is enhanced in the presence of a relative deficiency of glucose, the

incomplete oxidation of the fatty acids and the generation of actyl CoA results in the production and accumulation of ketones of which B-hydroxybutyrate is the most quantitatively important.

Recent evidence[8] has suggested that ketones acquired by the fetus from the mother either during starvation or associated with poorly controlled diabetes, may prove detrimental to the later motor-mental performance of the offspring. Since maternal ketonuria commonly occurs during the latter part of pregnancy if the daily caloric intake becomes less than 1600 calories and since starvation of the pregnant woman for twelve hours in late pregnancy also results in a significant increase in plasma ketones[7] it is important to learn more about the metabolism of ketones by the fetus.

In addition to the acquisition of ketones transplacentally, it is possible the fetus may generate such compounds. Whether the fetus under normal or abnormal circumstances is capable of catabolizing his own fat stores and thereby inducing a potential mechanism for ketone production, has been the subject of much controversy. Undoubtedly the enzymatic potential for lipolysis is present in the fetus[9] and it has been previously shown that lipolysis in brown adipose tissue is accelerated in the fetal rabbit during post-term nutritional deprivation.[10] Twenty years ago Popjak[11] noted the rapid incorporation of minor quantities of ketones injected into the mother, but concluded that under normal circumstances, glucose represented the exclusive fetal substrate. In spite of this evidence, it is possible that the "normal" fetus to whom it has always been assumed the availability of glucose is continuously abundant, may be exposed to frequent episodes of relative glucose deficiency during the usual overnight fast of the mother. The fact that the slow infusion of glucose into the laboring mother subjected to starvation results in a significant reduction of maternal plasma ketone concentration would tend to support this proposal. With this background suggesting that the human fetus may frequently be exposed to a ketone challenge, we elected to study the fetal metabolism of radio labelled C^{14} B-hydroxybutyrate that was injected into the mother, using the rat as our model.

The Incorporation of B-hydroxybutyrate into the
Lipids of Fetal Tissues

On the day prior to expected delivery, approximately 25 microcuries of C^{14} B-hydroxybutyric acid was injected into the tail vein of the pregnant rat under light ether anesthesia. The disposition of the radioactive ketone in the mother and fetus during the following three hours was analyzed. The tissues examined included brown adipose tissue, pancreas, liver, brain, lung, placenta and maternal and fetal blood. Radioactivity excreted through the maternal lung and kidney was also determined.

RESULTS

Of the fetal tissues, brown adipose tissue incorporated B-hydroxybutyrate into lipids at a much greater rate than any of the other tissues studied (Figs. 6-4 & 6-5). Its closest rival, lung, incorporated one-fourth the quantity of ketone per gram of tissue into lipid during the three hours as compared to brown adipose tissue. The remaining tissues in descending order of incorporation into lipids were pancreas, liver, brain and placenta. Extraction of fetal blood yielded very few counts and the activity present resided in the water soluble component and appeared to represent nonmetabolized B-hydroxybutyrate. As yet it is uncertain what proportion of the radioactivity in fetal plasma was associated with CO_2.

In brown adipose tissue, the greatest activity was within the triglyceride fraction followed by the phospholipid fraction (Figs. 6-6 & 6-7). In other tissues, the major portion of the extracted counts appeared in the phospholipid fraction, probably as a membrane component. It is of interest to note that in the case of liver, brain and pancreas, the next highest activity was found in the diglyceride fraction. Diglyceride probably represents a precursor substrate for phospholipid synthesis. In tissues other than adipose tissue, the phospholipid pattern showed maximum incorporation into phosphatidyl choline and to a lesser extent phosphatidyl ethanolamine; whereas, in adipose tissue,

The Mammalian Fetus

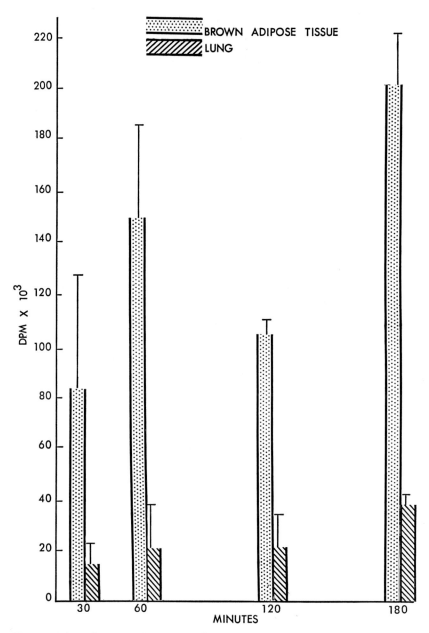

Figure 6-4. The incorporation of maternally injected DL-β-hydroxy-butyrate-3-C[14] into BAT and lung of the term fetal rat over 3 hours (radioactivity/gm wet weight).

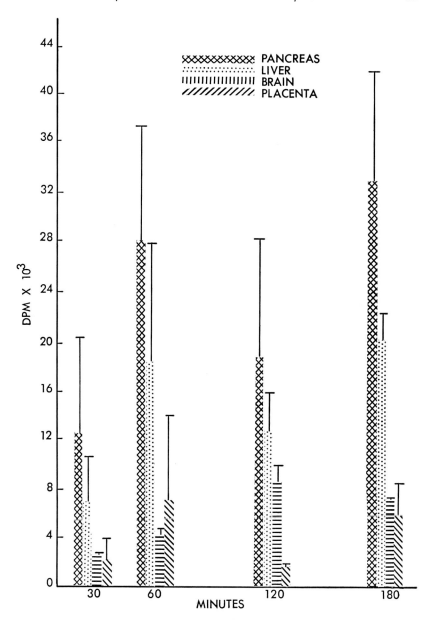

Figure 6-5. The incorporation of maternally injected DL-β-hydroxy-butyrate-3-C[14] into fetal pancreas, liver, brain and placenta over 3 hours (radioactivity/gm wet weight).

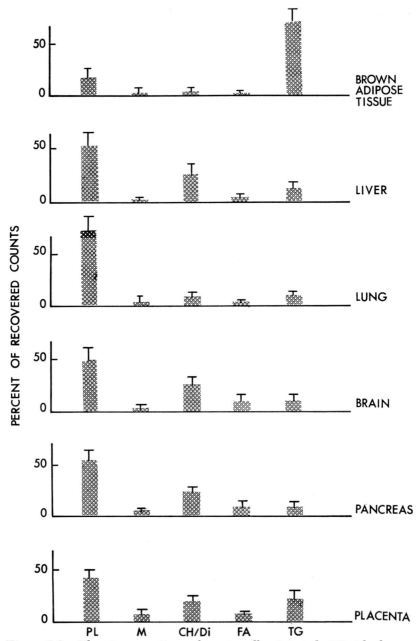

Figure 6-6. The incorporation of maternally injected DL-β-hydroxy-butyrate-3-C^{14} into the lipid fractions of fetal tissues expressed as a % of total radioactivity recovered (Mean = S.D.): Term fetal rat. PL—phospholipid: M—monoglyceride: CH/DI—cholesterol and diglyceride: FA—fatty acid: TG—triglyceride.

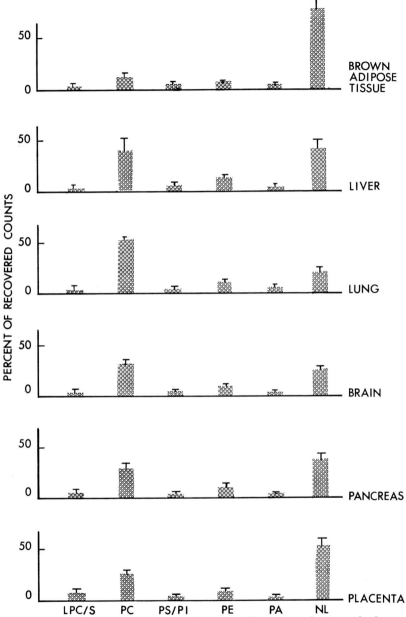

Figure 6-7. The incorporation of maternally injected DL-β-hydroxy-butyrate-3-C[14] into the phospholipid fractions of fetal tissues expressed as a % of total radioactivity recovered (Mean + S.D.): Term fetal rat. LPC/S—lysophosphatidyl choline + sphingomyelin: PS/PI—phosphatidylserine + phosphatidyl inositol: PE—phosphatidyl ethanolamine: PA—phosphatidyl glycerol and phosphatidic acid: NL—neutral lipid.

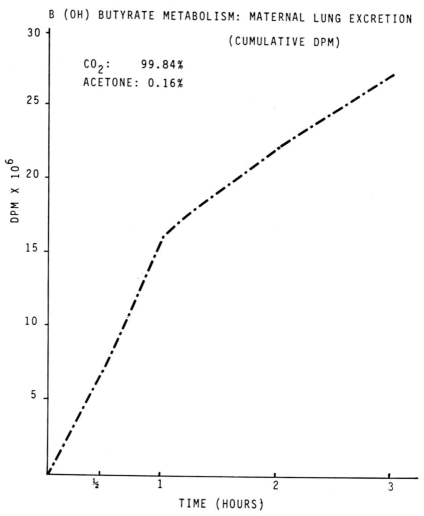

Figure 6-8. Maternally expired $^{14}CO_2$ collected during 3 hours following injection of DL-β-hydroxybutyrate-3-C^{14} (32 μCi). (Mean radioactivity + S.D.)

phospholipid incorporation was minimal compared to that into triglyceride.

During the three hour study period, the maternal loss of radio-activity through lung approximated slightly less than 35 percent of the total injected activity (Fig. 6-8). The major, if not total portion of lung loss would be the result of oxidation by either maternal or fetal tissues of the D-isomer subsequently yielding radioactive CO_2. It has been assumed that the L-isomer of B-hydroxybutyrate is not metabolized to any physiologic extent although red blood cells are capable of oxidizing this isomer to a minor degree and a fraction of the lung excretion of radioactive CO_2 may be due to this source. The amount of radioactive acetone excreted in lung and the overall radioactivity in urine was negligible. Assuming the D-isomer to be the major active metabolite, approximately 7 percent of the maternally injected dose of B-hydroxybutyrate was incorporated into fetal tissue lipid within the three hour period. As far as the quantitative lipid synthesis within the total organ was concerned, brown adipose tissue, liver and lung were by far the principal consumers of the ketone substrate.

The foregoing data would suggest that the most concentrated ketone in plasma, B-hydroxybutyric acid, rapidly traverses the placenta in the rat (and other evidence would suggest a similar situation exists in the human) and that a significant proportion of the ketone quickly becomes incorporated into fetal lipid both neutral and phospholipid. Whether maternally acquired ketones are utilized preferentially over glucose by specific fetal tissues, or under certain circumstances such as maternal starvation or whether ketones produced within the fetus itself are metabolized in the same way are still open, yet valid and practical questions.

Ketone Metabolism in the Human Fetus and the Diagnosis of Fetal Malnutrition

It has been suggested that during a relative deficiency of glucose, the human fetus may resort to the hydrolysis and oxidation of his own lipid reserves thereby establishing the mechanism for ketone production. Presumably during an acute process of lipolysis, the water soluble ketones would appear in fetal plasma and possibly in amniotic fluid via fetal excretion. A correlation between ketone production by the fetus and other complications of pregnancy has been suggested by the evidence that an elevated level of B-hydroxybutyrate is found in the blood of newborn infants who have experienced fetal distress during labor or, who have been subjected to a pre-eclamptic environment *in utero*.[13] This would imply that, in addition to nutritional stress, intrauterine hypoxia may induce significant lipolysis in the fetus as well.

There would appear to be two components to the origin of fetal ketones:

1. Under normal circumstances there exists a maternal to fetal ketone gradient that is probably established by the elevated maternal ketone plasma level associated in part with the strong lipolytic potential attributed to placental lactogen. This maternal component is most marked after fasting and can be abolished by maternal glucose infusion.

2. A fetal source that occurs during a state of metabolic fetal "stress" presumably initiates fetal lipolysis and ketonemia. This may abolish or even reverse the normal ketone gradient from mother to fetus, to a fetus to mother situation.

The clinical application of ketone metabolism by the fetus has been advanced by several recent studies demonstrating a correlation between maternal and fetal plasma and amniotic fluid ketones both during and prior to labor.[7, 14, 15]

The following data from our obstetrical intensive care unit supports the hypothesis that an elevated ketone concentration in umbilical cord blood is present in the "metabolically stressed" infant. Of eighty confinements analyzed in the Unit, twenty-three resulted in "abnormal" infants as defined by a trained neonatalogist present at the time of delivery. These included small for gestational age infants, infants of diabetic mothers and those showing evidence of acute fetal distress on the basis of a monitored deceleration in fetal heart rate, acidosis at birth or a five minute Apgar score of six or less (Fig. 6-9). All infants in the study population were delivered vaginally and the mothers routinely receive 5 percent glucose infusion during the labour.

The "abnormal" infants demonstrated elevated cord blood ketone concentrations when compared with normal infants of comparable birth weight and gestational age. It is apparent that the relative significance of the cord blood ketone concentration

CORD BLOOD B (OH) BUTYRATE WITH COMPLICATIONS

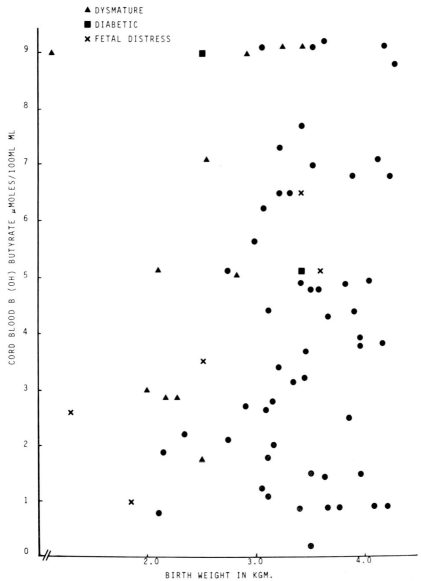

Figure 6-9. The concentration of β-hydroxybutyrate in mixed umbilical cord blood from normal, dysmature, diabetic and hypoxic newborn infants as related to birth weight.

is dependent on the weight and/or gestational age of the infant. This reflects the reduced fat substrate available for lipolysis in the smaller infant compared to the heavier infant who possesses both advantages in substrate availability and presumably the effectiveness of mature metabolic mechanisms for lipolysis. The ability to synthesize ketones thus appears to reflect both maturity and the availability of triglyceride reserves and both parameters must be taken into account in assessing the clinical significance of ketone levels in the fetus. Studies are presently under way to determine whether the same principle applies to amniotic fluid ketones in view of the wide scatter in this assay shown in the data of Smith and Scanlon.[12]

CONCLUSION

The aforementioned evidence allows the following points to be made:

1. Fetal insulin although not acutely sensitive to changes in fetal glucose, nonetheless serves an important anabolic role in the promotion of fetal adipose tissue lipid in particular. Beyond this one might speculate as to the possibility that a failure of adipose tissue to respond to insulin may represent part of the defect occurring during intrauterine growth retardation. The evidence that the fetal central nervous system is involved in peripheral lipid metabolism also supports the hypothesis that growth retardation may not necessarily result solely from a fetal deficiency of glucose.

2. Ketone bodies and in particular B-hydroxybutyrate can function as a significant substrate for a number of fetal tissues, especially adipose tissue and lung even in the presence of apparently adequate amounts of glucose. It is valid to ask whether the tissue pattern of ketone utilization by the fetus is altered either quantitatively or qualitatively during the short episodes of maternal fasting that are sufficient to produce maternal ketonemia. Whether ketone utilization by the fetus represents an advantage or indeed potential disadvantage to ultimate development is an important subject for further investigation.

REFERENCES

1. Manchester, K. L.: Protein metabolism. In Ellenberg, M. (Ed.): *Diab Mell Theory Practice*. New York, McGraw-Hill, 1970, p. 28.
2. Salter, J., and Best, C. H.: Insulin as a growth hormone. *Br Med J,* 2:354, 1953.
3. Shelley, H.: Fetal and Neonatal Physiology, Proceedings of the Barcroft Symposium. Cambridge U P, 1973, p. 360.
4. Chez, R. A.; Mintz, D. H., and Hutchinson, D. L.: Effect of theophylline on glucagon and glucose-mediated plasmia insulin responses in subhuman primate fetus and neonate. *Metabolism,* 20:805, 1971.
5. Shimak, T.; Price, S., and Foa, P.: Serum insulin concentration and birth weight in human infants. *Proc Soc Exp Biol Med, 121*:55, 1966.
6. Jack, P. M. B., and Milner, R. D. G.: Foetal decapitation and the development of insulin secretion in the rabbit. Foetal and Neonatal Physiology: Proc. Barcroft Symposium, 1973, p. 346.
7. Paterson, P.; Sheath, J.; Taft, P., and Wood, C.: Maternal and fetal ketone concentrations in plasma and urine. *Lancet, 1*:862, 1967.
8. Churchill, J. A., and Berendes, H. W.: Perinatal factors affecting human development. *W H O, 30*: 1969.
9. Roux, J. F.; Yoshioka, T., and Myers, R. E.: Conversion of palmitate to respiratory CO_2 by fetal tissue of man and monkey. *Nature* (London), *227*:963, 1970.
10. Harding, P., and Ralph, E. D.: Effects of chronic hypoxia on lipolysis in brown adipose tissue in the foetal rabbit. *Am J Obstet Gynecol, 106*:907. 1970.
11. Popjak, G.: Gold Spring Harbor Symposium. *Quant Biol, 19*:200, 1954.
12. Smith, A. L., and Scanlon, J.: Amnionic fluid β-hydroxybutyrate and the dysmature fetus. *Am J Obstet Gynecol, 115*:569, 1973.
13. Persson, B., and Tunell, R.: *Acta Paediat Scand, 60*:385, 1971.
14. Rubaltelli, F. F.: Maternal and foetal ketone levels. *Lancet, 1*:1103, 1967.
15. Szabota, V.; Wolf, H., and Lausman, S.: *Biol Neonate, 13*:7, 1968.
16. Yeomans, C., and O'Hea, K.: *In vitro* and *in vivo* effects of insulin on fetal rabbit tissue. *Can J Physiol Pharmacol,* 1974, in press.
17. ――――: The pancreatic insulin response of fetal rabbits to acute and chronic hyperglycaemia. *Can J Physiol Pharmacol,* 1974, in press.

Chapter 7

PERINATAL ENERGY METABOLISM

J. C. Sinclair, and J. B. Warshaw

ENERGY BALANCE

In describing energy balance in the perinatal period, we should consider that energy intake is balanced by the sum of various modes of energy expenditure.

After Birth

There are two sources of energy on the input side: caloric stores and caloric value of ingested food. In respect to body composition and caloric stores, important differences exist between newborn babies of differing birth weight. In small premature babies, water content is high due to a large extracellular water compartment. Fat, on the other hand, is virtually absent in babies under 1500g. With increasing fetal weight, the fat content of the body progressively increases; in normally-grown babies at term, it may comprise 16 percent of body weight. Glycogen stores in fetal liver accumulate mostly during the last weeks of gestation. Thus, the baby who is small at birth has a considerable limitation of caloric stores as compared with the large baby. Moreover, this deficiency applies both to the small pre-term baby and to the small-for-dates infant; in the latter, slow fetal growth is associated both with the failure to lay down fat at the normal rate and with failure to accumulate normal hepatic glycogen stores.

On the output side of the balance, we should consider the

following: fecal loss of ingested calories, basal metabolism, increments above basal imposed by thermal stress, activity, or the calorigenic response to ingested food (specific dynamic action), and caloric requirement for growth. Fecal loss of calories is mainly due to unabsorbed dietary fat. In babies fed a cow milk formula containing butter fat, 25 percent or more of the fat may be unabsorbed. However, when human breast milk or vegetable oils (as used in most proprietary formulas) are fed, term infants fail to absorb only about 5 percent of the fat, and premature babies only about 10 percent. Protein and carbohydrate are almost completely absorbed, even by the premature infant. Thus, it is unlikely that "metabolizable energy" will amount to less than 90 percent of ingested calories, except in the presence of malabsorption or the feeding of an inappropriate fat.

Using the technique of indirect calorimetry,[1] we have measured the minimal metabolic rate of fed, thriving low birthweight infants at weekly intervals during the nursery course. The measurements are obtained in a warm environment (thermoneutral) with the baby quietly asleep, within ninety minutes after feeding. Thus, the result obtained includes the contribution of SDA. The minimal metabolic rate, defined in this way, rises from 50 to 60 Cal/kg. day with increasing postnatal age beyond the first week of postnatal life (Table 7-I). Values within the first week are about 25 percent less. Most babies who are

TABLE 7-I

MINIMAL METABOLIC RATE IN LOW BIRTH-WEIGHT BABIES[*]

AGE (days)	MEAN (kCal/kg/day)	S.D.
8-14	49.4	6.2
15-21	52.0	7.1
22-28	55.2	5.7
29-35	55.1	7.4
36-42	55.0	5.9
43-49	58.6	6.1
50-56	60.8	6.2
57-63	60.4	10.6

[*] J. C. Sinclair, and W. A. Silverman, Longitudinal measurements of oxygen consumption and heat flux in infants of low birth weight, *Am Ped Soc and Soc Pediatr Res*, 1970, p. 246.

small for gestational age tend to have higher metabolic rates per kg. Experimental observations of others show increments above basal metabolic rate due to the effects of cold, activity and food in newborn babies.

The number of calories available for growth will depend on the caloric intake, and the caloric expenditures via the routes described. Studies of Fomon, *et al.*[2, 3, 4] provide for full-term infants, good quantitative descriptions of energy intake and growth in infancy. As might be expected, these studies showed that a higher caloric intake was associated with a more rapid rate of weight gain. Infant formulas believed to be nutritionally adequate were fed to normal full-term infants from 8 to 112 days of age. Weight of each food consumed by every infant during each day of study was recorded. Volume of intake and caloric intake were calculated for standardized post-natal age intervals, as were body weight and length. Performance of formula-fed babies was given by the 10th, 50th, and 90th percentiles for weight and length, by sex, up to 112 days. Males exceeded females both in caloric intake and growth increments; however, there was no sex difference in weight gain per unit calorie intake.

Fomon, *et al.* speculated about the partition of energy between growth and maintenance (defining the latter as metabolizable calories minus calories for growth). To calculate the energy cost of growth, two estimates are needed: the amount of fat and protein deposited in growing tissue, and the total energy cost of depositing each gram of fat and protein. The first estimate is derived from a consideration of body composition changes in infancy. Over the first four months of life, it can be calculated that weight gain consists of 40.8 percent lipid and 11.4 percent protein.[5] The second estimate is derived from energy balance trials in infant pigs (slaughter technique), where the total energy cost of synthesizing fat and protein was estimated at 11.6 and 7.5 Cal/g respectively.[6] The energy requirement for growth was calculated as 5.5 Cal/g. The energy partition of the growing normal infant, calculated in this way, indicates that about one third of the total caloric intake is used for growth.

We now return to the caloric intake and neonatal growth of low birth-weight babies whose metabolic rates were discussed earlier. Each infant had serial determinations of metabolic rate at approximately weekly intervals. Figure 7-1 shows a typical infant. The total basal energy expenditure over the postnatal age interval of study was calculated, subtracted from the total caloric intake, and related to the rate of weight gain. As shown in Figure 7-2, there is a significant tendency for the quantity (caloric intake minus basal expenditure) to rise as daily weight gain rises. This conclusion is similar to that of Fomon in full size infants, but here we have controlled one additional factor in energy balance, namely basal caloric expenditure.

By taking into account literature values for composition of weight gain in the low birth-weight infant, the caloric cost of weight gain in our low birth-weight infants can be calculated. Figure 7-3 shows a comparison between the energy partition

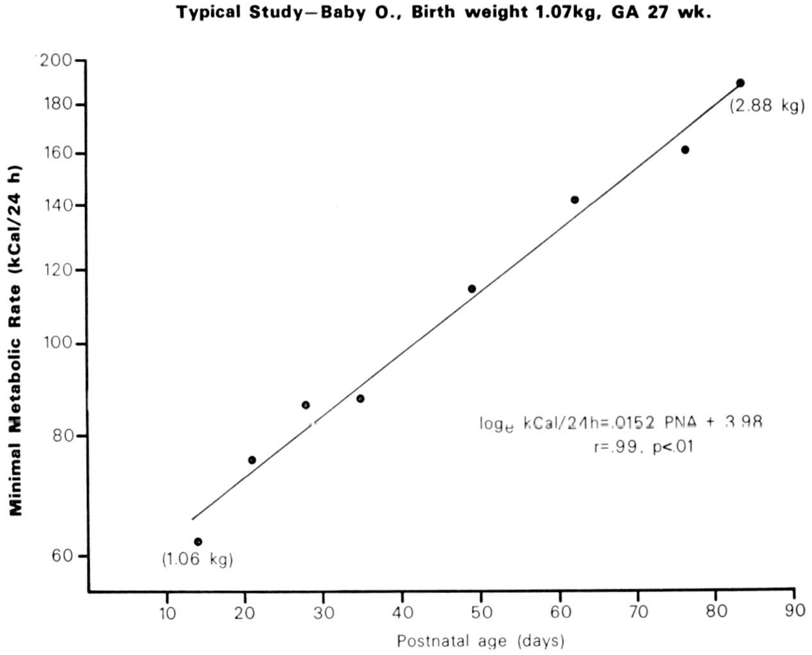

Typical Study—Baby O., Birth weight 1.07kg, GA 27 wk.

$$\log_e \text{kCal/24h} = .0152 \text{ PNA} + 3.98$$
$$r = .99, \ p < .01$$

Figure 7-1. Serial measurement of minimal metabolic rate in a single low birth-weight infant. J. C. Sinclair, and W. A. Silverman, Longitudinal measurements of oxygen consumption and heat flux in infants of low birth weight. *Am Ped Soc and Soc Pediatr Res* (Abstract), 1970, p. 246.

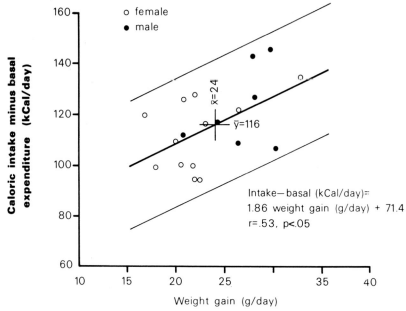

Figure 7-2. Relation between caloric intake, basal caloric expenditure and weight gain, in nineteen low birth-weight infants. J. C. Sinclair, and W. A. Silverman, Longitudinal measurements of oxygen consumption and heat flux in infants of low birth weight. *Am Ped Soc and Soc Pediatr Res* (Abstract), 1970, p. 246.

of a low birth-weight infant and a full-size infant, at comparable post-natal age (8-55 days). Over this age interval, gain in weight per 100 Cal intake averages 11.5 g/100 Cal for the low birth-weight infant and 7.2 g/100 Cal for the full size baby. Yet the comparison shown in Figure 7-3 suggests that the low birth-weight infant directs only about 25 percent of his intake to growth, versus 43 percent by the full size infant of comparable post-natal age. This is an apparent paradox, since a plane of nutrition in which the large majority of ingested calories go for maintenance costs would be expected to produce only a small weight gain per unit of calorie intake. The resolution of the paradox apparently resides in the calculated difference in composition of weight gain—lipid-rich in the case of the full size infant, and lipid-poor in the case of the low birth-weight infant.

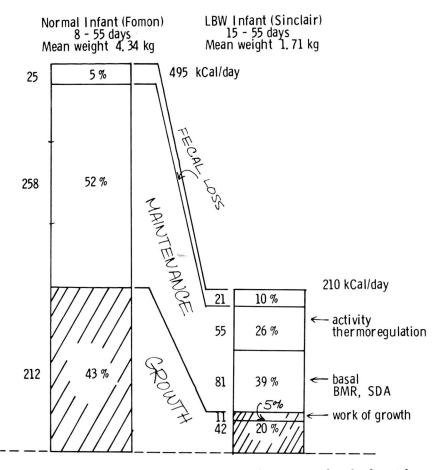

Figure 7-3. The postnatal energy balance of a growing low birth-weight infant is contrasted with that of a full size infant. The figures for the full size baby are derived from the report of Fomon and co-workers.[4] The figures for the low birth-weight infant were derived as follows: the total caloric intake, measured basal energy expenditure, and growth increments were experimentally determined for the infants described in Table 7-I. A fecal loss of 10 percent of ingested calories was assumed. Composition of weight gain was estimated from values given in the literature for fetal weight range 1 to 2.5 kg. The total energy cost of laying down fat and protein was estimated at 11.6 and 7.5 Cal/g respectively,[6] but the caloric equivalent of growth was calculated in addition on the heat of combustion of fat and protein. The difference was identified as the "work" of growth, and included part of the measured resting metabolism.

The caloric equivalent of weight gain is two to three times greater in the case of the full size baby.

Therefore, it might be postulated that weight gain by low birth-weight infants may be quite sensitive to changes in the various factors of the energy balance, because: 1) at a plane of nutrition which they are commonly able to achieve a relatively small proportion of intake is directed to weight gain, and a relatively large proportion to maintenance costs, and 2) the caloric equivalent of weight gain is low.

Studies of the effect of thermal environment on the growth of low birth-weight neonates[7, 8] demonstrate that the increased metabolic demand of a sub-thermoneutral environment slows growth when caloric intake is held constant. Thus, we have experimental confirmation that neonatal growth rate is a function of at least one factor determining energy expenditure, as well as being dependent on the level of energy intake.[2]

Before Birth

Sources of energy for the fetus are derived transplacentally. Quantitatively important nutrient intake via fetal swallowing does not occur, because the caloric value of amniotic fluid is low. It is of interest, however, that an attempt to increase fetal caloric intake by this route has been reported in cases where human fetal growth retardation was diagnosed antenatally; this method involved the repeated intra-amniotic injection of amino acids (protein hydrolysate).[9]

Fuels made available to the fetus from maternal circulation include glucose, amino acids, fatty acids and ketone bodies. Glucose and amino acids cross the placenta readily, fatty acids and ketones less readily. Considerable evidence has evolved suggesting glucose as the preferred metabolic fuel of the mammalian fetus. For example, the respiratory quotient of the human newborn is 1.0 at birth but by twelve to eighteen hours of age has fallen to 0.8, suggesting that the neonate only then begins to adapt to fatty acid oxidation. If one were to calculate the relationship between glucose uptake and oxygen consumption of the fetus, it might be predicted that all of the substrate for aerobic metabolism would be supplied by glucose. James, *et al.*[10]

investigated this possibility in fetal sheep. Using a chronic preparation, these authors found that the fetal glucose/O_2 quotient, at a normal maternal blood glucose concentration, was approximately 0.41. It would appear that in normal sheep umbilical glucose uptake accounts, at most, for 50 percent of fetal O_2 consumption. When the ewe is starved, fetal glucose uptake is diminished more than fetal oxygen uptake, and the glucose/O_2 quotient falls.[11] Under these circumstances, umbilical glucose uptake would appear to account for considerably less than half of fetal O_2 consumption. Thus, in the sheep, some other metabolic fuels must be crossing the placenta in significant amounts. They do not appear to be medium or long chain fatty acids or glycerol[12] or fructose.[13] Because amino acids rapidly cross the placenta, they may be a quantitatively important fetal substrate. In fact, the sheep fetus does show an active oxidation of amino acids and a high urea production rate.[14]

It has been shown[15] that the brain of the fetal lamb has a glucose/O_2 quotient of approximately one when the mother is in the fed state. Boyd, *et al.*[11] suggest that the organs of the fetal sheep may in fact consume glucose predominantly as a metabolic fuel despite the apparently low umbilical glucose uptake. This hypothesis implies the occurrence of gluconeogenesis from transplacentally derived amino acids or other substrates by the fetus. On the other hand, a number of investigators have shown, in other species, that key regulatory enzymes of gluconeogenesis such as pyruvate carboxylase and phosphoenolpyruvate carboxykinase are virtually absent from the fetal liver, and increase in activity only after birth (see below).

Overall energy expenditure, in the fetal lamb, amounts to about 6 ml of oxygen per kg per minute[10] (approximately 42 Cal per kg per 24h). This figure is only slightly below the basal metabolic rate after birth in this species. In addition to a basal metabolism, the fetus must have increments in expenditure associated with activity. Neither this cost, nor the theoretical possibility of fetal metabolic thermoregulation have been investigated. The proportion of the fetal fuel uptake that is directed to growth rather than maintenance can be inferred, at least for the fetal sheep, from the studies of the Denver group. Of

the total carbon and nitrogen crossing the placenta from mother
to fetus in late pregnancy, about 40 percent of the carbon, and
60 percent of the nitrogen, are retained in the normally growing
fetus.[10, 14]

BIOCHEMICAL PATHWAYS OF ENERGY
TRANSFORMATION—PERINATAL ADAPTATIONS

In man and other species, glycogen accumulates in organs
such as heart, liver, and kidney throughout much of the latter
half of gestation. Coincident with birth, the large glycogen
depot, which in the liver may be as great as 5 percent of hepatic
weight, drops precipitously, and only during the ensuing days
does it reach levels found in the adult. This large reservoir of
glucose in the form of glycogen is an important available source
of energy during the intra-partum period when the fetus is likely
to be exposed to hypoxic stress. Indeed, hypoxia itself in the
asphyxiated newborn provides a potent stimulus for glycogen
breakdown to glucose. Abnormally rapid depletion or failure
of glycogen deposition may be associated with neonatal hypoglycemia, as in the cases of small-for-dates or pre-term infants.

Glycolysis

Fetal tissues have an active anaerobic glycolysis. Glycolytic
enzyme activity during fetal and postnatal development reflects
the differences in fuels provided to the organisms at these times.
For example, pyruvate kinase activities in the rat are high in
fetal tissues but decrease at birth, probably in association with
the high fat content of milk; they increase again at the time of
weaning when carbohydrate intake of the rat increases.[16]

Embryonic and fetal tissues also have an enhanced capacity
for glucose utilization via the pentose phosphate pathway. In
general, this activity shows a gradual decrease after birth.[16]

Gluconeogenesis

A number of investigators have shown, in the rat and other
species, that key regulatory enzymes of gluconeogenesis such as
pyruvate carboxylase and phosphoenolpyruvate carboxykinase
are virtually absent from the fetal liver, and increase in activity

only after birth when glucose is no longer available from the maternal circulation and the animal switches to the high fat intake of milk. Hepatic gluconeogenesis occurs mainly in the post-natal rat and is virtually absent from the fetal liver, although three of the four enzymes required in the system are already present in late fetal life.[17] The last enzyme to make its appearance is PEP carboxykinase, which can be detected within a few hours of birth in the rat. Experiments on the incorporation of ^{14}C pyruvate into glucose by liver slices in such animals indicate the appearance of this enzyme initiates the overall process of gluconeogenesis.[17] Gluconeogenesis is prevented by anoxia with either lactate or aspartate as precursor.[18]

Oxidative Phosphorylation

Of far greater importance to the fetus than glycolysis is energy derived from glucose via citric-acid cycle oxidations and oxidative phosphorylation. A number of investigators have suggested that oxidative phosphorylation becomes quantitatively more important after birth when the newborn is exposed to a more aerobic environment. Indeed, increases in both mitochondrial number and in specific components of the citric acid cycle have been described in the immediate postnatal period.

Fatty Acid Oxidation

In the suckling animal, large quantities of fatty acids are available as metabolic fuels for the first time. Indeed, fatty acids are made available from endogenous stores as well as from the high fat intake of milk feeding. In the first hours of life, there is a surge in serum catechol levels and a rapid increase in the concentration of serum free fatty acids. As hepatic glycogen is depleted, fatty acids become important substrates, reflected by the fall of the respiratory quotient of the newborn from 1.0 to 0.7 to 0.8 during the first day of life. In contrast to their virtually absent oxidation during fetal development, fatty acids become the preferred substrates of adult tissue with high energy demands such as the heart, renal cortex and small intestinal mucosa. In those tissues fatty acid oxidation generates far more energy than would be obtained from the complete oxidation of glucose.

Development of the capacity to carry out long chain fatty acid oxidation also may be important because oxidation of fatty acids by tissues such as heart and muscle may spare glucose for brain metabolism where its availability during the postnatal period may be critical.

Figure 7-4 summarizes the sequence of events associated with the transport, cellular uptake, and mitochondrial oxidation of long chain fatty acids. Fatty acids are released from adipose tissue stores in response to B-adrenergic stimulation and are carried to the liver complexed to albumin. In the liver, the fatty acids are transported into the cell complexed to anionic binding protein. Once in the cytoplasm of the cell, the fatty acids are converted to coenzyme A esters in an energy-requiring reaction. Since fatty acid oxidation occurs in the mitochondria, the acyl-coenzyme A esters must be transported to the sites of mito-chondrial B-oxidation. However, the inner mitochondrial membrane is impermeable to coenzyme A esters of fatty acids and the palmityl-CoA must be converted to a palmitylcarnitine which

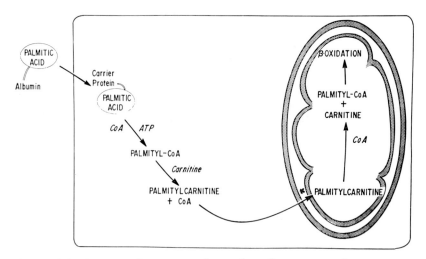

Figure 7-4. Fatty acids transported into the cell are activated to coenzyme A esters, and then are converted to carnitine esters so they can permeate the mitochondrial membrane. Inside the mitochondrion, they are recon-verted to the coenzyme A form and B-oxidation proceeds. The asterisk indicates where the initial formation of palmitylcarnitine is thought to occur.

gains rapid access to the mitochondria. The enzyme, palmityl-carnitine transferase catalyzes the equilibrium reaction between palmityl-CoA and palmitylcarnitine. Once transport has been effected, the palmitylcarnitine is reconverted to palmityl-CoA and B-oxidation proceeds. B-oxidation involves the repetitive cleavage of two carbon units of acetyl-CoA from the long chain fatty acids; the acetyl-CoA then can participate in citric acid cycle oxidations and oxidative phosphorylation.

The failure of fetal tissues to actively oxidize long chain fatty acids may relate to low activities of controlling enzymes such as palmityl-CoA synthetase, palmitylcarnitine transferase, or the enzymes of B-oxidation. Perinatal changes in these activities have been studied.[19] In the rat, activities of palmityl-CoA synthetase and palmitylcarnitine transferase were low in fetal rat liver and heart, but rose markedly during the first days after birth. There was a large rise after birth in fatty acid oxidation by rat heart (Fig. 7-5).[19]

A very special adaptation of fatty acid oxidation which is important for thermogenesis and for maintaining early survival, relates to the oxidation of fatty acids by brown adipose tissue. Brown adipose tissue is found in many species, including human infants, and is closely associated with major blood vessels where heat can be effectively transduced to the rest of the organism. Cold exposure of the newborn results in B-adrenergic stimulation of brown adipose tissue lipases in brown adipocytes. This results in an accumulation of intracellular free fatty acids in the brown fat cells. The fatty acids are then oxidized by brown fat mitochondria. The high intracellular concentration of free fatty acids is thought to uncouple oxidative phosphorylation so that heat instead of ATP is generated. This affords the newborn an early effective mechanism for temperature regulation.

Ketone Utilization

Another adaptation important for newborn metabolic homeostasis relates to the capacity of a variety of fetal and newborn tissues to oxidize ketones. It has been recognized for a number of years that serum ketone concentrations of normal newborns reach high levels during the first days of life. It appears that

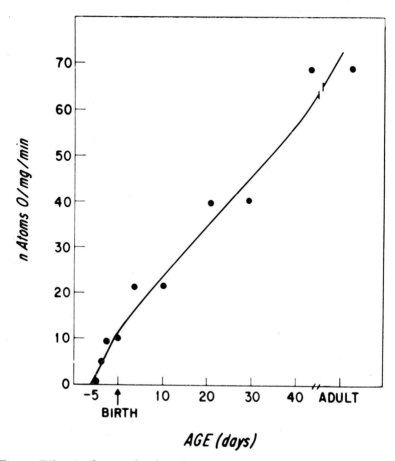

Figure 7-5. Oxidation of palmityl-Co A plus carnitine by rat heart homogenates. (J. B. Warshaw, Cellular energy metabolism during fetal development. IV. Fatty acid activation, acyl tranfer and fatty acid oxidation during development of the chick and rat, *Develop Biol, 28*:537, 1972.)

fetal and newborn brains can utilize ketone bodies as oxidative fuel quite effectively.[20] The three key enzymes for ketone body utilization, acetoacetyl-CoA thiolase, B-hydroxybutyrate dehydrogenase, and CoA transferase, all increase during the suckling period of rats to levels considerably higher than those observed in adults. Enzyme activity reaches a peak about the time of weaning and then decreases in response to higher carbohydrate intake.[21] Thus, ketone utilization is another perinatal metabolic adaptation which can effectively support newborn energy needs at a time when serum glucose may be low or restricted.

SUMMARY

Factors contributing to energy balance in the late fetal and immediate postnatal period have been reviewed. Metabolism of the fetus reflects its dependence on maternally derived substrates. Fetal energy needs are met largely, but not completely, by transplacentally derived glucose. Growth, dependent on an active incorporation of amino acids into protein, and an active capacity for lipogenesis, accounts for a large share of fetal energy uptake. After birth, a large proportion of energy uptake continues to be directed to growth; however, in the case of the low birth-weight infant, neonatal growth rate is particularly sensitive to the thermal (and probably other) demands of the extra-uterine environment. Catabolic pathways such as gluconeogenesis and fatty acid oxidation appear to be important only after emergence of the fetus from its nutritionally protected intra-uterine environment. Early metabolic adaptation of the newborn reflects changes in its substrate supply such as the sudden availability of fatty acids from adipose tissue and dietary sources. It is extremely important that the considerable amount of information obtained from animal experiments be extended to the human, where information bearing on metabolic control and integration are fragmentary at best, but of great importance.

REFERENCES

1. Sinclair, J. C., and Silverman, W. A.: Longitudinal measurements of oxygen consumption and heat flux in infants of low birth weight. *Am Pediatr Soc and Soc Pediatr Res* (abstract), 1970, p. 246.
2. Fomon, S. J.; Filer, L. J., Jr.; Thomas, L. N.; Rogers, R. R., and Proksch, A. M.: Relationship between formula concentration and rate of growth of normal infants. *J Nutr*, 98:241, 1969.
3. Fomon, S. J.; Filer, L. J., Jr.; Thomas, L. N., and Rogers, R. R.: Growth and serum chemical values of normal breastfed infants. *Acta Paediatr Scand*, (Suppl. 202), 1970.

4. Fomon, S. J.; Thomas, L. N.; Filer, L. J.; Jr.; Zeigler, E. E., and Leonard, M. T.: Food consumption and growth of normal infants fed milk-based formulas. *Acta Paediatr Scand* (Suppl. 223), 1971.

5. Fomon, S. J.: Body composition of the male reference infant during the first year of life. *Pediatrics, 40*:863, 1967.

6. Kotarbinska, M., and Kielanowski, J.: In Baxter, K. L.; Kielanowski, J., and Thorbek, G. (Eds.): *Energy Metabolism of Farm Animals.* Proc. 4th Symp. Energy Metab. Jablonna, 1967. Newcastle, Oriel Press. 1969, pp. 229-311.

7. Glass, L.; Silverman, W. A., and Sinclair, J. C.: Effect of the thermal environment on cold resistance and growth of small infants after the first week of life. *Pediatrics, 41*:1033, 1968.

8. Glass, L.; Silverman, W. A., and Sinclair, J. C.: Relationship of thermal environment and caloric intake to growth and resting metabolism in the late neonatal period. *Biol Neonat, 14*:324, 1969.

9. Renaud, R.; Vincendon, G.; Boog, G.; Brettes, J. P.; Schumacher, J. C.; Koehl, C.; Kirchstetter, L., and Gandar, R.: Injections intra-amniotiques d'acids amines dans les cas de malnutrition foetale. *J Gynecol Obstet Biol Reprod* (Paris), *1*:231, 1972.

10. James, E. J.; Raye, J. R.; Gresham, E. L.; Makowski, E. L.; Meschia, G., and Battaglia, F. C.: Fetal oxygen consumption, carbon dioxide production and glucose uptake in a chronic sheep preparation. *Pediatrics, 50*:361, 1972.

11. Boyd, R. D. H.; Morriss, F. H., Jr.; Meschia, G.; Makowski, E. L., and Battaglia, F. C.: Growth of glucose and oxygen uptakes by fetuses of fed and starved ewes. *Am J Physiol, 225*:897, 1973.

12. James, E.; Meschia, G., and Battaglia, F. C.: A-V differences of free fatty acids and glycerol in the ovine umbilical circulation. *Proc Soc Exper Biol Med, 138*:823, 1971.

13. Tsoulos, N. G.; Colwill, J. R.; Battaglia, F. C.; Makowski, E .L., and Meschia, G.: Comparison of glucose, fructose and O_2 uptakes by fetuses of fed and starved ewes. *Am J Physiol, 221*:234, 1971.

14. Gresham, E. L.; James, E. J.; Raye, J. R.; Battaglia, F. C.; Makowski, E. L., and Meschia, G.: Production and excretion of urea by the fetal lamb. *Pediatrics, 50*:372, 1972.

15. Tsoulos, N. G.; Schneider, J. M.; Colwill, J. R.; Meschia, G.; Makowski, E. L., and Battaglia, F. C.: Cerebral glucose utilization during aerobic metabolism in fetal sheep. *Pediatr Res, 6*:182, 1972.

16. Vernon, R. G., and Walker, D. G.: Changes in activity of some enzymes involved in glucose utilization and formation in developing rat liver. *J Biochem, 106*:321, 1968.

17. Yeung, D., and Oliver, I. R.: Development of gluconeogenesis in neonatal rat liver. Effect of premature delivery. *Biochem J, 105*:1229, 1967.

18. Ballard, F. J.: Regulation of gluconeogenesis during exposure of young rats to hypoxic conditions. *Biochem J, 121*:169, 1971.

19. Warshaw, J. B.: Cellular energy metabolism during fetal development. IV. Fatty acid activation, acyl transfer and fatty acid oxidation during development of the chick and rat. *Develop Biol, 28*:537, 1972.

20. Hawkins, R. A.; Williamson, D. H., and Krebs, H. A.: Ketone-body utilization by adult and suckling rat brain *in vivo*. *Biochem J, 122*:13, 1971.

21. Page, M. A.; Krebs, H. A., and Williamson, D. H.: Activities of enzymes of ketone-body utilization in brain and other tissues of suckling rats. *Biochem J, 121*:49, 1971.

Chapter 8

FETAL RENAL FUNCTION AND WATER AND ELECTROLYTE BALANCE

L. I. KLEINMAN

INTRODUCTION

THE EXCHANGE OF water between mother and fetus can be viewed as taking place within a three compartment fluid system as outlined by the scheme in Figure 8-1. The direct exchange between fetus and mother is through the placenta and the indirect

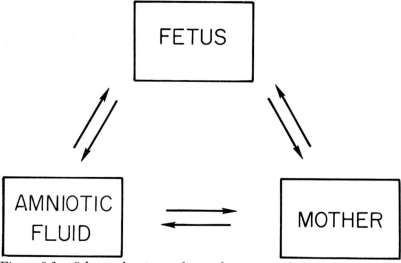

Figure 8-1. Scheme showing pathways for water and electrolyte exchange between mother and fetus.

120

maternal fetal exchange is through the amniotic fluid (in some species a fourth compartment, the allantoic fluid, should be included). One of the routes of exchange between fetus and amniotic fluid is the fetal kidney. This chapter will deal primarily with a description of the potential of the fetal kidney for excretion of water and solutes. Perinatal renal function will be emphasized not because the kidney is the primary regulator of water and electrolyte balance in the fetus, but rather because the laboratory investigation of the author has centered around the maturation of the immature kidney. This chapter, therefore, will contain the results obtained in our laboratory during the past few years, including some yet unpublished data, and a discussion of the relationships between these results and the mechanisms involved in water and electrolyte excretion by the immature kidney. In addition, a review of pertinent investigations dealing with perinatal renal physiology and background information about water compartments in the fetus will be presented in order to place the role of the fetal kidney in the appropriate perspective.

FETAL WATER COMPARTMENTS

Composition of Fetal Fluids

The total water content of the human fetus at term constitutes approximately seventy percent of the total body weight. Although the absolute volume of body water increases as the fetus matures the relative volume decreases (Fig. 8-2). At twelve weeks gestation 90 to 95 percent of the fetus is water, at twenty-four weeks this percentage drops to 85, at thirty-two weeks to 80 and finally to approximately 70 percent at birth.[35, 38, 49] Body water percentage continues to fall slowly postnatally, until it finally reaches the adult value of 55 percent. There is a great deal of variability in the measurement of total body water from fetus to fetus and this is largely related to the variability in body fat found among fetuses. The variability of the values diminishes if body water is calculated in terms of fat-free or lean body weight. Since there is a rapid increase in the percentage of

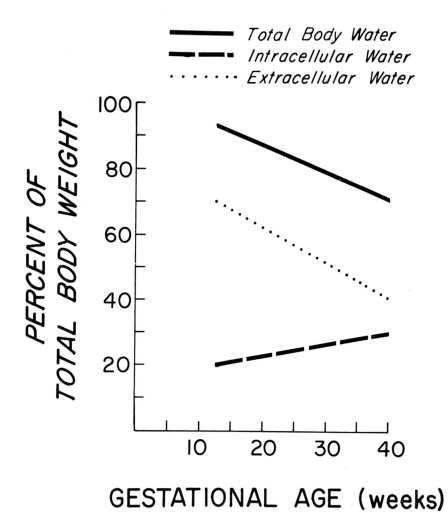

Figure 8-2. Changes in total body water, extracellular water, and intra-cellular water of the fetus during gestation. Water compartments are expressed as percentage of total body weight. Lines were derived from data of various investigators. (B. A. Fee, and W. B. Weil, Jr., Body composition of infants of diabetic mothers by direct analysis, *Ann NY Acad Sci,* *11*:869, 1963. M. H. Givens, and I. G. Macy, The chemical composition of the human fetus, *J Biol Chem, 102*:7, 1933. V. Iob, and W. W. Swanson, Mineral growth of the human fetus, *Am J Dis Child,* 47:302, 1934.)

fat after twenty-four weeks gestation the fall in percentage of water to fat-free body weight is much less during this period than that mentioned above for total body weight. At term the body water content is about 80 percent of lean body mass.[35, 93]

Most of the measurements on fetal body water content were made by direct analysis of postmortem or aborted specimens. Isotopic dilutional studies on live newborn infants, however, yield similar results to the direct body analyses.[32, 93]

Most of the water in the young fetus is found in the extra-cellular space. Extracellular water (measured as the chloride space) decreases from 65 percent of the total body weight (70% of the total body water) at twelve weeks gestation to 40 percent of the total body weight (55% of the total body water) at forty weeks gestation (Fig. 8-2). During this period of time intracellular water is increasing from 20 percent of the total body weight (30% of the total body water) at sixteen weeks to 30 percent of the total body weight (45% of the total body water) at term (Fig. 8-2). Thus, in the fetus most of the water is in the extracellular space but the relative proportion of intracellular to extracellular water increases as the fetus matures. This relative increase in intracellular water continues postnatally so that the adult has approximately 60 percent of his total body water intracellularly.

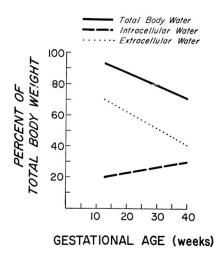

As mentioned previously, extracellular water in the fetus is usually measured as the chloride space using direct analyses of postmortem specimens. In the newborn infant extracellular water has been measured as either a) chloride space, b) corrected bromide space (corrected for intracellular chloride), c) thiocyanate space, d) inulin space, e) mannitol space, or f) thiosulfate space. Techniques using d, e, or f usually give values less than techniques using a, b, c in the adult, but in the newborn infant there is usually much closer agreement among the various techniques.[37, 51] Intracellular water is measured as the difference between total body water and extracellular water.

Since intracellular water is increasing with gestation, it is not surprising to find that total body potassium is also increasing during this time. At term, the concentration of potassium in the fat-free body tissue reaches a level about 77 percent of that of the adult value.[93] Total body sodium per unit body weight decreases during early fetal life, along with the decrease in extracellular water, but after twenty-four weeks gestation the total body sodium remains relatively constant. This is due to a balancing of two opposite effects; the tendency for sodium to decrease along with the decreasing extracellular water and the tendency for body sodium to increase along with the formation of bone.[95] Total body sodium is always much higher than total body potassium in the fetus.[93, 95]

The concentration of sodium and chloride in the extracellular space remains relatively constant throughout gestation and is nearly equal to that of maternal values. Extracellular potassium on the other hand is high in the immature fetus and decreases with maturation. The extracellular potassium concentration has been found to be 10.2 mEq/liter for a fetus of twenty to twenty-four weeks gestation, 8.0 mEq/liter for a term fetus and 4.9 mEq/liter for adults.[94] The high extracellular potassium concentration, and the relatively large extracellular water volume in the young fetus creates a situation wherein 19 percent of the total body potassium in the twenty to twenty-four week fetus is found in the extracellular space (compared to 8% for the term fetus and 2% for the adult).

Amniotic Fluid

An average 3.5 kg human fetus at term has about 700 ml of fluid in his amniotic sac. The amniotic fluid in the human fetus begins accumulating at about eight weeks gestation, reaches a maximum of about 1 liter at thirty-eight weeks gestation and then begins to decline. If parturition is delayed the volume of amniotic fluid can be expected to fall below 500 ml at forty-two weeks.[78] In contrast to fetal water volume, amniotic fluid volume is quite variable. The values given above are average values and volumes of amniotic fluid at term vary from 400 to 1500 ml. Values below this range are felt to represent conditions of oligohydramnios and values above the range represent conditions of polyhydramnios.

Early in gestation the amniotic fluid has concentrations of sodium, chloride, urea, and total osmoles similar to that of extracellular fluid. Later in gestation the concentrations of sodium, chloride and total osmoles decrease and urea rises.[78]

The origin and disposal of the amniotic fluid have still not been determined with certainty. Since the early amniotic fluid content is similar to that of extracellular fluid most investigators believe that amniotic fluid during this period of time is derived as a dialysate of maternal or fetal plasma. In this earlier period of pregnancy amniotic fluid solute concentrations are more closely related to fetal than maternal plasma concentrations.[56] In addition, fetal skin is freely permeable to water and sodium early in gestation, but the rate of diffusion of solutes through the skin decreases as the fetus matures. These observations have led Lind, *et al.*[56] to conclude that the fetus is the primary source of the amniotic fluid and that early in pregnancy amniotic fluid represents an extension of the fetal extracellular space.

In the latter half of pregnancy sources other than fetal and maternal plasma dialysates contribute to the amniotic fluid. Since fetal urine is hypotonic to plasma and has a concentration of urea greater than that of plasma,[4, 17, 39, 80] and since amniotic fluid in later pregnancy is hypotonic to plasma and has a urea concentration greater than that of plasma, it is held by most investigators that the fetal urine contributes a significant volume to the amniotic fluid. In addition, those cases associated with abnormalities of the urinary tract are often associated with abnormalities of amniotic fluid.[10]

Another source of amniotic fluid during the later part of pregnancy is the secretions of the tracheobronchial tree.[3, 74] These secretions have a sodium and osmolar concentration similar to that of plasma but a chloride and hydrogen ion concentration a good deal higher.[3] Evidence suggests that this fluid originates in the pulmonary system and moves up the tracheobronchial tree where it is either swallowed or excreted into the amniotic sac.

Since urine and pulmonary secretions are continuously being produced during the latter half of pregnancy, a source of disposal for the amniotic fluid must exist. Since fetal swallowing is known to occur,[27, 70] the gastrointestinal tract has been considered a major conduit for amniotic fluid disposal. It is hypothesized that the fetus swallows the amniotic fluid, water and solutes are absorbed into the blood stream across the intestinal mucosa, and from there carried by the blood stream to the placenta where they are returned to the mother. This hypothesis is supported by results from experiments in sheep and rabbits which revealed that the fetal gastrointestinal tract can absorb amniotic fluid.[97, 98] One of the major sources of evidence for the role of the GI tract in amniotic fluid disposal has been the association of polyhydramnios with fetuses having congenital anomalies of the GI tract (esophageal atresia, for example) or abnormalities of the swallowing mechanism (thought to be associated with anencephaly).[77]

Although the fetal kidney, respiratory tract, skin, and gastro-intestinal tract all play a role in the maintenance of the amniotic water content, other factors must also be contributory. This is based on the clinical observation that although fetuses with abnormalities of the urinary, respiratory, or gastrointestinal tracts often have abnormalities of amniotic fluid, there are instances of fetuses with renal agenesis or esophageal atresia without amniotic fluid abnormalities.[2, 24, 84] Therefore, many investigators have proposed that exchange of fluid between amnion and maternal circulation contribute to the maintenance of the amniotic fluid volume. Although there have been many studies showing the large amount of diffusional exchange of water and solutes[47, 48, 65, 68] between these two compartments, there have been few studies quantitating the bulk flow of water and solutes. Thus, although exchange of water and solutes between mother and amniotic cavity probably contribute to the regulation of amniotic fluid volume, its role relative to that of the kidney, respiratory tract, and GI tract still needs to be determined.

RENAL FUNCTION OF THE FETUS

Techniques Used to Study Fetal Renal Function

Analysis of renal function in the human fetus may be performed by investigating the human fetus directly, by studying renal function in a fetal animal model or by studying renal function postnatally in a newborn animal model with renal maturational characteristics of the human fetus. Studies of renal function dealing directly with the human fetus have been semiquantitative at best, since they have been limited to analyses of bladder urine obtained from aborted fetuses. Studies utilizing non-human fetuses have been performed with chronic *in situ* preparations[15, 20, 39, 72] or in acute experiments with the fetuses exteriorized.[6, 71, 80] The major advantage of the former technique is that results are more likely to represent the true physiological condition of the fetus since there has been minimal interference with his natural intrauterine environment. In addition, the same fetus can be utilized many times to study maturation of renal function in individual animals. The advantage of the latter technique is that more sophisticated studies may be performed (exteriorization of the fetus permits placement of catheters in almost any vessel desired). Studies in newborn animals may be done in anesthetized or unanesthetized animals and permit studies of renal function as sophisticated as any performed in adult animals. Newborn animals that may be appropriately used as models for the study of renal function in the human fetus are the dog, rat, and pig since nephrogenesis in these species is not complete until after birth.[8, 54, 91] Nephrogenesis in the human fetus is complete at thirty-five to thirty-six weeks gestation,[57, 69] and in the dog, for example, is complete two weeks after birth.[54]

Anatomical Development of the Kidney

The kidneys of most vertebrates develop through three successive but overlapping stages—the pronephros, the mesonephros, and the metanephros. The functional significance of the three stages of renal development is not the same in all animals. The mesonephros, for example, is a functional organ in cattle, sheep, pigs, cats, opossum, and rabbits.[59, 81] In rodents and man, on the other hand, the mesonephros never becomes functional. Moreover, the mesonephros persists for varying periods of time in different mammalian species. In the pig degeneration occurs in the first half of gestation; whereas, in the rabbit degeneration takes place in the second half.

The definitive mammalian kidney, the metanephros, develops from the union of the cranial part of the ureteral bud with the metanephric blastema. The ureteral bud arises from an offshoot of the mesonephric duct and ultimately forms the ureters, renal pelves, major and minor calyces, and collecting ducts. The nephroblastic cells of the metanephric blastema, upon contact with the ureteral bud, eventually develop into the glomerulus, proximal convoluted tubule, loop of Henle, and distal convoluted tubule.

The first glomeruli to develop are those which will be found in the juxtamedullary region of the mature kidney. Potter[69] has shown that at twenty-two weeks gestation all the glomeruli in the human fetus are juxtamedullary glomeruli. Since glomerular development starts in the juxtamedullary region and progresses toward the capsule, at any time during development there is a greater percentage of mature nephrons in the juxtamedullary region than there is in the outer cortex.

Glomerular Function

Glomerular filtration rate (GFR) is usually measured using a substance which is freely filterable and not reabsorbed or secreted by the tubules. Clearance of this substance, defined as UV/P, where U is the concentration of the substance in urine, P is the concentration of the substance in plasma, and V is the rate of urine flow, is equal to the GFR. Inulin has been shown in adult species to fulfill these requirements,[41, 81] and has been used frequently in perinatal renal studies. However, many studies of glomerular function in the perinatal animal have utilized substances such as creatinine, fructose, or mannitol which are not ideal glomerular markers. Some of the discrepancies in the reported values of glomerular filtration rate may be related to the use of these indicators.

Regardless of which indicator is used to measure glomerular function, all investigators have found that glomerular filtration rate is lower in the perinatal animal of all species studied than in the adult. This is true whether comparisons are made on the basis of body weight, body surface area, extracellular fluid volume or kidney weight.[5, 17, 25, 34, 42, 44, 45, 52, 62, 92] Moreover, all investigators agree that there is a progressive increase in glomerular filtration as the animal matures postnatally. Early studies in fetal lambs did not show a progressive rise in glomerular filtration rate with maturation,[5] but more recent investigations utilizing the chronic fetal sheep preparation reveal that in the latter part of gestation, at least, glomerular filtration rate increases as the fetus matures.[20] In addition, studies revealing maturational increase in glomerular filtration rate in newborn dogs[52] and rats[44] suggest that similar progressive changes probably occur in the fetus as well.

Physiological factors affecting the maturational increase in glomerular filtration rate have been studied only in newborn animal models. One important factor involved in the maturation of glomerular filtration in newborn dogs is the progressive rise in blood pressure that occurs as the animals mature (Fig. 8-3). Renal function studies were done on newborn dogs during the first month of life and a close correlation between GFR (expressed in terms of gram kidney weight) and blood pressure was found (Fig. 8-4). In addition, when the blood pressure of the puppy was acutely increased or decreased, there was a parallel increase or decrease in GFR (Fig. 8-5). When similar changes in blood pressure were made in adult animals there was no change in GFR. The effect of blood pressure changes becomes less important in more mature animals because of the phenomenon of autoregulation. At blood pressures above 80

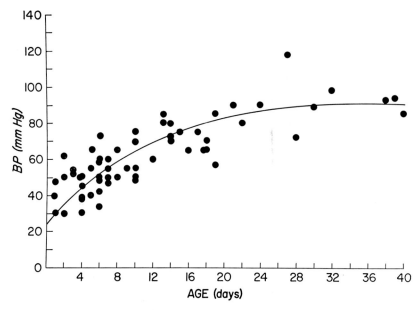

Figure 8-3. Maturation of mean arterial blood pressure in newborn dogs. (L. I. Kleinman, and J. H. Reuter, Maturation of glomerular blood flow distribution in the newborn dog, *J Physiol*, 228:91, 1973.)

mm Hg changes in blood pressure produce little or no changes in GFR.[1, 64] However, when the blood pressure is lowered below 80 mm Hg in adult animals, GFR falls, and values of GFR for adult and newborn dogs are similar at equivalent blood pressures.[52, 64] Blood pressure is low in the fetus, and rises progressively as the fetus matures.[29] Thus, it is likely that the progressive rise in glomerular filtration rate may be related to the progressive increases in blood pressure with fetus maturation.

Arterial blood pressure is not the only controlling factor in the maturation of glomerular filtration rate in the perinatal animal. At any given arterial blood pressure GFR increases as the animal matures (Fig. 8-6). A possible explanation may be found in the studies of Arturson, *et al.*[9] who found that there is an increase in the porosity of the human glomerular membrane as infants mature. Again, this change is a progressive one suggesting that similar changes may have been occurring *in*

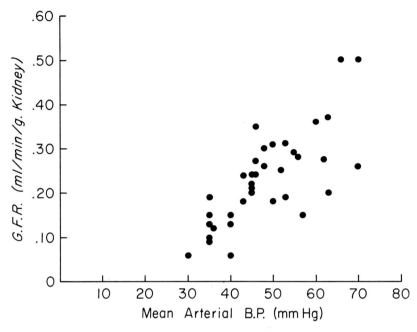

Figure 8-4.   Relationship between mean arterial blood pressure and glomer-ular filtration rate (GFR) in newborn dogs. GFR is expressed in terms of kidney weight to normalize differences in size between animals. (L. I. Kleinman, and R. J. Lubbe, Factors affecting the maturation of glomerular filtration rate and renal plasma flow in the newborn dog, *J Physiol*, 223:395, 1972.)

utero, contributing to the progressive rise in glomerular filtration.

Glomerular filtration rate is closely allied with renal blood or plasma flow and it is not surprising, therefore, that renal blood flow increases progressively as the perinatal animal matures. Earlier investigations used the clearance of para-aminohippurate (PAH) or similar substances as an estimate of renal plasma flow. PAH clearance, however, may be used as an indicator of renal plasma flow only under those circumstances in which renal extraction of PAH is essentially complete (i.e. all of the substance arriving via the renal artery is extracted by the kidney and excreted in the urine, so that none appears in the renal vein). In the adult animal about 90 percent of the PAH is usually

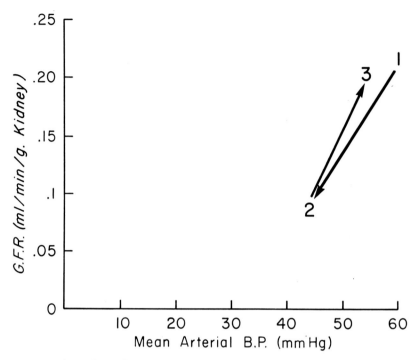

Figure 8-5. Effect of acute change in arterial blood pressure on glomerular filtration rate in a newborn dog. Arterial blood pressure was lowered from period 1 to period 2 and then raised from period 2 to period 3. Note that GFR changed in the same direction as the blood pressure. (L. I. Kleinman, and R. J. Lubbe, Factors affecting the maturation of glomerular filtration rate and renal plasma flow in the newborn dog, *J Physiol, 223*:395, 1972.)

extracted and PAH clearance has been used as a reliable indicator of renal plasma flow. In the newborn animal, however, much less PAH is extracted (approximately 50%),[21, 44, 53] and PAH clearance by itself may not be utilized for the measurement of renal plasma flow. However, simultaneous measurement of PAH clearance and renal PAH extraction permit the use of the Fick principle for the calculation of renal plasma flow.[96] Using this technique in the newborn dog we found that renal blood flow is low at birth and increases with a maturational pattern similar to that for GFR. Renal vascular resistance, however, did not change during the first month of life indicating that

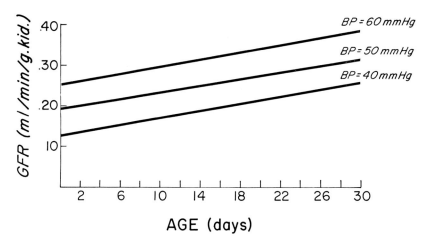

Figure 8-6. Maturation of glomerular filtration rate (GFR) in newborn dogs. GFR is expressed in terms of kidney weight to normalize differences in size between animals. Regression lines were calculated from data published by Kleinman and Lubbe. Note that at any blood pressure there is a rise in GFR as the animal matures ($p < 0.01$). Also, at any age GFR is higher at the higher blood pressure ($< p0.01$).

this factor, in the dog at least, plays a relatively minor role in controlling maturation of renal hemodynamics.[52] In the newborn pig, however, there is a fall in renal vascular resistance as the animal matures[40] suggesting that there are species differences in factors affecting the maturation of renal hemodynamics.

More recently, interest in renal blood flow has shifted to the distribution of the blood flow to the various regions of the kidney. As mentioned previously maturation of the kidney progresses outwards, i.e. the more mature nephrons are found in the inner part of the kidney and the less mature ones in the outer cortex. Therefore, we were interested to see if intrarenal blood flow distribution matched maturational patterns in the immature kidney. If radioactive microspheres of appropriate size are injected into the circulation they will be trapped in the capillaries and will be distributed in proportion to the blood flow to any region of the body or organ. By measuring the distribution of radioactivity in any organ it is possible to estimate the distribu-

tion of blood flow to that organ. In the kidney the microspheres
are trapped in glomerular capillaries and, thus, measure glomerular blood flow distribution. When this was done in the newborn
dog it was found that during the first two weeks of life glomerular
blood flow distribution was changing progressively so that as
the animal matured a greater fraction of the flow was going to
more peripheral (outer cortical) glomeruli (Fig. 8-7). After
two weeks the distribution remained relatively constant. The
change in intrarenal blood flow distribution was due largely to
the increase in outer cortical flow.[54]

The change in blood flow distribution parallels the anatomic
maturation of nephrons in the kidney. During the first two weeks
of life in the dog new nephrons are being formed in the outer

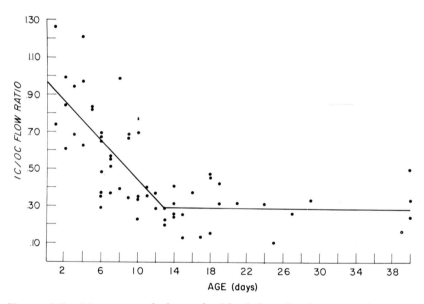

Figure 8-7. Maturation of glomerular blood flow distribution in the newborn dog. IC/OC flow ratio represents the ratio of blood flow to inner
cortical (IC) glomeruli divided by the flow to outer cortical (OC) glomeruli.
During the first two weeks of life flow to outer cortical glomeruli was
increasing relative to that of inner cortical glomeruli (IC/OC ratio was
decreasing). After two weeks there was no change in blood flow distribution. (L. I. Kleinman, and J. H. Reuter, Maturation of glomerular blood flow
distribution in the newborn dog, *J Physiol*, 228:91, 1973.)

cortical region of the kidney and increasing amounts of blood are being distributed to this region. Upon completion of nephrogenesis blood flow to both the inner and outer cortical nephrons are increased proportionately.

Tubular Function

The tubules of most animals begin functioning early in gestation. Tubule cells from a human fetus of three months gestation, growing in tissue culture, have been observed to transport phenol red from the environment into the tubular lumen.[22] Perry and Stanier[67] found that pig fetuses as early as fifty-five days gestation had no glucose in the urine, indicating that reabsorption must have taken place in the tubule. Alexander and Nixon[5] demonstrated significant active reabsorption of glucose in the seventy-day sheep fetus.

Although tubular transport takes place in the fetus there is evidence, anatomically as well as physiologically, that it is not as efficient as that in the more mature animal. For example, Fetterman and coworkers[36] found that the ratio of glomerular surface area divided by proximal tubular volume was greater in the newborn than in the adult, signifying that in the newborn animal the anatomic potential for glomerular filtration appears to be greater than that for proximal tubule transport. Since glomerular function has been found to be limited in the perinatal animal, as discussed previously, it is not surprising that tubular function is also depressed. However, it is difficult to discuss tubular function, particularly, proximal tubular function, without simultaneously looking at glomerular function.

Classically, tubular function has been evaluated by measuring rates of transport of various substances across the tubular cells. Certain substances appear to be limited by a transport maximum (T_m); so measurement of the T_m of these substances has been utilized as an index of tubular function. The T_m of glucose, a substance transported from proximal renal tubule to peritubular capillary (reabsorption), and the T_m of PAH, a substance transported from peritubular capillary to proximal renal tubule (secretion), have both been used as a measure of renal tubular potential. However, more recent studies have indicated that the

T_m of both these substances is a function of the GFR, i.e. T_m increases as GFR increases.[30, 55, 76, 86, 90] In the case of glucose this relationship applies to the perinatal animal as well.[11] The relationship between T_{mPAH} and GFR has not yet been studied in the perinatal animal.

Absolute values for T_{mPAH} have been found to be low in newborn dogs[43] and humans.[75] In addition the ratio of T_{mPAH} to GFR is lower in newborns than adults.[75] Glucose T_m is lower in the newborn human than the adult[88, 89] and glucose T_m is lower per unit GFR in the newborn than the adult dog.[11, 12] Therefore, these studies suggest that the depression of proximal tubular function is more than can be explained by the depressed GFR.

The matching of glomerular with tubular function is known as glomerular tubular balance. Glomerular tubular balance occurs in the kidney as a whole i.e. total tubular activity, reabsorption or secretion, is related to GFR for the whole kidney, and also individually among different nephrons i.e. some nephrons have poor glomerular function but their tubules also have relatively poor transport ability and vice versa. If all the well-functioning glomeruli are matched with well-functioning tubules and all the poorly functioning glomeruli are matched with poorly functioning tubules then there is homogeneity of glomerular tubular balance among the nephrons. However, if the well functioning glomeruli go with the poorly functioning tubules (and vice versa), then there is nephron heterogeneity in terms of glomerular tubular balance. Analysis of glomerular tubular nephron homogeneity may be made by examining a titration curve of a substance such as glucose which has a transport maximum (Fig. 8-8). If all the nephrons were alike, all glucose would be reabsorbed until the T_m was reached and then reabsorption would cease. This is portrayed by the solid straight lines in Figure 8-8 which shows a continuing increase in glucose reabsorption equal to that of the load (the line has an angle of 45°), and then a cessation of reabsorption when the T_m is reached (the line is horizontal). If some tubules have lower transport ability per unit GFR than others, then glucose reabsorption will cease in these tubules before the others, and there will be a deviation

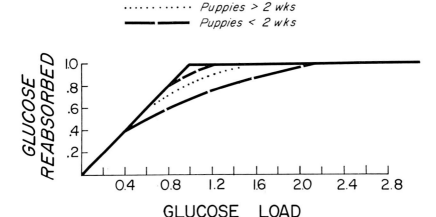

Figure 8-8. Relationship between filtered glucose load and tubular reabsorption of glucose. Both glucose load and glucose reabsorbed are divided by glucose T_m. The 45° line is a hypothetical line which occurs when all the glucose load is reabsorbed. The horizontal line represents the theoretical line which occurs when no glucose is reabsorbed, i.e. when the load is greater than T_m. The various dashed lines represent the actual titration curves for puppies and adults.

from the two straight lines. This deviation is referred to as splay, and is shown in Figure 8-8 as the dashed curved lines connecting the two straight lines. The degree of splay is a function of nephron heterogeneity.[82] As can be seen from Figure 8-8 there is a progressive decline in the degree of splay as the newborn dog matures. Thus, the immature kidney demonstrates a large degree of glomerular tubular heterogeneity, and as the kidney matures it becomes more homogeneous.

The nephron heterogeneity found in the perinatal animal can influence water and electrolyte metabolism in many ways. As soon as glucose reabsorption ceases in the tubule the glucose that is filtered must be excreted in the urine. Thus, as soon as the function in Figure 8-8 deviates from the forty-five degree straight line, it represents the point at which glucose appears in the urine. This is made more apparent in Figure 8-9, which plots urinary glucose excretion against plasma glucose. The plasma glucose level at which glucose first appears in the urine

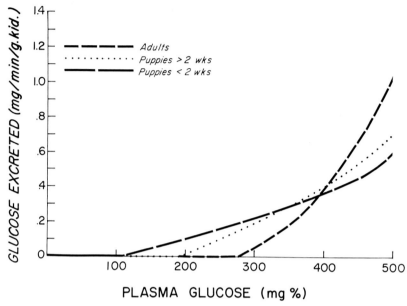

Figure 8-9. Relatonship between plasma glucose and glucose excreted in the urine. The plasma level at which glucose first appears in the urine is referred to as the plasma threshold for glucose.

is known as the plasma threshold for glucose. In the adult dog no glucose appears in the urine until plasma glucose is well above 200 mg%. However, in puppies less than two weeks of age (the fetal model), glucose is spilled when the glucose in the plasma is only 100 mg%. This degree of depression of the glucose threshold in the perinatal animal means that the immature kidney will excrete glucose at a blood level only slightly above the physiological level for the adult. Plasma glucose levels in the fetus are lower than those in the mother but changes in maternal blood glucose are reflected in the fetal plasma.[79] Thus, any situation that would elevate the maternal plasma glucose (diabetes mellitus, glucose infusions), would also elevate fetal blood glucose and might cause the fetus to excrete glucose in the urine.

The effect of glucose excretion on water and sodium excretion is shown in Figures 8-10 and 8-11. As urinary glucose excretion

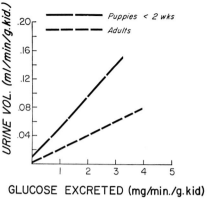

Figure 8-10. Relationship between glucose excretion and urine volume for puppies less than two weeks of age and adult dogs. The lines are regression equations based on data from experiments in which a glucose load was given to puppies and adults. The slope of the line for the puppy was significantly greater ($p < 0.01$) than that for the adult, indicating that for any degree of glucose excretion more water was excreted by the puppy.

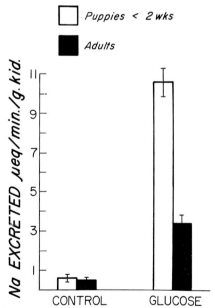

Figure 8-11. Sodium excretion in puppies less than two weeks of age and adult dogs before and after a glucose load. During the control period puppies and adults excreted small but equivalent amounts of sodium. Following the glucose load, puppies increased sodium excretion to a greater extent than did the adult ($p < 0.01$).

increases water excretion increases, but the water excretion is much greater in the perinatal animal than in the adult (Fig. 8-10). During control conditions, when there was no glucosuria, both adult and newborn dogs excreted similar (and very small), amounts of sodium (Fig. 8-11). However, when glucosuria was present, the newborn dog excreted about three times as much sodium as did the adult. Thus, the immature kidney is exquisitely sensitive to the osmotic effects of glucose.

Since the immature kidney is likely to spill glucose at relatively low plasma glucose levels, and since the immature kidney will lose a relatively large amount of water and electrolytes for any amount of glucose excreted, the fetus should be extremely susceptible to water and electrolyte depletion if the mother has an elevated blood glucose. These aspects of the immature kidney probably account for the polyhydramnios found in infants of diabetic mothers and might also contribute to the decreased body water content per unit body weight also found in these infants.[35] Further investigation into the water and electrolyte composition of infants of mothers receiving large volumes of glucose containing intravenous fluids seems warranted in view of these findings on the immature kidney.

Glucose and PAH are not the only substances regulated by glomerular tubular balance. Tubular reabsorption of sodium has been known for a long time to be related to glomerular filtration rate or filtered sodium load. In fact, the bulk of investigation dealing with sodium excretion has involved studies of the mechanism of this relationship. Under most conditions, as GFR is increased or decreased, sodium reabsorption is increased or decreased, respectively (in the proximal tubule at least), so that the fraction of filtered sodium that is reabsorbed remains relatively constant. Under conditions of antidiuresis in the adult animal this fraction is usually greater than 0.99. However, if the animal's extracellular volume is expanded by a saline load then glomerular tubular balance is upset, and the animal reabsorbs only approximately 90 percent rather than 99+ percent of the filtered sodium. This decrease in fractional sodium reabsorption (fraction of filtered sodium reabsorbed) occurs in both the proximal (proximal convoluted tubule) and distal (loop of Henle, distal convoluted tubule, collecting duct) nephron.[26, 28, 46]

The immature kidney reabsorbs as high a fraction of the filtered sodium load as does the adult under conditions of antidiuresis.[73] This does not by itself indicate that tubular sodium transport is as efficient in the immature as in the mature kidney since the sodium load presented to the tubules is much less in the immature kidney due to the low glomerular filtration rate. The micropuncture studies of Capek, *et al.*[23] demonstrated that proximal tubules of newborn rats have lower intrinsic sodium transport capacities than those of more mature rats. Under conditions of antidiuresis and long transit times this decreased transport capacity would not affect fractional sodium reabsorption. However, under conditions of high tubular urine flows (osmotic diuresis for example) with shortened transit times, the reduced transport capacity would limit sodium reabsorption. This may account for the greater susceptibility of the immature kidney to a glucose diuresis in terms of sodium and water loss.

Glomerular tubular balance in the proximal tubule, in terms of sodium reabsorption, probably applies to the immature kidney as well as to the mature kidney. Horster and Valtin,[45] using micropuncture techniques, found that fractional sodium reabsorption was the same in the proximal tubule of the very young newborn dog, whose GFR was very low, as it was in the slightly older puppy whose GFR was higher. Thus, as GFR increased proximal sodium reabsorption increased, so that fractional sodium reabsorption remained relatively constant.

In our laboratory proximal tubular reabsorption was estimated by blocking distal nephron sodium reabsorption with ethacrynic acid and chlorothiazide, and measuring total sodium reabsorption. Under the assumption that these drugs completely inhibit distal nephron sodium reabsorption and do not significantly interfere with proximal tubular sodium transport, we calculated the proximal tubular sodium reabsorption as being equal to the total sodium reabsorption. The linear relationship between GFR and proximal tubular sodium reabsorption in the immature kidney verifies the existence of some degree of glomerular tubular balance (Fig. 8-12).

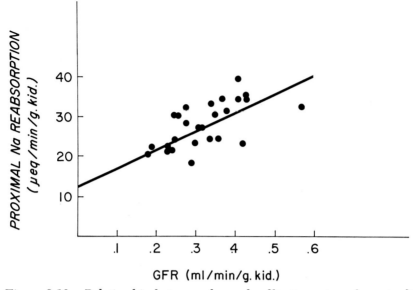

Figure 8-12. Relationship between glomerular filtration rate and proximal tubular sodium reabsorption in the newborn dog. The correlation between the two functions is significant (p<0.01). The line is a statistical regression line.

When an adult is given a large sodium load there is an immediate expansion of the extracellular fluid space which stimulates the kidney to respond by increasing glomerular filtration rate and decreasing tubular sodium reabsorption resulting in an increase in sodium excretion and a relatively rapid return of the extracellular fluid space to the preload condition. McCance and Widdowson[63] observed that both newborn infants and piglets were unable to excrete a dietary sodium load rapidly. The newborns had a rise in sodium levels, abnormal increases in weight and generalized edema.

When newborn dogs in our laboratory were given an intravenous sodium load they excreted only 10 percent of the infused load after two hours compared to adult dogs which excreted 32 percent of a similar load in the same time.[73, 83] The major difference between the adult and immature kidney was that the adult kidney excreted 6.5 percent of the filtered sodium while the immature kidney excreted only 2.5 percent (Fig. 8-13). Thus, the immature kidney is hampered in its ability

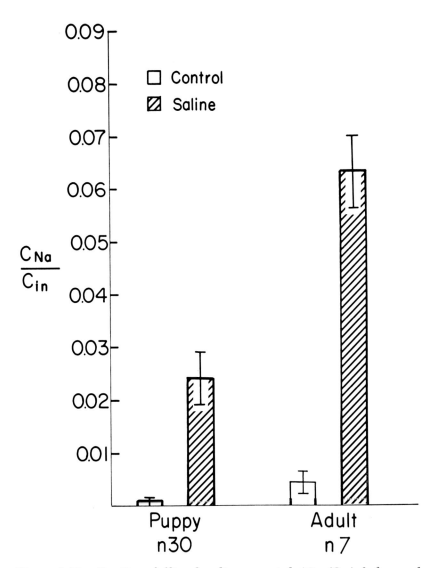

Figure 8-13.   Fraction of filtered sodium excreted (C_{Na}/C_{in}) before and after a sodium load for newborn and adult dogs. Note that both adult and newborn dogs excreted less than 0.5 percent of the filtered sodium during the control period, and there was no statistical difference between them. During saline loading adults excreted a significantly ($p < 0.01$) greater fraction of the filtered sodium than did the newborn dog.

to excrete a salt load not only by its low GFR but also by its inability to lower fractional sodium excretion. When the distal tubules of newborn dogs were blocked with diuretics (as discussed previously) and were then given a sodium load, there was a significant increase in fractional sodium excretion following the saline load (Table 8-I). These results indicate that the proximal tubules were capable of decreasing its sodium reabsorption rate following a salt load, but that the distal nephron increased its sodium reabsorption (in contradistinction to the situation in the adult where both proximal and distal reabsorption is depressed) so that the fractional reabsorption of sodium for the kidney as a whole was not significantly lowered.

TABLE 8-I

SODIUM REABSORPTION IN NEWBORN DOGS

	% of filtered		Eq/min/g kidney	
	Control	Saline Load	Control	Saline Load
Total	99.7	97.5*	37.5	52.6*
Proximal	71.2	52.0*	28.2	27.8
Distal	28.5	45.5*	9.3	24.8*

* Difference between control and saline statistically different ($p < 0.01$).

Water Excretion

All mammalian fetuses studied excrete urine hypotonic to plasma,[4, 17, 39, 80] and the minimal solute concentration of the urine (under conditions of water loading) is comparable in the perinatal and adult animal.[13] However, the perinatal animal is not able to excrete a water load as well as the adult can.[7, 13, 31, 60, 61] The ability to excrete a water load is a function of the amount of water presented to the diluting segment (ascending limb of the loop of Henle and early distal convoluted tubule), and the ability of this segment to dilute the urine. Diluting ability in turn is a function of the ability of the loop of Henle to transport sodium against a concentration gradient, and the ability of the collecting duct to remain impermeable to water. The amount of water presented to the diluting segment is a function of the GFR and proximal water reabsorption. The immature kidney can dilute the urine to the same extent as the adult so that the basic reason for the poor response of the perinatal animal is the decreased load presented to the diluting segment, which in turn is a function of the low GFR.

Conversely, the perinatal animal is not capable of responding to dehydration or hypertonic solute loading by excreting as concentrated a urine as the adult.[31, 34, 58] The following factors may contribute to the poor concentrating ability of the immature kidney; a) since the ability of the kidney to produce a concentrated urine is a function of the ability of the loops of Henle to generate and maintain a countercurrent solute concentration gradient from medullary tissue to cortico medullary junction, and since this ability is in turn a function of the length of the loops, the shorter loops found in the immature kidney[16, 31] may contribute to the poor concentrating ability in the perinatal animal; b) since urea is necessary for enhancing the countercurrent medullary solute gradient, the low urea excretion (due primarily to the positive nitrogen balance) and the anatomical immaturity of the loop of Henle which retards urea recycling in medulla,[31, 87] probably play a role in the poor urinary concentrating ability of the perinatal animal;[33] c) since a large blood flow through the medullary region of the kidney may dissipate the countercurrent solute gradient, the intrarenal distribution of blood flow in the immature kidney[54] with a higher fraction going to deeper renal structures (as discussed previously), may contribute to the poor concentrating ability of the perinatal animal; d) since the ability to concentrate urine is a function of antidiuretic hormone (ADH) activity in plasma and the responsiveness of the collecting duct to this hormone it is possible that a diminution of either of these factors may play a role in the poor concentrating ability of the perinatal animal.[31, 50]

IMPORTANCE OF THE KIDNEY TO THE MAINTENANCE OF WATER AND ELECTROLYTE HOMEOSTASIS

As discussed previously, the immature kidney does not filter as well nor do its tubules have the capacity to function as efficiently as those from the more mature kidney. Thus, when placed under the stress of a glucose load, sodium load, water

load, or water deprivation the neonatal animal experiences alterations in body water and electrolyte content. This is understandable in the postnatal animal, since the kidney is the prime
regulator of water and electrolyte metabolism. The fetus, however, has an alternative mechanism to regulate the imposed
stress; namely placental regulation. It would appear at first
thought that under most conditions the kidneys are relatively
superfluous to maintenance of water and electrolyte balance in
the fetus. Moreover, some infants are born without any kidneys
at all and have no major abnormalities in water and electrolyte
composition at birth. However, the kidneys would be superfluous
only if the water and electrolyte stress came from the fetus, and
the placenta were capable of regulating the water and electrolyte
imbalance. If the stress came from the mother, and the placenta
was acting as the agent imposing the stress on the infant, then
the fetal kidney would be the primary organ to regulate water
and electrolyte imbalance.

Alterations in maternal water and electrolyte balance produce
similar changes in the fetus. When pregnant women were infused
with large amounts of 5% glucose solutions (in essence giving a
water load), the fetuses of the mothers responded as if they
too had received a load, since their serum osmolalities and
sodium concentrations fell to the level of the mother. When the
mothers received a hyperosmotic infusion the fetuses responded
by transferring water to the mother, producing a situation of
hypertonic dehydration in the fetus.[14] Similar studies in rabbits[19]
and primates[18] confirmed these studies in humans, indicating
that a water load or a dehydrating stress can be given to the
fetus via the mother. The renal response to these stresses was
not studied in any of the experiments but the kidney might be
expected to respond similarly to the kidney of neonatal animals
receiving equivalent stresses.

There have been few physiological studies of water and
electrolyte metabolism in the fetuses or infants of mothers who
might have a clinical disorder which would affect water and
electrolyte balance in the infant. One such condition is maternal
diabetes, which can produce fetal hyperglycemia and glucose
diuresis. As mentioned previously infants of diabetic mothers

have decreased body water content per unit body weight. Although the low ratio of body water to body weight is due largely to the high body fat content of these infants, fetal dehydration may also be present. Renal vein thrombosis, a syndrome associated with extracellular fluid dehydration, is more common in infants of diabetic mothers than in other infants.[66, 85] In addition, further work is clearly called for to ascertain whether the immaturity of the fetal kidney affects the water and electrolyte balance in infants of mothers who have been put on diuretics, or placed on a high or low salt diet, or who have any condition that might produce an abnormality in their water and electrolyte metabolism.

REFERENCES

1. Abe, Y.; Dixon, F., and McNay, J. L.: Dissociation between auto-regulation of renal blood flow and glomerular filtration rate. *Am J Physiol, 219*:986, 1970.
2. Abramovich, D. R.: Fetal factors influencing the volume and composition of liquor amnii. *J Obstet Gynaecol Br Commonw, 77*: 865, 1970.
3. Adams, F. H.; Fujiwara, T., and Rowshan, G.: The nature and origin of the fluid in the fetal lamb lung. *J Pediatr, 63*:881, 1963.
4. Alexander, D. P., and Nixon, D. A.: The foetal kidney. *Br Med Bull, 17*:112, 1961.
5. Alexander, D. P., and Nixon, D. A.: Reabsorption of glucose, fructose, and meso-inositol by the foetal and postnatal sheep kidney. *J Physiol, 167*:480, 1963.
6. Alexander, D. P.; Nixon, D. A.; Widdas, W. F., and Wohlzogen, F. X.: Renal function in the sheep fetus. *J Physiol, 140*:14, 1958.
7. Ames, R. G.: Urinary water excretion and neurohypophysical function in full term and premature infants shortly after birth. *Pediatrics, 12*:272, 1953.
8. Arataki, M.: Post-natal growth of kidney with special reference to number and size of glomeruli (albino rat). *Am J Anat, 36*:399, 1926.
9. Arturson, G.; Groth, T., and Grotte, G.: Human glomerular membrane porosity and filtration pressure: Dextran clearance data analysed by theoretical models. *Clin Sci, 40*:137, 1971.
10. Bain, A. D., and Scott, J. S.: Renal agenesis and severe urinary tract dysplasia. *Br Med J, 1*:841, 1960.

11. Baker, J. T., and Kleinman, L. I.: Glucose reabsorption in the newborn dog kidney. *Proc Soc Exp Biol Med, 142*:716, 1973.

12. Baker, J. T., and Kleinman, L. I.: Renal glucose and sodium excretion in the newborn dog. *Pediatr Res, 7*:412, 1973.

13. Barnett, H. L.; Vesterdal, J.; McNamara, H., and Lauson, H. D.: Renal water excretion in premature infants. *J Clin Invest, 31*:1069, 1952.

14. Battaglia, F.; Prystowsky, H.; Smisson, C.; Hellegers, A., and Bruns, P.: The effect of the administration of fluids intravenously to mothers upon the concentrations of water and electrolytes in plasma of human fetuses. *Pediatrics, 25*:2, 1960.

15. Bernstine, R. L.: A chronic renal model for the fetus. *Lab Anim Sci, 20*:949, 1970.

16. Boss, J. M.; Dlouha, H; Kraus, M., and Krecek, J.: The structure of the kidney in relation to age and diet in white rats during the weaning period. *J Physiol, 168*:196, 1963.

17. Boylan, J. W.; Colbourn, E. P., and McCance, R. A.: Renal function in the foetal and new-born guinea-pig. *J Physiol, 141*:323, 1958.

18. Bruns, P. D.; Hellegers, A. E.; Seeds, A. E., Jr.; Behrman, R. E., and Battaglia, F. C.: Effects of osmotic gradients across the primate placenta upon fetal and placental wtaer contents. *Pediatrics, 34*:407, 1964.

19. Bruns, P. D.; Linder, R. O.; Drose, V. E., and Battaglia, F.: The placental transfer of water from fetus to mother following the intravenous infusion of hypertonic mannitol to the maternal rabbit. *Am J Obstet Gynecol, 86*:160, 1963.

20. Buddingh, F.; Parker, H. R., Ishizaki, G., and Tyler, W. S.: Long term studies of the functional development of the fetal kidney in sheep. *Am J Vet Res, 32*:1993, 1971.

21. Calcagno, P. L., and Rubin, M. I.: Renal extraction of PAH in infants and children. *J Clin Invest, 43*:1632, 1963.

22. Cameron, G., and Chambers, R.: Direct evidence of function in kidney of an early human fetus. *Am J Physiol, 123*:482, 1938.

23. Capek, K.; Dlouha, H.; Fernandez, J., and Popp, M.: Regulation of proximal tubular reabsorption in early post-natal period of infant rats: Micropuncture study. *Proc Int Union Physiol Sciences, Washington, D.C. Abstracts of Volunteer Papers, 7*:72, 1968.

24. Carter, C. O.: *Congenital Malformations. Ciba Foundation Symposium.* London, Churchill, 1960, p. 264.

25. Chez, R. A.; Smith, F. G., and Hutchinson, D. L.: Renal function in the intrauterine primate fetus. I. Experimental technique; rate of formation and chemical composition of urine. *Am J Obstet Gynecol, 90*:128, 1964.

26. Davidman, M.; Alexander, E.; Lalone, R., and Levinsky, N.: Nephron function during volume expansion in the rat. *Am J Physiol, 223:* 188, 1972.

27. Davis, M. E., and Potter, E. L.: Intrauterine respiration of the human fetus. *JAMA, 131:*1194, 1946.

28. Davis, B. B.; Walter, M. J., and Murdaugh, H. V., Jr.: Renal response to graded saline challenge. *Am J Physiol, 217:*1604, 1969.

29. Dawes, G. S.: *Foetal and Neonatal Physiology.* Chicago, Year Book Medical Publishers, 1968.

30. Deetjen, P., and Sonnenberg, H.: Der tubuläre Transport van PAH. Microperfusionsversuche am Einzelnephron der Rattennier *in situ. Pflüegers Arch, 285:*35, 1965.

31. Dicker, S. E.: *Mechanisms of Urine Concentration and Dilution in Mammals.* Baltimore, Williams & Wilkins Company, 1970.

32. Edelman, I. S.; Haley, H. B.; Schloerb, P. R.; Sheldon, D. B.; Friis-Hansen. B. J.; Stoll, G., and Moore, F. D.: Further observations on total body water: Normal values throughout the life span. *Surg Gynecol Obstet, 95:*1, 1952.

33. Edelmann, C. M., Jr.: *Maturation of the Neonatal Kidney.* Proc. Third Int. Congr. Nephrol., Washington, 1966, 1967, Vol. 3, pp. 1-12.

34. Falk, G.: Maturation of renal function in adult rats. *Am J Physiol, 181:*157, 1955.

35. Fee, B. A., and Weil, W. B., Jr.: Body composition of infants of diabetic mothers by direct analysis. *Ann N Y Acad Sci, 110:*869, 1963.

36. Fetterman, G. H.; Shuplock, N. A.; Philipp, F. J., and Gregg, H. S.: The growth and maturation of human glomeruli and proximal convolutions from term to adulthood: Studies by microdissection, *Pediatrics, 35:*601, 1965.

37. Friis-Hansen, B.: Body water compartments in children: Changes during growth and related changes in body composition. *Pediatrics, 28:*169. 1961.

38. Givens, M. H., and Macy, I. G.: The chemical composition of the human fetus. *J Biol Chem, 102:*7, 1933.

39. Gresham, E. L.; Rankin, J. H. G.; Makowski, E. L.; Meschia, G., and Battaglia, F. C.: An evaluation of fetal renal function in a chronic sheep preparation. *J Clin Invest, 51:*149, 1972.

40. Gruskin, A. B.; Edelmann, C. M., Jr., and Yuan, S.: Maturational changes in renal blood flow in piglets. *Pediat Res, 4:*7, 1970.

41. Gutman, Y.; Gottschalk, C. W., and Lassiter, W. E.: Micropuncture study of inulin absorption in the rat kidney. *Science, 147:*753, 1965.

42. Heller, J., and Capek, K.: Changes in body water compartments and

inulin and PAH clearance in the dog during postnatal development. *Physiol Bohemoslov, 14*:433, 1965.

43. Hook, J. B.; Williamson, H. E., and Hirsch, G. H.: Functional maturation of renal PAH transport in the dog. *Can J Physiol Pharmacol, 48*:169, 1970.

44. Horster, M., and Lewy, J. E.: Filtration fraction and extraction of PAH during neonatal period in the rat. *Am J Physiol, 219*:1061, 1970.

45. Horster, M., and Valtin, H.: Postnatal development of renal function: Micropuncture and clearance studies in the dog. *J Clin Invest, 50*:779, 1971.

46. Howards, S. S.; Davis, B. B.; Knox, F. G.; Wright, F. S., and Berliner, R. W.: Depression of fractional soduim reabsorption by the proximal tubule of the dog without sodium diuresis. *J Clin Invest, 47*:1561, 1968.

47. Hutchinson, D. L.; Gray, M. J.; Plentl, A. R.; Alvarez, H.; Caldeyro-Barcia, R.; Kaplan, B., and Lind, J.: The role of the fetus in the water exchange of the amniotic fluid of normal and hydramniotic patients. *J Clin Invest, 38*:971, 1959.

48. Hutchinson, D. L.; Hunter, L. B.; Nelsen, E. D., and Plentl, A.: The exchange of water and electrolytes in the mechanism of amniotic fluid formation and the relationship to hydramnics. *Surg Gynecol Obstet, 100*:391, 1955.

49. Iob, V., and Swanson, W. W.: Mineral growth of the human fetus. *Am J Dis Child, 47*:302, 1934.

50. Janovsky, M.; Martínek, J., and Stanincová, V.: Antidiuretic activity in the plasma of human infants after a load of sodium chloride. *Acta Pediat, 54*:543, 1965.

51. Kerpel-Fronius, E.: Electrolyte and water metabolism. In Stave, U. (Ed.): *Physiology of the Perinatal Period,* Vol. 2. New York, Appleton, 1970.

52. Kleinman, L. I., and Lubbe, R. J.: Factors affecting the maturation of glomerular filtration rate and renal plasma flow in the new-born dog. *J Physol, 223*:395, 1972.

53. Kleinman, L. I., and Lubble, R. J.: Factors affecting the maturation of renal PAH extraction in the new-born dog. *J Physiol, 223*:411, 1972.

54. Kleinman, L. I., and Reuter, J. H.: Maturation of glomerular blood flow distribution in the new-born dog. *J Physiol, 228*:91, 1973.

55. Kurtzman, N. A.; White, M. G.; Rodgers, P. W., and Flynn, P. P. III.: Relationship of sodium reabsorption and glomerular filtration rate to renal glucose reabsorption. *J Clin Invest, 51*:127, 1972.

56. Lind, T.; Kendall, A., and Hytten, F. E.: The role of the fetus in the

formation of amniotic fluid. *J Obstet Gynaecol Br Commonw,* 79:289, 1972.

57. MacDonald, M. S., and Emery, J. L.: The late intrauterine and post-natal development of human renal glomeruli. *J Anat, 93*:331, 1959.

58. McCance, R. A.: Renal function in early life. *Physiol Rev, 28*:331, 1948.

59. McCance, R. A.: Age and renal function. In Black, D. A. K. (Ed.): *Renal Disease.* Oxford, Blackwell Scientific Publications, 1962, pp. 157-170.

60. McCance, R. A.; Naylor, N. S. B., and Widdowson, E. M.: The response of infants to a large dose of water. *Arch Dis Child, 29*:104, 1954.

61. McCance, R. A., and Widdowson, E. M.: The response of puppies to a large dose of water. *J Physiol, 129*:628, 1955.

62. McCance, R. A., and Widdowson, E. M.: Metabolism, growth and renal function of piglets in the first days of life. *J Physiol, 133*:373, 1956.

63. McCance. R. A., and Widdowson, E. M.: Hypertonic expansion of the extracellular fluids. *Acta Paediatrica, 46*:337, 1957.

64. Navar, L. G.: Minimal preglomerular resistance and calculation of normal glomerular pressure. *Am J Physiol, 219*:1658, 1970.

65. Nelsen, E. D.; Hunter, C. B., and Plentl, A. A.: Rate of exchange of sodium and potassium between amniotic fluid and maternal system. *Proc Soc Exp Biol Med, 86*:432, 1954.

66. Oppenheimer, E. H., and Esterly, J. R.: Thrombosis in the newborn: Comparison between infants of diabetic and nondiabetic mothers. *J Pediatr, 67*:549, 1965.

67. Perry, J. S., and Stanier, M. W.: The rate of flow of urine of foetal pigs. *J Physiol, 161*:344, 1962.

68. Plentl, A. A.: The dynamics of the amniotic fluid. *Ann NY Acad Sci, 75*:746, 1959.

69. Potter, E. L.: Development of the human glomerulus. *Arch Path, 80*:241, 1965.

70. Pritchard, J. A.: Deglutition by normal and anencephalic fetuses. *Obstet Gynecol, 25*:289, 1965.

71. Rahill, W. J., and Subramanian, S.: The use of fetal animals to investigate renal development. *Lab Anim Sci, 23*:92, 1973.

72. Rankin, J. H. G.; Gresham, E. L.; Battaglia, F. C.; Makowski, E. L., and Meschia, G.: Measurement of fetal renal insulin clearance in a chronic sheep preparation. *J Appl Physiol, 32*:129, 1972.

73. Reuter, J. H., and Kleinman, L. I.: Sodium excretion and the glomerular blood flow distribution in the newborn dog. *Physiologist, 15*:247, 1972.

74. Reynolds, S. R. M.: A source of amniotic fluid in the lamb: The naso-pharyngeal and buccal cavities. *Nature, 172*:307, 1953.

75. Rubin, M. I.; Bruck, E., and Rapoport. M.: Maturation of renal function in childhood: Clearance studies. *J Clin Invest, 28*:1144, 1949.

76. Schultze, R. G., and Berger, H.: The influence of GFR and saline expansion on T_{mG} of the dog kidney. *Kidney Int, 3*:291, 1973.

77. Scott, J. S., and Wilson, J. K.: Hydramnios as an early sign of oesophageal atresia. *Lancet, 2*:569, 1957.

78. Seeds, A. E., Jr.: Water metabolism of the fetus. *Am J Obstet Gynecol, 92*:727, 1965.

79. Shelley, H. J., and Neligan, G. A.: Neonatal hypoglycemia. *Br Med Bull, 22*:34, 1966.

80. Smith, F. G., Jr.; Adams, F. H.; Borden, M., and Hilburn, J.: Studies of renal function in the intact fetal lamb. *Am J Obstet Gynecol, 96*:240, 1966.

81. Smith, H. W.: *The Kidney.* New York, Oxford U P, 1951.

82. Smith, H. W.; Goldring, W.; Chasis, H.; Ranges, A., and Bradley, S. E.: The application of saturation methods to the study of glomerular and tubular function in the human kidney. *J Mt Sinai Hosp, 10*:59, 1943.

83. Steichen, J., and Kleinman, L. I.: Influence of dietary Na on renal maturation in unanesthetized puppies. *J Pediat, 84*:914, 1974.

84. Sylvester, P. E., and Hughes, D. R.: Congenital absence of both kidneys; Report of four cases. *Br Med J, 1*:77, 1954.

85. Takeuchi. A., and Benirschke, K.: Renal vein thrombosis of the newborn and its relation to maternal diabetes. *Biol Neonate, 3*:237, 1961.

86. Torelli, G.; Milla, E.; Kleinman, L. I., and Faelli, A.: Effect of hypothermia on renal sodium reabsorption. *Pflüegers Arch, 342*: 219, 1973.

87. Trimble, M. E.: Renal response to solute loading in infant rats: relation to anatomical development. *Am J Physiol, 219*:1089, 1970.

88. Tudvad, F.: Sugar reabsorption in prematures and full term babies. *Scand J Clin Lab Invest, 1*:281, 1949.

89. Tudvad, F., and Vesterdal, J.: The maximal tubular transfer of glucose and para-amino-hippurate in premature infants. *Acta Paediat Scand, 42*:337, 1953.

90. VanLiew, J. B.; Deetjen, P., and Boylan, J. W.: Glucose reabsorption in the rat kidney. *Pflüegers Arch, 295*:232, 1967.

91. Vogh, B., and Cassin, S.: Stop-flow analysis of renal function in newborn and maturing swine. *Biol Neonat, 10*:153, 1966.

92. Weil, W. B., Jr.: Evaluation of renal function in infancy and childhood. *Am J Med Sci, 229*:678, 1955.

93. Widdowson, E. M.: Growth and composition of the fetus and newborn. In Assali, N. S. (Ed.): *Biology of Gestation,* Vol. II, *The Fetus and Neonate.* New York, Acad Pr, 1968.

94. Widdowson, E. M., and McCance, R. A.: The effect of development on the composition of the serum and extracellular fluids. *Clin Sci, 15*:361, 1956.

95. Widdowson, E. M., and Spray, C. M.: Chemical development in utero. *Arch Dis Child, 26*:205, 1951.

96. Wolf, A. V.: Total renal blood flow at any urine flow or extraction fraction. *Am J Physiol, 133*:496, 1941.

97. Wright, G. H.: Absorption and secretion of electrolytes in the stomach of the rabbit foetus. *J Physiol, 155*:24P, 1960.

98. Wright, G. H., and Nixon, D. A.: Absorption of amniotic fluid in the gut of foetal sheep. *Nature, 190*:816, 1961.

Chapter 9

PSYCHOBIOLOGICAL ASPECTS OF FETAL AND INFANTILE MALNUTRITION

Francine Wehmer and E. S. E. Hafez

INTRODUCTION

ONE OF THE MOST serious problems facing the human race today is the effect of developmental malnutrition. Whether the problem is conceptualized in terms of human suffering, or the stunting of human potential, or as the danger to stable relations between governments, there is no greater need for research and intervention than in this area.

This chapter shall review some of the data related to maternal and fetal malnutrition, including low birthweight in man. Some techniques used in studies of experimental fetal malnutrition will be briefly examined. Major neurobiological consequences will then be discussed including reversibility or irreversibility of effect following dietary rehabilitation. Finally, the major behavioral consequences will be reviewed, including the effects of early malnutrition on the development of intelligence in man.

CAUSES OF LOW BIRTHWEIGHT IN MAN

In any study of the effects of maternal malnutrition on birthweight, the simultaneous influences of all factors associated with lower birthweight must be taken into account, and if possible, controlled.

Length of Gestation: In man, as in other primate species, there is variability in the length of normal gestation.[1] Added to this is the factor of actual prematurity. Holding all other factors constant, one week's decrease in gestation length is associated with a 130 gram decrease in birthweight.[2] Prematurity is differentially found among the socioeconomic groups most likely to be malnourished.[3]

Maternal Genetic Factors: Classical animal cross breeding studies have shown that birthweight reflects the size of the maternal strain.[4, 5, 6] More recent ova-transplantation studies have supported these findings (Fig. 9-1). The maternal-genetic aspect of low birthweight may also exist in man. In one study, holding all other factors constant, each previous delivery of a low birthweight neonate was associated with a decreased expectation of 113 grams in the prediction of birthweight in the index pregnancy.[2] The tendency towards repeated low birthweight parities was also found in other study populations.[8] Since the Collaborative Study did not find that socioeconomic factors could entirely

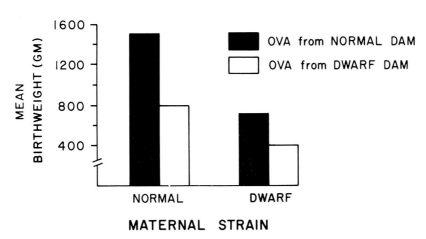

Figure 9-1. Maternal regulation of birthweight of piglets of genetically normal and dwarf strains. Maternal size modifies the genetic relationship. (D. Smidt; J. Steinbach, and B. Scheven, Die beeninflussung der pra-und postnatalen enswicklung durch gorsse und korpergewicht dur mutter, dargestellt on ergebaissen reziproker eitransplantation zwischen zwergschweinen und grossen hausschweinen, *Mschr Kinderheilk,* 115:533, 1967.)

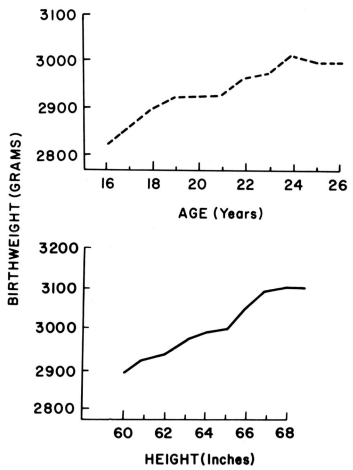

Figure 9-2a. The long known relationships between maternal age, maternal height, and birthweight.

explain birthweight differences between Negroes and whites, the suggestion has been made that these birthweight differences may reflect maternal-genetic tendencies.[9] Evidence derives from analyses indicating that low birthweight in Negro neonates does not necessarily reflect only an increase in pathologic pregnancy since low birthweight Negro neonates experience lower perinatal death rates than low birthweight whites.[10, 11]

Low Pre-Pregnancy Weight: Low pre-pregnancy weight entirely accounts for relationships between maternal age, height, parity and birthweight.[2] Young women, short women, and low parity women all tend to have lower pre-pregnancy weight than older, taller, or high parity women (Fig. 9-2a, b, and c). The Collaborative Study contained numerous women who had more than one pregnancy during the Study period. If there was no difference in pre-pregnancy weight or pregnancy weight gain between the two pregnancies, there was no difference in birthweight.[12]

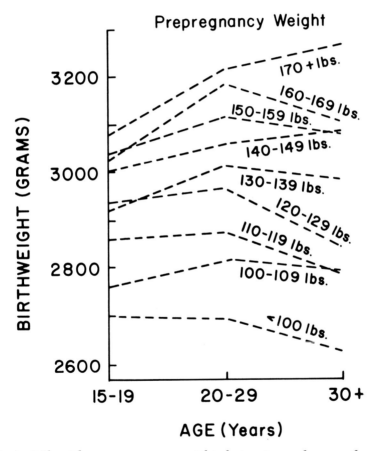

Figure 9-2b. The prepregnancy weight factor imposed upon the age relationship. Age is an artifact of lower prepregnancy weights typically found in younger women.

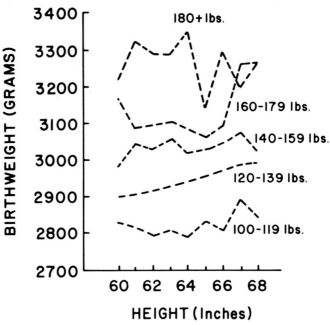

Figure 9-2c. The prepregnancy weight factor imposed upon the height relationship. Height is an artifact of the lower prepregnancy weights typically found in short women. (Courtesy of Dr. D. Rush.)

Weight Gain During Pregnancy: Low weight gain during pregnancy is associated with low birthweight, the only exception being that obese women give birth to high birthweight neonates even if there is a net weight loss during pregnancy.[2, 11, 13] Eastman and Jackson[11] found that low pre-pregnancy weight (<120 pounds) combined with low pregnancy weight gain (<11 pounds) in term pregnancies produced a 5.8 percent incidence of low birthweight in whites, and a 16 percent incidence in Negroes. Their data additionally imply that high pregnancy weight gain may have disproportionately desirable effects among Negroes. Predicting from their multiple regression data, they suggest that if the low pre-pregnancy weight group had, in fact, gained thirty pounds during pregnancy, the incidence of low birth weight in whites and Negroes would have been reduced to 1.5 percent and 3.5 percent, respectively.

Multiple Birth: The human uterus is adapted to the gestation of a singleton fetus. Multiple births are associated with both intrauterine growth retardation and prematurity with mono-chorionic twins showing greater growth retardation than dichorionic twins.[14]

Rates of Intrauterine Growth: A commonly accepted definition of low birthweight is 2,500 gm. or less. However, this birthweight reflects anything from extreme growth retardation at term to extreme growth acceleration combined with prematurity (Table 9-I). There is little likelihood that these various

TABLE 9-I

BIRTHWEIGHT OF 2,500 GRAMS BY WEEK OF GESTATION*

Week of Gestation	Relative Weight for Gestation Length	Implication
40	—2 S.D.	extreme growth retardation at term
37	—1 S.D.	small infant born at term
35	Mean	average size premature
33	+1 S.D.	large premature infant
31	+2 S.D.	extreme growth acceleration in a premature infant

* P. Gruenwald, *Growth of the Human Fetus,* A. McLaren, ed. Advances in reproductive physiology. (New York, Academic Press, 1967).

conditions will reflect either a single cause or a single consequence. In man, from one-third to three-fifths of low birthweight neonates are born at term.[16, 17, 18]

Pathologies of Pregnancy: Various pathologies of pregnancy can produce fetal malnutrition in the absence of maternal malnutrition. Among these are toxemia of pregnancy, gestation over forty-three weeks, major placental abnormalities and maternal hypertension.[16, 19] Between thirty-three to forty weeks of gestation, 30 percent of all cases of perinatal death are two standard deviations below the mean birthweight for living infants born during this period, the greatest numbers being found associated with maternal hypertension.[20] One half of all full term growth retarded neonates who die display the elevated brain weight:

liver weight weight ratio associated with intrauterine malnutrition.[19] The sparing of the brain and the severe reduction in liver weight is also found in experimental malnutrition (Table 9-II).

Maternal Malnutrition During Gestation: Of all the species studied, the effects of gestational malnutrition on birthweight are least in pig, primate, and man. In the pig, this reflects the abundant nutritional reserves of the sow.[22] In primate and man, the resistance of birthweight to malnutrition reflects slow rates

TABLE 9-II

EFFECTS OF MALNUTRITION DURING THE LATTER HALF OF
GESTATION ON ORGAN WEIGHTS OF THE SHEEP FETUS,
EXPRESSED AS A PERCENTAGE OF CONTROLS*

Magnitude of Weight Loss	*Organs*
mild (0-15%)	brain and spinal cord
moderate (40-60%)	pancreas, skeleton, heart lungs, *fetus*, kidneys, alimentary system
severe (80-85%)	spleen, heart thymus, neck thymus
very severe (90%)	liver

* L. R. Wallace, The growth of lambs before and after birth in relation to the level of nutrition, *J Agr Sci*, 38:93, 1948.

of uterine growth and the minimal nutritional demands made by a singleton fetus[23, 24] (Fig. 9-3). Pregnancy associated with anorexia nervosa gives the clearest indication of the resistance of birth weight to maternal malnutrition. Dr. H. E. Fox[26] reports of an anorexic gravida one, para one Negro woman in her early twenties whose prepregnancy weight was eighty-five pounds. She lost seven to eight pounds during pregnancy and after a gestation length of thirty-eight weeks, gave birth to a vigorous male infant who weighed 2,600 grams. Several studies of the effects of war-time famine have also demonstrated birth-weight reductions. Birthweights in Rotterdam during its World War II famine of 1944 to 1945 fell 300 gm compared to the control city of Heerlen.[27] Bergner and Susser's analysis indicated that the lowest median weights occurred when exposed to famine affected the second half of gestation, and exposure earlier in gestation led to no additional decrease.[10] The World War II Leningrad famine lasted two and one-half years, and was most

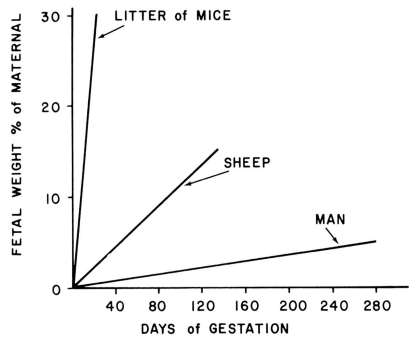

Figure 9-3.   The relationship of fetal and maternal weight in man, mouse, and sheep. The low fetal: maternal weight ratio and the slow rate of intrauterine growth may partly explain the relative resistance of the human fetus to growth retardation due to maternal malnutrition during gestation. (C. A. Smith, Prenatal and neonatal nutrition. *Pediatrics, 30*:145, 1962.)

severe between September, 1941 and February, 1942. Fifty percent of the neonates born during the first half of 1942 weighed less than 2,500 gm.[28] In the sub-human primate, birthweight reductions of 12 percent and a neonatal mortality rate of 50 percent are produced by extremely low protein diets.[29]

Life Long Maternal Malnutrition: Socioeconomic measures are available as epidemiological indices of presumptive life long maternal malnutrition. The average birthweight in developing nations varies between 2.7 and 3.0 kg, compared to 3.3 kg in Western populations. Low socioeconomic status within these developing nations further reduces birthweight by 200 to 600 gm (Fig. 9-4). The particularly low birthweights among the poor in India reflects the Calcutta data. Thirty-three percent

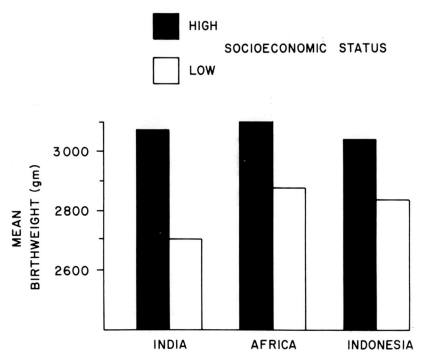

Figure 9-4.   Socioeconomic status and birthweight in developing areas of
the world. (S. T. Achar, and A. Yankauer, Studies on birth weight of South
Indian infants, *Indian J Child Health*, 11:57, 1962. M. G. Hollingsworth,
The birth weights of African and European babies born in Ghana, *W Afr
Med J*, 9:256, 1960. C. Jans, The weight increase of the pygmy infant,
Am Soc, Belg Med Trop, 39:851, 1959. S. Mukherjee, and S. Biswas,
Birthweight and its relationship to gestation period, sex, maternal age,
parity and socio-economic status, *J Indian Med Assoc*, 32:389, 1959.
M. Timmer, Prosperity and birthweight in Javanese infants, *Trop Geogr,
Med*, 13:316, 1961. P. M. Udani, Physical growth of children in different
socio-economic groups in Bombay, *Indian J Child Health*, 12:593, 1963.
P. S. Venkatachalm, Maternal nutritional status and its effects on the new-
born bull, *WHO*, 26:193, 1962.)

of neonates born to the poor in Calcutta are 2,500 gm or less,
compared to a 10 percent incidence in the United States.[36]
Increases in birthweight averaging 10 percent have been reported
as a consequence of industrialization.[37] Animal models of
endemic malnutrition have been produced. The mean birth-

weights in a rat colony maintained for seven generations on low protein diets is 20 percent less than controls, and 43 percent of the seventh generation have birthweights two standard deviations below the mean of the control colony.[38] Interestingly, it is the "firm impression" of the laboratory personnel that the extremely small pups in the seventh generation have a higher probability of survival than like sized small pups in the first generation, indication that a genetic shift may be in progress. Several laboratories have now shown that reversibility of the effects of malnutrition may require more than one generation on an adequate diet.[38, 39]

EXPERIMENTAL TECHNIQUES TO INDUCE FETAL MALNUTRITION

Some workers have suggested that a distinction should be made between undernutrition and malnutrition. Undernutrition reflects inadequate amounts of an otherwise well balanced diet. Malnutrition reflects imbalance in dietary constituents. However, there may be no real distinction between undernutrition and malnutrition, since the extent to which protein is metabolized to provide energy depends upon the number of other calories available. Thus, a well balanced diet with inadequate calories (undernutrition) is also a protein deficient diet (malnutrition) since its lower absolute protein content is effectively further reduced to provide calories. For example, an adequate diet, when fed in amounts which satisfy only 70 percent of energy requirements (a restriction of 30%) will cause a reduction of nearly 60 percent in the protein value of the diet.[24]

Types of Restriction

Inadequate amounts of maternal diet: Experimental females are matched in pre-pregnancy weight with controls and fed a reduced percentage of ad libitum intake of commercial chow. Typically this has been a fixed amount of chow, approximately 10 grams a day.[40, 41, 42] An improved technique is to increase amounts slightly during the latter states of gestation, since females eat more during this period.

Restriction of Maternal Dietary Protein: In most experiments, maternal diet is altered by lowering percent protein.[44, 45, 46, 47] The experimental diet should be iso-caloric with the control diet.[48] Pair fed good diet controls should be used, in addition to ad libitum good diet controls, since rats tend to eat less of these low protein diets, perhaps because of reduced palatability or food neophobia.[44, 45] Effective dietary protein availability may also be lowered by diluting commercial chow with sugar.[49] Only a few investigators have studied the effects of diets equal in total percent protein, but differing in protein quality.[50, 51]

Onset of Experimental Diets

Most investigators begin dietary restriction on the day of mating and continue this throughout gestation.[41, 44, 52] There are some studies on the effects of malnutrition initiated at the mother's own weaning[49, 53] or a few weeks before mating.[48] The effects of dietary restriction during only parts of gestation have also been reported.[54, 55] An increasing number of investigators have reported transgenerational effects in the F_2,[39] F_3,[56] and F_7[38] generations.

Surgical Techniques

In rodents, ligation of one uterine horn prior to mating reduces the number of fetuses and increase their rate of intra-uterine development with results opposite to those produced by maternal protein deficiency (Table 9-III). Mid-gestation clamping of the arteries feeding the secondary placenta has been used to produce experimental growth retardation in the subhuman primate.[58]

Control Groups

In addition to paired feeding of experimental and controls, one should insure that experimental and control females are not inadvertently exposed to differential handling or environments. Handling or stressing pregnant females affects characteristics of the F_1[59] and F_2 generation.[60] For a review see Archer and Blackman.[61]

TABLE 9-III

THE EFFECTS OF PRE-MATING UNILATERAL UTERINE HORN
LIGATION (PRENATAL OVERNUTRITION) ON NEONATAL BRAIN
WEIGHT, DNA CONTENT, BRAIN PROTEIN CONTENT AND BIRTH
WEIGHT, COMPARED TO THE EFFECTS PRODUCED BY
PRENATAL UNDERNUTRITION*

Measure	Prenatal Overnutrition (Percent Increase of Experimental Compared to Control)	Prenatal Undernutrition (Percent Decrease of Experimental Compared to Control)
Birthweight	7	30
Brain Weight	15	10
Brain DNA	13	10
Brain Protein	11	20

* S. Zamenhof; E. van Marthens, and F. L. Margolis, DNA (cell number)
and protein in neonatal brain: alteration by maternal dietary protein restriction,
Science, 160:322, 1968. E. van Marthens; S. Zamenhof, Deoxyribonucleic acid
of neonatal rat cerebrum increased by operative restriction of litter size, *Exp
Neurol, 23*:214, 1969.

NEUROBIOLOGICAL EFFECTS

Brain Weight: In the rat and guinea pig, severe protein or
calorie reductions in the maternal diet reduces fetal brain weight
at birth.[45, 46, 47, 48, 62, 63] Milder restrictions do not affect brain
weight at birth, but reductions appear as postnatal growth
continues, even when dietary rehabilitation is initiated at
birth.[43, 46] This stunting cannot be overcome with supraoptimal
feeding.[46] The weight of the brain is reduced less than body
weight, e.g. an elevated brain weight body weight is found in
both animal[64, 65] and man.[66] This limited reduction in brain
weight is remarkable, given that the brain grows faster than
the body during development, and thus might be expected
to be more affected by malnutrition than the slower growing
body. However, this sparing of the brain may be less important
in influencing long term effects than the recent finding that the
brain is more resistant to dietary rehabilitation than other organs,
producing, in adulthood, a true micro-cephaly, e.g. smaller brain
for body size than in controls.[67]

Brain DNA (cell number): DNA is constant within diploid
cells, and the amount of DNA in an organ can be used to estimate

the number of cells in that organ. In the rat, 10 percent of brain DNA is present at birth, with synthesis stopping at seventeen days while in the human, 67 percent of brain DNA is present at birth, synthesis stopping five months after birth.[68]

Severe protein or calorie deficiency in the diets of pregnant rats reduces brain cell number and mitotic activity.[42, 47, 48, 69] This has also been found in the guinea pig[62] and in runt piglets.[64] Zeman[46] found that neither fostering at birth to a well nourished dam nor supraoptimal post-natal feeding could alter the deficit. In the guinea pig, rehabilitation at birth will restore cerebral DNA levels, but cerebellar DNA is still reduced.[62] Reductions in brain DNA may last beyond one generation of rehabilitation.[39]

In man, the brains of infants of normal birthweight who subsequently died of marasmus during the first year of life showed a 15 percent reduction in expected brain DNA, while infants of low birthweight dying of marasmus showed a 60 percent reduction. Infants breast fed during the first year, but who died of kwashiokor during the second year showed no reduction in brain DNA.[70] These data expecially emphasize the importance of *in utero* malnutrition in prediction of the effect of postnatal malnutrition. Reductions in brain DNA are also found in intra-uterine growth retarded subhuman primates at birth, with the cerebellum contributing most to this deficit.[58]

Brain Lipids: Concentration of lipids per gram of wet weight becomes asymptotic in rat brain by twenty-five days of age. Myelin lipids are metabolically stable, and are sensitive measures of the effects of malnutrition.[71] Lipogenesis in the brain is a largely post-natal phenomenon,[66] and there are only a few studies on prenatal influences. In the dog, combining pre- and post-natal malnutrition histologically results in decreased white matter in brain and thinner myelin sheaths in the spinal cord.[72] In the guinea pig, severe prenatal malnutrition results in lower concentrations of brain cholesterol and myelin specific cerebrosides and sulfatides.[62] Marked reductions in these myelin specific lipids have also been found as a consequence of intrauterine growth retardation in man.[73]

Brain Protein: The rat brain cortex reaches adult protein concentration by day fourteen postnatal, the cerebellum not until day thirty postnatal. Protein in neonatal brain at birth is reduced with severe maternal protein deprivation.[39, 46, 48] Rehabilitation at birth does not restore deficits, nor does supra-optimal feeding instituted within the first postnatal week.[46]

Cerebellum: The brain is not a homogenous organ, thus different parts of the brain are differentially affected by prenatal malnutrition. The cerebellum is disproportionately sensitive. In animal and man, malnutrition induced brain weight loss is greatest in the cerebellum.[62, 66] Cerebellar DNA is reduced by prenatal malnutrition more than cerebral DNA in man,[66] guinea pig,[62] rat,[74] and subhuman primate.[58] Similarly, cerebellar protein is reduced more than cerebral protein.[68] Reduction in brain lipids seems to affect the entire brain.

BEHAVIORAL CONSEQUENCES OF EARLY MALNUTRITION

Although malnutrition has been experimentally imposed on young animals for varying lengths of time during varying ages, the data do not demonstrate the existence of behavioral critical periods. The results seem to be additive, with prolonged malnutrition producing more severe effects than malnutrition during shorter periods.[75, 76, 77]

Infant Development: Since, of all brain regions studied, the cerebellum is disproportionately affected by early malnutrition, it would be expected that the development of motor reactions and complex balancing and righting would be impaired in malnourished animals. Rats whose mothers were malnourished during gestation, lactation, or during both gestation and lactation showed behavioral evidence of cerebellar and generalized C.N.S. damage, including circling, tremor, twitching, twitching and convulsions, and retardation in neuromotor development, including onset of complex reflex behavior and locomotion.[77, 78, 79] Young malnourished dogs show head and tongue tremors, walk with a wide-based waddling gait and stiff hind legs. If weaned to a good diet, abnormalities regress, if weaned to a poor diet, the tremors intensify. Gentle exercise leads to agitation, often convulsions.[80, 81] Table 9-IV summarizes some of the indices of

TABLE 9-IV

INDICES OF RETARDED NEONATAL DEVELOPMENT IN
EARLY MALNOURISHED RODENTS*

Category	Index of Retardation
Anatomic	opening of external ear, appearance of upper incisors, opening of eyeslits, opening of vagina and descent of testes
Reflexive	startle, righting, free-fall righting
Neuromotor	spontaneous activity, motor strength
Social	increased aggression and isolation, disturbed mother-infant interaction

* M. Simonson; R. W. Sherwin; J. K. Anilane; W. Y. Yu; B. F. Chow, Neuromotor development in progeny of underfed mother rats, *J Nutr*, 98:18, 1969. J. L. Smart; J. Dobbing, Vulnerability of developing brain. II. Effects of early nutritional deprivation on reflex ontogeny and development of behavior in the rat, *Brain Res*, 28:85, 1971. J. Altman; K. Sudarsham, G. D. Das; N. McCormick; D. Barnes, The influence of nutrition on neural and behavioral development: III. Development of some motor, particularly locomotor patterns during infancy, *Devel Psychbiol*, 4:97, 1971. S. Frankova, Effect of protein-calorie malnutrition on the development of social behavior in rats, *Develop Psychobiol*, 6:33, 1973.

retarded development that have differentiated normal from early malnourished rats. These indices relate to several parameters of growth and development. The opening of the external ear, the appearance of the upper incisors and the opening of the eyeslits and age of puberty are anatomic landmarks of delayed development. Retardation in the emergence of complex reflexive behavior such as free fall righting and startle reflects neurophysiological immaturity in response to potentially life threatening stimuli. Spontaneous open field activity, and searching of the environment by head lifting, and rearing up on hind legs are the forerunners of environmental exploration, an important part of an animal's behavioral repertoire of responses to new inanimate environments. Even the rats earliest social responses to conspecifics are altered. Preweaning homing behavior is disrupted by severe postnatal malnutrition. Progeny of females on low protein diets engage in less play with each other or the mother, and aggregate less than controls. In a pair behavior test, litter mates are slow to approach each other, and engage in less social grooming when contact is made. In fact, the deprived pups responded with aggression towards the second animal when contact was made; a type of response not seen in any pairs of normal animals. Similarly, infant primates on low protein diets spend only a fraction of the time in social play that high protein diet in which infants engage. The social behavior of low protein primates is characterized by marasmus-like self stimulation and indifference towards the social environment.[83, 84] Thus, at many levels of analysis, the malnourished infant animal begins life at a great deficit, which is most probably predictive of maladaption as an adult.

Social Behavior in Adulthood: Rehabilitated malnourished rodents are aggressive in initial encounters with early well-nourished conspecifics.[106] However, with repeated testing, well nourished adults eventually establish dominance, and when placed in group living cages, early malnourished animals are lower on the dominance hierarchy than early well nourished controls.[86]

Emotionality in Adulthood: A major characteristic of the behavior of early undernourished rodents is their high level of emotionality. Their heightened excitability affects every behavior engaged in. Early malnourished rodents are slow to leave their home cage;[87] and when they do it it is accompanied by high rates of defecation[88] and fear of new stimuli.[89] Exploratory behavior is depressed,[82, 88, 90] and latency to initiate exploration in a new environment is prolonged.[86] Increased emotionality has also been found in early malnourished cats,[91] pigs[92] and dogs.[81]

Learning Ability in Adulthood

Learning can never be measured directly, but can only be assayed through observation of responses, i.e. performance. In normal animals under most circumstances one can expect a reasonable correlation between learning and performance, however, problems arise when examining early malnourished animals. Rehabilitated rats are inferior to controls in learning a water maze when the water is warm (35°C), but when it is cooled (15°C) they perform as well as well nourished controls.[93] The increased sensitivity of early malnourished animals to aversive stimulation makes it difficult to attribute either improved performance or poor performance to changes in learning ability *per se*.[94, 95] Attempts have been made to reduce pre-learning emotionality levels of early malnourished animals, so as to better study learning ability.

Hebb-Williams Maze: The procedures involved in using the Hebb-Williams maze require an extensive pre-training period. When used properly, the maze is insensitive to subject difference in level of food motivation and emotionality.[96, 97] The maze is considered to be a test of animal intelligence and has successfully discriminated between normal and brain damaged animals.[97, 98] Zimmerman and Wells[99] found that pre-training reduced the early malnourished animals' emotional responses to the maze as reflected in very short latencies to enter the start box. However, despite this pre-training, early malnourished animals made more errors than controls.

Discrimination Reversal Learning: Reversal learning follows extensive acquisition learning, during which time initial differences between malnourished groups in their fear responses to novelty[89] or level of emotionality[85] should be washed out. However, malnourished animals are still inferior to controls in learning to reverse the original training stimuli.[100]

Latent Learning: The typical technique in maze learning is to place an animal in a maze, the goal box of which contains an appropriate reinforcer. In the presence of reinforcement, performance over trials quickly improves. As has been well documented, early malnourished animals make more errors while learning a maze than controls.[54, 95] In the latent learning procedure, an animal is allowed to freely explore a maze for several trials in the absence of reinforcers for learning. There is no improvement in performance during this initial period. At the end of this period a reinforcer is placed in the goal box and "discovered" by the rat. On the next trial behavior is examined for evidence of any "latent" learning that may have occurred during the previous free exploration period, since the animal now will rush directly to the goal box, i.e. perform. Use of this technique avoids many of the problems of emotionality, since animals have an opportunity for adaption to the maze prior to formal testing. Introduction of food reinforcement reduces errors in the maze by only one-half in early malnourished rats, compared to a two-thirds reduction in controls.[100]

Specific Protein Hunger and Food Motivation: Infant primates on low protein diets show evidence of a specific protein hunger. When infant monkeys receive only half-strength milk formula, they will double their fluid intake and grow normally. When the formula is diluted to one-fourth strength, ad libitum fluid intake increases to nearly four times normal volume, although this degree of fluid intake impairs growth.[83] Malnourished infant monkeys readily choose high protein pellets in an assortment containing low protein pellets and nonfood objects, while controls choose equally among the various objects and pellets.[101]

Long term food motivation is altered in the rehabilitated adult rodent. Such animals work faster to obtain food,[102] eat it more rapidly,[103] and hoard more of it[104] than controls. Similar findings have been reported for the early malnourished dog,[105] cat[91] and pig.[92]

Effects of Environment: Rearing of animals in isolation increases rat emotionality. Rearing in enriched environments reduced the deleterious effects of early malnutrition on behaviors such as activity, aggression, and exploration,[106] and reduces errors on the Hebb-Williams maze.[145]

In summary, the effects of malnutrition on animal behavior are so severe that they are reflected in almost every facet of its existence from earliest development, and seem largely resistant to substantial modification after dietary rehabilitation.

INTELLIGENCE IN MAN

Low Birthweight and Intelligence: The greater the time between birth and behavioral testing, the greater the likelihood that intervening events will influence reductions in intelligence which may be incorrectly attributed to low birthweight. Socioeconomic factors play an important moderator role in this regard, since they independently correlated with incidence of low birthweight and low intelligence.[107, 108, 109] For example, low birthweight children get poorer reports on their school behavior than high birthweight children. However, this turns out to be a reflection of over-representation of low socioeconomic group children, and not a birthweight factor per se.[110, 111]

In the higher socioeconomic groups, rearing conditions are typically optimal for the development of intelligence (stable families, adequate education, absence of disease). Thus, studies of the effects of low birthweight in children from high socioeconomic groups may offer the clearest direct indication of the influence of low birthweight *per se* on intelligence (Table 9-V). The comprehensive studies conducted by the Department of Population and Family Health, John Hopkins University[109, 112-116] clearly indicated that socioeconomic factors, positive maternal attitudes and race were each more strongly related to IQ than was low birthweight. Low birthweight was related to impaired general intelligence and poor school achievement only when clinical neurological signs were observed during the first year. However, although general intelligence was not impaired when

TABLE 9-V

PERCENTAGE OF CHILDREN IN EACH SOCIOECONOMIC GROUP AND BIRTHWEIGHT CATEGORY WHO ARE BELOW NORMAL IN INTELLIGENCE. CHILDREN WERE BETWEEN FIVE AND SEVEN YEARS OLD AT TESTING*

Socioeconomic Group	Birthweight (gm.)		
	⩽2,000	2,000-2,500	⩾2,500
Highest	15.8	3.2	1.0
Lowest	51.5	40.6	25.9

* C. M. Drillen, *Growth and Development of the Prematurely Born Infant.* Baltimore, Williams and Wilkins, 1964.

the neurological data were controlled for, other specific tests for organicity (incomplete or rotated drawings, perseveration, overly concrete thinking) did continue to discriminate between the high and low birthweight groups. Length of gestation associated with very low birthweight was not a factor, although intelligence and school achievement was impaired in normal birthweight children who experienced either short or long gestation periods. Complex findings reported by Drillien[117] suggest that studies of birthweight-intelligence relationships must take absolute birthweight, gestational age and socio-economic status into account to clearly predict consequence. For a review see Caputo and Mandell.[118]

Multiple Birth and Intelligence

When there are significant differences in birthweight between twins, the lower birthweight twin has the lower IQ.[119, 120, 121] Further analysis indicates that this may be true only for monozygous twins, with monochorionic twins being particularly at risk.[122] Other behavioral pathologies have been associated with low birthweight in multiple births. In pairs of twins discordant for schizophrenia, the lower birthweight twin is more likely to be the schizophrenic.[123] There exists an extensive case report from the National Institute of Mental Health of identical quadruplet girls, all of whom became schizophrenic. The earliest onset and the poorest prognosis occurred in the lowest birthweight quad, and the progression thereafter was directly related to birthweight, the heaviest at birth having the latest onset and most mild form of schizophrenia.[124]

In summary, the relationship between birthweight and reproductive casualty, including impaired intelligence may be best exemplified by Yerushalmy's[8] analysis of perinatal mortality in New York City by birthweight and gestation length (Figure 9-5). The continuum of casualty steeply rises below birthweights of 2,500 grams, with impairment most severe in birthweights below 1,500 grams. Behavioral impairments in the survivors in each birthweight class most likely reflect the same type of continuum.

Malnutrition and Intelligence

The specific effects of malnutrition on intelligence in man are still largely unknown. General research problems have not yet been satisfactorily resolved, particularly with regard to the influence of the non-nutritional social and biological factors that in the human situation are almost inextricably interwoven with the presence of malnutrition. As the late Dr. Herbert Birch has stressed, the same context that impairs the development of the individual as a biological entity, also impairs him as a cultural entity.[125] Since there are no intelligence tests that can satisfactorily distinguish between "biological" and "cultural" intelligence, caution should be exercised in imputing causality to one or the other factor. Moreover, performance on intelligence tests

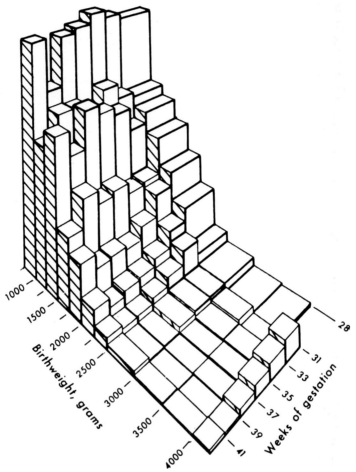

Figure 9-5. Prenatal mortality by birthweight and gestational age for single white births in New York City, 1957-1959. (Courtesy of Harper & Row Publishers).

may be impaired for various reasons. Zimmerman,[126] working with malnourished primates, and Canosa,[127] working with malnourished children have both observed that ability to maintain sustained attention during testing, rather than ability to learn the task differentiates malnourished from control subjects.

Adding to the problem is the fact that, in man, protein malnutrition is not a clear-cut deficiency state. Protein deficient diets may be poor in both quantity and quality of protein, deficient in fat, excessive in starch, poor in vitamins. Where malnutrition is endemic, other biological problems are present, including various debilitating diseases.[128]

Short-Term Malnutrition: There is little evidence that maternal malnutrition during pregnancy has adverse effects on the later intelligence of children. The best studies of the effects of gestational malnutrition derive from examination of the effects of short-term famine on otherwise well nourished, socially well-organized societies. The Rotterdam famine of World War II lasted less than a year, and resulted in a significant reduction in birthweight.[129] A comprehensive epidemiological study of nineteen-year-old males born or conceived during the famine revealed no reduction in intelligence, no increase in rates of mild or severe mental retardation, or any narrowing of differences in intelligence as a function of socioeconomic status.[27]

Long-Term Malnutrition: In the typical situation the child or adult being tested has suffered from malnutrition for most of his life, and has been reared in a poor social and biological environment by relatives who, during their lifetimes, have also lived with cultural and biological handicaps. Only after the most careful use of appropriate controls can one state that only the presence of malnutrition was instrumental in reducing intelligence, all other biological and social factors being equal. Unfortunately, significant discrepancies between experimental and control groups are typically found. Stoch and Smythe[130, 131] in their long term studies of severely malnourished South African children, found EEG and behavioral (motor and perceptual) evidence of organic brain damage which was related to the low IQ's of their group. However, they also believe that lack of energy and inactivity, characteristic of malnourished children, decreased their responsivity to the social environment which, in turn, affected intellectual growth. They also admitted that their control groups were not adequate. Their malnourished groups lived in inadequate housing with no sanitary facilities, come from broken homes and were generally neglected, while controls lived in neat houses, came from intact families, and went to nursery. In other studies in which malnourished children were matched with controls, significant differences on important variables were found between groups, despite all attempts to eliminate them.[132, 133, 134] One approach used to better match groups has been the use of sibling controls. Children who had been hospitalized for clinical malnutrition prior to the age of two were compared to their own nearest sibling and matched unrelated children. All IQ measures were lower in the malnourished children than in the matched controls, and Fall Scale and Verbal IQ were lower in the malnourished index cases than in their siblings.[135]

The most extensive series of studies are those of Cravioto and his colleagues, investigating intellectual development of rural populations in Central America.[136, 137, 138] Impaired intellectual performance was strongly related to inadequate nutrition, and not related to other factors such as personal cleanliness, monetary or crop income, or education of parents. Performance of the malnourished children on intellectual tests was correlated with height, shorter children being more retarded than larger children.[1] This unusual correlation has been found by others.[132, 139] Anthropometric analysis indicated that height of the malnourished children reflected nutritional rather than genetic influences.[138]

In summary, the overwhelming body of research implicates a strong association between malnutrition and retarded intelligence, but the casual chain is still under question.[140] Intervention research currently underway may answer more questions.[127, 141, 142]

REFERENCES

1. Fujikura, T., and Niemann, W. H.: Birthweight, gestational age, and type of delivery in rhesus monkeys. *Am J Obstet Gynecol,* 97:76, 1967.
2. Rush, D.; Davis, H., and Susser, M.: Antecedents of low birthweight in Harlem, New York City. *Int J Epidemiology,* 1:375, 1972.
3. Birch, H. G., and Gussow, J. D.: Disadvantaged Children: *Health, Nutrition and School Failure.* New York, Harcourt, Brace & World, 1970.
4. Hunter, G. L.: The maternal influence on size in sheep. *J Agric Res,* 48:36, 1956.
5. Venge, O.: Studies of the maternal influence on the birth weight in rabbits. *Acta Zool, 31:1,* 1950.

6. Walton, A., and Hammond, J.: The maternal effects on growth and conformation in Shire horse and Shetland pony crosses. *Proc R Soc Med, 125*:311, 1938.

7. Smidt, D.; Steinbach, J., and Scheven, B.: Die Beeinflussung der prä-und postnatalen Enswicklung durch Grösse und Korpergewicht der Mutter, dargestellt on Ergebaissen reziproker Eitransplantation zwischen Zwergschweinen und grossen Hausschweinen. *Mschr Kinderheilk, 115*:533, 1967.

8. Yerushalmy, J.: Relation of birth weight, gestational age, and the rate of intrauterine growth to perinatal mortality. In Gold, E. M. (Ed.): *Perinatal Mortality.* New York, Harper Row, 1970.

9. Naylor, A. F., and Myrianthropoulos, N. C.: The relation of ethnic and selected socioeconomic factors to human birthweight. *Ann Hum Genet, 31*:71, 1967.

10. Bergner. L., and Susser, M. W.: Low birthweight and prenatal nutrition: an interpretive review. *Pediatrics, 46*:946, 1970.

11. Eastman, N. J., and Jackson, E.: Weight relationships in pregnancy I. The bearing of maternal weight gain and pre-pregnancy weight on birth weight in full term pregnancies. *Obstet Gynecol Survey, 23*:1003, 1968.

12. Weiss, W.; Jackson, E. C.; Niswander, K., and Eastman. N. J.: Influence on birthweight of change in maternal weight gain in successive pregnancies in the same woman. *Int J Gyn Obstet, 7*:210, 1969.

13. Niswander, K. R.; Singer, J.; Westphal, M., and Weiss, W.: Weight gain during pregnancy and pre-pregnancy weight: Association with birth weight of term gestation. *Obstet Gynecol, 33*:482, 1969.

14. Gruenwald, P.: Growth of the human fetus. In McLaren, A. (Ed.): *Advances in Reproductive Physiology.* New York, Acad Pr, 1967.

15. Gruenwald, P.: Growth and maturation of the foetus and its relationtion to perinatal mortality. In Butler, N. R., and Alberman, E. D. (Eds.): *Perinatal Problems.* Edinburgh & London, Livingstone, 1969.

16. Gruenwald, P.: Fetal malnutrition. In Waisman, H. A., and Kerr, G. R. (Eds.): *Fetal Growth and Development.* New York, McGraw, 1970.

17. Naeye, R. L.: Structural correlates of fetal undernutrition. In Waisman, H. A., and Kerr, G. R. (Eds.): *Fetal Growth and Development.* New York, McGraw, 1970.

18. Van den Berg, B. J., and Yerushalmy, J.: The statistical approach to fetal growth. In Waisman, H. A., and Kerr, G. R. (Eds.): *Fetal Growth and Development.* New York, McGraw, 1970.

19. Naeye, R. L.; Benirschke, K.; Hagstrom, J. W. C., and Marcus, C. C.: Intrauterine growth of twins as estimated from liveborn birth-weight data. *Pediatrics, 37*:409, 1966.
20. Gruenwald, P.: Chronic fetal distress and placental insufficiency. *Biol Neonat, 5*:215, 1963.
21. Wallace, L. R.: The growth of lambs before and after birth in relation to the level of nutrition. *J Agr Sci, 38*:93, 1948.
22. Pond, W. G.: Influence of maternal protein and energy nutrition during gestation on progeny performance in swine. *J Amin Sci, 36*:175, 1973.
23. Payne, P. R., and Wheeler, E. F.: Comparative nutrition in pregnancy. *Nature, 215*:1134, 1967.
24. Platt, B. S.: Congenital protein calorie deficiency. *Proc R Sc Med, 59*:1077, 1966.
25. McCance, R. A., and Widdowson, E. M.: The chemistry of growth and development. *Br Med Bull, 7*:297, 1951.
26. Fox, H. E.: Dept. Ob/Gyn. U of Rochester School of Medicine, Rochester, New York (Personal communication).
27. Stein, Z.; Susser, M.; Saenger, G., and Marolla, F.: Nutrition and mental performance. *Science, 178*:708, 1972.
28. Antonov, A. N.: Children born during the siege of Leningrad in 1942. *J of Pediatrics, 30*:250, 1947.
29. Kohrs, M. B.: Effects of low protein diet on reproductive performance of the rhesus monkey. *Fed Proc, 32*:901, 1973.
30. Achar, S. T., and Yankauer, A.: Studies on the birth weight of South Indian infants. *Indian J Child Health, 11*:57, 1962.
31. Hollingsworth, M. G.: The birth weights of African and European babies born in Ghana. *W Afr Med J, 9*:256, 1960.
32. Jans. C.: The weight increase of the pygmy infant. *Am Soc Belg Med Trop, 39*:851, 1959.
33. Mukherjee, S., and Biswas, S.: Birthweight and its relationship to gestation period, sex, maternal age, parity and socio-economic status. *J Indian Med Assoc, 32*:389, 1959.
34. Timmer, M.: Prosperity and birthweight in Javanese infants. *Trop Geogr Med, 13*:316, 1961.
35. Udani, P. M.: Physical growth of children in different socio-economic groups in Bombay. *Indian J Child Health, 12*:593, 1963.
36. Venkatachalam, P. S.: Maternal nutritional status and its effects on the newborn bull. *WHO, 26*:193, 1962.
37. Gruenwald, P.; Funakawa, H.; Mitani, S.; Nishimura, T., and Takeuchi, S.: Influence of environmental factors on foetal growth in man. *Lancet, 1*:1026, 1967.
38. Stewart, R. J. C.: Small-for-dates offspring: an animal model. *Pan Am Health Org, 251*:33, 1972.

39. Zamenhof, S.; van Marthens, E., and Grauel, L.: DNA (cell number) in neonatal brain: Second generation (F_2) alternation by maternal (F_0) dietary protein restriction. *Science, 172*:850, 1971.

40. Adlard, B. P. F., and Dobbing, J.: Vulnerability of developing brain, V. Effects of fetal and postnatal undernutrition or regional brain enzyme activities in three week old rats. *Pediatr Res, 6*:38, 1972.

41. Chow, B. F., and Lee, C. J.: Effect of dietary restriction on pregnant rats on body weight gain of offspring. *J Nutr, 82*:10, 1964.

42. Patel, A. J.; Bálazs, R., and Johnson, A. L.: Effect of undernutrition on cell formation in the rat brain. *J Neurochem, 20*:1151, 1973.

43. Barnes, D., and Altman, J.: Effects of different schedules of early undernutrition on the preweaning growth of the rat cerebellum. *Exp Neurol, 38*:406, 1973.

44. Nelson, N. M., and Evans, H. M.: Relation of dietary protein levels to reproduction in the rat. *J Nutr, 51*:71, 1953.

45. Zeman, F.: Effect on the young rat of maternal protein restriction. *J Nutr, 93*:167, 1967.

46. Zeman, F.: Effect of protein deficiency during gestation on the postnatal cellular development in the young rat. *J Nutr, 100*:530, 1970.

47. Zeman, F., and Stanbrough, E.: Effect of maternal protein deficiency on cellular development in the fetal rat. *J Nutr, 99*:274, 1969.

48. Zamenhof, S.; van Marthens, E., and Margolis, F. L.: DNA (cell number) and protein in neonatal brain: Alteration by maternal dietary protein restriction. *Science, 160*:322, 1968.

49. Widdowson, E. M., and Cowen, J.: The effect of protein deficiency and calorie deficiency on the reproduction of rats. *Br J Nutr, 27*:85, 1972.

50. Barnes, R. H.; Kwong, E.; Morrissey, L.; Vilhjalms-dottir, L., and Levitsky, D. A.: Maternal protein deprivation during pregnancy on lactation in rats and the efficiency of food and nitrogen utilization of the progeny. *J Nutr, 103*:273, 1973.

51. Chow, B. F.; Blackwell, R. Q; Blackwell, B. N.; Sherwin, R. W.; Hsueh, A. M., and Lee, C. J.: Studies on the progeny of underfed mothers. *Proc of the VIIth Int Cong of Nutr, 4*:238, 1967.

52. Hsueh, A. M.; Agustin, C. E., and Chow, B. F.: Growth of young rats after differential manipulation of maternal diet. *J Nutr, 91*:195, 1967.

53. Turner, M. R.: Perinatal mortality, growth, and survival to weaning in offspring of rats reared on diets moderately deficient in protein. *Br J Nutr, 29*:139, 1973.

54. Caldwell, D. F., and Churchill, J. A.: Learning ability in the progeny of rats administered a protein deficient diet during the second half of gestation. *Neurology, 17*:95, 1969.

55. Zemenhof, S.; van Marthens, E.. and Grauel, L.: DNA (cell number) in neonatal brain: alteration by maternal dietary caloric restriction. *Nutr Int, 4*:269, 1971.

56. Cowley, J. J., and Griesel, R. D.: Effect on growth and behavior of rehabilitating first and second generation low protein rats. *Anim Behav, 14*:506, 1966.

57. van Marthens, E., and Zamenhof, S.: Deoxyribonucleic acid of neonatal rat cerebrum increased by operative restriction of litter size. *Exp Neurol, 23*:214, 1969.

58. Hill, D. E.; Myers, R. E.; Holt, A. B.; Scott, R. E., and Cheek, D. B.: Fetal growth retardation produced by experimental placental insufficiency in the rhesus monkey. *Biol Neonate, 19*:68, 1971.

59. Porter, R., and Wehmer, F.: Maternal and infantile influences upon exploratory behavior and emotional reactivity in the albino rat. *Develop Psychobiol, 2*:19, 1969.

60. Wehmer, F.; Porter, R., and Scales. B.: Premating and pregnancy stress affects behavior of grandpups. *Nature, 227*:622, 1970.

61. Archer, J. E., and Blackman, D. E.: Prenatal psychological stress and offspring behavior in rats and mice. *Develop Psychobiol, 4*:193, 1971.

62. Chase, H. P.; Dabiere. C. S.; Welch, N. N., and O'Brien, D.: Intra-uterine undernutrition and brain development. *Pediatrics, 3*:491, 1971.

63. Zamenhof, S.; van Marthens, E., and Grauel, L.: Prenatal cerebral development: Effect of restricted diet, reversal by growth hormone. *Science, 174*:954, 1971.

64. Dickerson, J. W. T.; Merat, A., and Widdowson, E. M.: Intra-uterine growth retardation in the pig III. The chemical structure of the brain. *Biol Neonate, 19*:354, 1971.

65. Dobbing, J.: Undernutrition and the developing brain. In W. Himwich (Ed.): *Developmental Neurobiology.* Springfield, Thomas. 1970.

66. Chase, W. P.: The effects of intrauterine and postnatal under-nutrition on normal brain development. *Annals NY Acad Sci, 205*:231, 1973.

67. Dobbing, J., and Sands, J.: Vulnerability of the developing brain IX. The effect of nutritional growth retardation on the timing of the brain growth spurt. *Biol Neonate, 19*:363, 1971.

68. Chase, H. P.; Lindsley, W. F. B., and O'Brien, D.: Undernutrition and cerebellar development. *Nature, 221*:554, 1969.

69. Winick, M.: Malnutrition and brain development. *Pediatrics, 74*:667, 1969.

70. Brasel, J. A., and Winick, M.: Maternal nutrition and prenatal growth. *Arch Dis Child, 47*:479, 1972.

71. Dickerson, J. W. T., and Dobbing, J.: The effect of undernutrition in early life in the brain and spinal cord in pigs. *Proc Nutr Soc, 26*:5, 1967.

72. Platt, B. S., and Stewart, R. J. C.: Effects of protein-calorie deficiency on dogs. 2. Morpohlogical changes in the nervous system. *Dev Med Child Neurol, 11*:174, 1969.

73. Chase, H. P.; Welch, N. N.; Dabiere, C. S.; Vasan, N. S., and Butterfield, L. J.: Alterations in human brain biochemistry following intrauterine growth retardation (In press). Reported in: Chase, H. P.: The effects of intrauterine and postnatal undernutrition on normal brain development. *Ann NY Acad Sci, 205*:231, 1973.

74. Winick, M.: Cellular growth in intrauterine malnutrition. *Pediatr Clin N Am, 17*:69, 1970.

75. Barnes, R. H.; Cunnold, S. R.; Zimmerman, R. R.; Simmons, H.; MacLeod, R. B., and Krook, L.: Influence of nutritional deprivations in early life on learning behavior of rats as measured by performance in a water maze. *J Nutr, 89*:399, 1966.

76. Vore, D. A., and Ottinger, D. R.: Maternal food restriction: Effects on offspring development, learning, and a program of therapy. *Develop Psychol, 3*:337, 1970.

77. Simonson, M.; Sherwin, R. W.; Anilane, J. K.; Yu, W. Y., and Chow, B. F.: Neuromotor development in progeny of underfed mother rats. *J Nutr, 98*:18, 1969.

78. Smart, J. L., and Dobbing, J.: Vulnerability of developing brain. II. Effects of early nutritional deprivation on reflex ontogeny and development of behavior in the rat. *Brain Res, 28*:85, 1971.

79. Altmarn, J.; Sudarshan, K.; Das, G. D.; McCormick, N., and Barnes, D.: The influence of nutrition on neural and behavioral development: III Development of some motor, particularly locomotor patterns durng infancy. *Devel Psychobiol, 4*:97, 1971.

80. Stewart, R. J. C.: The influence of protein calorie deficiency on the central nervous system. *Proc Nutr Soc, 27*:95, 1968.

81. Stewart, R. J. C., and Platt, B. S.: Nervous system damage in experimental protein-calorie deficiency. In Scrimshaw, N. S., and Gordon, J. E. (Eds.): *Malnutrition Learning and Behavior.* Cambridge, M.I.T. Press, 1968.

82. Frankova, S., and Barnes, R. H.: Effect of malnutrition in early life on avoidance conditioning and behavior of adult rats. *J Nutr, 96*:485, 1968.

83. Kerr, G. R., and Waisman, H. A.: A primate model for the quantitative study of malnutrition. In Scrimshaw, N. S., and Gordon, J. E. (Eds.): *Malnutrition, Learning, and Behavior.* Cambridge, M.I.T. Press, 1968.

84. Zimmermann, R. R.; Steere, P. O.; Strobel, D. A., and Hom, H. L.:

Abnormal social development of protein malnourished rhesus monkeys. *J Abn Soc Psychol, 80*:125, 1972.

85. Levitsky, D. A., and Barnes, R. H.: Effect of early malnutrition on the reaction of adult rats to aversive stimuli. *Nature, 225*:468, 1970.

86. Ryan, R., and Wehmer, F.: The effect of litter size on aggression, competition for food and home cage dominance in the laboratory mouse. (In preparation).

87. Cowley, J. J., and Grisel, R. D.: Low protein diet and emotionality in the albino rat. *J Genet Psychol, 104*:89, 1964.

88. Simonson, M.; Stephan, J. K.; Hanson, H. M., and Chow, B. F.: Open field studies in offspring of underfed mother rats. *J Nutr, 101*:331, 1971.

89. Zimmermann, R. R., and Zimmermann, S. J.: Responses of protein malnourished rats to novel objects. *Percept Motor Skills, 35*:319, 1972.

90. Lat, J.; Widdowson, E. M., and McCance, R. A.: Some effects of accelerating growth: III. Behavior and nervous activity. *Proc R Soc Biol, 1953B*:347, 1960.

91. Seitz, P. F. D.: Infantile experience and adult behavior in animal subjects. II age of separation from the mother and adult behavior in the cat. *Psychosom Med, 21*:353, 1959.

92. Barnes, R. H.; Moore, A. U., and Pond, W. F.: Behavioral abnormalities in young adult pigs caused by malnutrition in early life. *J Nutr, 100*:149, 1970.

93. Geist, C. R.: Performance of rats raised on low protein diets in a water maze. Paper presented at the Montana Psychological Association, 1973.

94. Hanson, H. M., and Simonson, M.: Effects of fetal undernourishment on experimental anxiety. *Nutr Reps International, 4*:307, 1971.

95. Simonson, M., and Chow, B. F.: Maze studies on progeny of underfed mother rats. *J Nutr, 100*:685, 1971.

96. Das, G., and Broadhurst, P. L.: The effect of inherited differences in emotitonal reactivity on a measure of intelligence in the rat. *J Comp Physiol Psycho, 52*:300, 1959.

97. Rabinovitch, M. S., and Rosvald, H. E.: A closed field intelligence test for rats. *Can J Psychol, 4*:122, 1951.

98. Hebb, D. O., and Williams, K. A.: A method of rating animal intelligence. *J of Genet Psycho, 34*:59, 1946.

99. Zimmerman, R. R., and Wells, A. M.: Performance of malnourished rats on the Hebb Williams closed-field maze learning task. *Percept Motor Skills, 33*:1043, 1971.

100. Levitsky, D. A., and Barnes, R. H.: Malnutrition and the Biology

of Experience. Paper presented to IX Int. Cong. of Nutrition, Mexico City, Mexico. Sept., 1972.

101. Peregoy, E.; Zimmermann, R. R., and Strobel, D. A.: Protein preference in protein malnourished monkeys. *Percept Mot Skills,* 35:495. 1972.

102. Mandler, J. M.: Effects of early food deprivation on adult behavior in the rat. *J Comp Physiol Psychol, 51:*513, 1958.

103. Marx, M. H.: Infantile deprivation and adult behavior in the rat: Retention of increased rate of eating. *J Comp Physiol Psychol,* 45:43, 1952.

104. Hunt, J. McV.: The effects of infant feeding—frustration upon hoarding in the albino rat. *J Abnorm Soc Psychol, 36:*338, 1941.

105. Elliott, O., and King, J. A.: Effect of early food deprivation upon later consummatory behavior in puppies. *Psychol Rep, 6:*391, 1960.

106. Levitsky, D. A., and Barnes, R. H.: Nutritional and environmental interations in the behavioral development of the rat: Long-term effects. *Science, 176:*68, 1972.

107. Benton, A.: Mental development of prematurely born children. *Am J Orthopsychiatry, 10:*719, 1940.

108. Rider, R. V.; Taback, M., and Knobloch, H.: Assocations between premature births and socioeconomic status. *Am J Public Health,* 45:1022, 1955.

109. Wiener, G.; Rider, R. R.; Oppel, W. C.; Fisher, L., and Harper, P. A.: Correlates of low birth weight: Psychological status at six to seven years. *Pediatrics, 35:*434, 1965.

110. Douglas, J. W. B.: Premature children at primary schools. *Br Med J, 1:*1008, 1960.

111. Drillen, C. M.: *Growth and Development of the Prematurely Born Infant.* Baltimore, Williams & Wilkins, 1964.

112. Harper, P. A.; Fisher, L. K., and Rider, R. V.: Neurological and intellectual status of prematures at three to five years of age. *J Pediatr, 55:*679, 1959.

113. Knobloch, H.; Rider, R.; Harper, P., and Pasamanick, B.: Neuropsychiatric sequaelae of prematurity. *JAMA, 161:*581, 1956.

114. Wiener, G.: Scholastic achievement at age twelve to thirteen of prematurely born infants. *J Spec Ed, 2:*237, 1968.

115. Wiener, G.: The relationship of birthweight and length of gestation to intellectual development at ages eight to ten years. *J Pediatr,* 76:694, 1970.

116. Wiener, G.; Rider, R. V.; Oppel, W. C., and Harper, P. A.: Correlates of low birthweight: Psychological status at eight to ten years of age. *Pediatr Res, 2:*110, 1968.

117. Drillien, C. M.: Intellectual sequelae of "fetal malnutrition." In Waisman, H. A., and Kerr, G. R. (Eds.): *Fetal Growth and Development*. New York, McGraw, 1970.

118. Caputo, D. V. ,and Mandell, W.: Consequences of low birth weight. *Develop Psychol, 3*:363, 1970.

119. Babson, S. G.; Kangas, J.; Young, N., and Bramhall, J. L.: Growth and development of twins of dissimilar size at birth. *Pediatrics, 33*:327, 1964.

120. Churchill, J. A.: The relationship between intelligence and birth weight in twins. *Neurology, 15*:341, 1965.

121. Willerman, L., and Churchill, J. A.: Intelligence and birth weight in identical twins. *Child Dev, 38*:623, 1967.

122. Kaelber, C. T., and Pugh, T. F.: Influence of intrauterine relations on the intelligence of twins. *N Engl J Med, 28*:1030, 1969.

123. Lane, E. A., and Albee, G. W.: Comparative birthweights of schizophrenics and their schlings. *J Psychol, 64*:227, 1966.

124. Rosenthal, D.: *The Genain Quadruplets*. New York, Basic Books, 1964.

125. Birch, H. G.: Malnutrition learning and intelligence. *Am J Public Health, 62*:773, 1972.

126. Zimmermann, R. R.; Geist, C. R.; Strobel, D. A., and Cleveland, T. J.: Attention deficiencies in malnourished monkeys. Paper presented to the Symposium on Early Malnutrition and Mental Development. Stockholm, Sweden. August, 1973.

127. Canosa, C. A.; Solomon, R. L., and Klein, R. E.: The intervention approach: The Guatemala study. In Moore, W. M.; Silverberg, M. M., and Read, M. S. (Eds.): *Nutrition Growth and Development of North American Indian Children*. Washingtons DHEW Pub. No. (NIH) 72-76, 1973.

128. Metcoff, J.: Biochemical effects of protein-calorie malnutrition in man. *Ann Rev Med, 18*:377, 1967.

129. Smith, C. A.: Effects of maternal undernutrition upon newborn infants in Holland (1944-1945). *J Pediatr, 30*:229, 1947.

130. Stoch, M. B., and Smythe, P. M.: The effect of undernutrition during infancy on subsequent brain growth and intellectual development. *S Afr Med J, 12*:345, 1967.

131. Stoch, M. B., and Smythe, P. M.: Does undernutrition during infancy inhibit brain growth and subsequent intellectual development? *Arch Dis Child, 38*:546, 1963.

132. Brockman, L. M., and Ricciuti, H. N.: Severe protein calorie malnutrition and cognitive development in infancy and early childhood. *Devel Psychol, 4*:312, 1971.

133. Chase, H. P., and Martin, H. P.: Undernutrition and child development. *N Engl J Med, 282*:933, 1970.

134. Fisher, M. M.; Killcross, M. C.; Simonsson, M., and Elgie, K. A.: Malnutrition and reasoning ability in Zambian school children. *Trans R Soc Trop Med & Hyg, 66*:471, 1972.

135. Hertzig, M. E.; Birch, H. G.; Richardson, S. A., and Tizard, J.: Intellectual levels of school children severely malnourished during the first two years of life. *Pediatrics, 49*:814, 1972.

136. Cravioto, J.: Malnutrition and behavioral development in the preschool child. In: *Preschool Child Malnutrition*. Washington, Nat. Health Sci. Publ. No. 1282, 1966.

137. Cravioto, J.: Nutritional deficiencies and mental performance in childhood. In Glass, D. C. (Ed.): *Environmental Influence*. New York, Rockefeller, 1968.

138. Cravioto, J., and Delicardie, E. R.: Intersensory development of school age children. In Scrimshaw, N. S., and Gordon, J. E. (Eds.): *Malnutrition, Learning and Behavior*. Cambridge, M.I.T. Press, 1968.

139. Monckëberg, F.; Tisler, S.; Toro, S.; Galtás, V., and Vega, L.: Malnutrition and mental development. *Am J Clin Nutr, 25*:766, 1972.

140. Warren, N.: Malnutrition and mental development. *Psychol Bull, 80*:324, 1973.

141. Rush, D.; Stein, Z., and Susser, M.: The rationale for, and design of, a randomized controlled trial of nutritional supplementation in pregnancy. *Nutr Rep Int, 7*:547, 1973.

142. National Academy of Science, National Research Council: Nutritional supplementation and the outcome of pregnancy. Washington, NTIS (NAS) U.S. Dept. of Commerce, 1973.

143. Frankova, S.: Effect of protein-calorie malnutrition on the development of social behavior in rats. *Develop Psychobiol, 6*:33, 1973.

144. McCance, R. A.: The effect of calorie deficiencies and protein deficiencies on final weight and stature. In McCance, R. A., and Widdowson, E. M. (Eds.): *Calorie Deficiencies and Protein Deficiencies*. Boston, Little, 1968.

145. Wells, A. M.; Geist, C. R., and Zimmermann, R. R.: Influence of environmental and nutritional factors on problem solving in the rat. *Percept Motor Skills, 35*:235, 1972.

SECTION III

METHODOLOGY AND INTERUTERINE DIAGNOSIS

Chapter 10_____

FETO-MATERNAL INCOMPATABILITY— CYTOTOXIC ANTIBODIES AGAINST HL-A TISSUE ANTIGENS

J. L. Sever and P. L. Terasaki

INTRODUCTION

Feto-maternal tissue differences result in the development of cytotoxic antibodies aaginst HL-A tissue antigens in 20 to 50 percent of females following repeat pregnancies.[4, 7] Transplacental passage of these antibodies to the fetus has been known for a number of years.[2] The possibility that this antibody may be of significance in the production of fetal abnormalities, disease, or mortality has been suggested by several reports. Injection of heterologous antibodies into pregnant female mice produced a wide range of congenital anomalies.[1] A study of Terasaki, et al.[5] indicated that women with cytotoxic HL-A antibody had significantly more infants with congenital abnormalities than those without antibodies. Also, the frequency of abortions was increased in one series of women with antibodies but not in another. They pointed out that there was nearly a ten-fold greater incidence of antibodies to HL-A than to Rh antigens.

To investigate further these possible important associations we selected specimens from the serum bank of over 300,000 sera which were collected prospectively from 50,000 pregnant women in the Collaborative Perinatal Project.[3] For our initial investigation several groups of patients were included: women who had spontaneous abortions, mothers of children with central

189

nervous system malformations, congenital heart disease, mongolism, and microcephaly. In each case matched controls were tested along with the study sera. For the first analysis of the study population, both white and black patients were included.[3] Unfortunately, however, the screening for antibodies was done using lymphocytes from a white population only. We realized that this would tend to miss antigens more predominant among Negroes. For the present report we have analyzed the data for the white patients only.

METHODS

Clinical and laboratory data were available for 50,000 pregnant women who were under study from 1959 through 1966. These women were registered in the Collaborative Perinatal Project at twelve university hospitals throughout the United States. Detailed longitudinal pediatric data were available for their offspring. Most children are now seven years of age or older.

Patients who registered in the collaborating institutions were largely an urban group and the majority were semi-indigent. Approximately 20 percent of the patients registered during the first trimester.

Blood specimens were taken at the time of registration, at approximately two-month intervals during pregnancy, at delivery, and at six weeks postpartum. Sera from these samples were obtained under uniform conditions using Vacutainers®, frozen and sent to the National Institutes of Health. They were kept at −20° C until used.

For the present tests, the great majority of sera was obtained during the first or second trimester of the pregnancies. In almost every case two controls were used for each patient. The matching of controls included age of the mother (± 5 years), race, geographic location, last menstrual period (± 6 weeks), date of the specimen (± 6 weeks), and gravidity (70% identical match and all within one pregnancy for gravidities of one, two or three; matching within one or two pregnancies for gravidities of four to six; multiparity of ⩾ 7 matched with similar high multiparity).

Sera were tested for cytotoxic activity against lymphocytes from a minimum of forty patients according to the methods previously described.[6] A given serum was considered positive for cytotoxic activity when it killed all 1000 test cells from at least six individuals at dosages of 0.001 ml. A serum found positive for 5 to 15 percent of the random cells tested was considered to have "possible antibody."

RESULTS

Gravidity and Cytotoxic Antibodies

The development of increasing frequency of cytotoxic antibodies with increasing gravidity is shown in Table 10-I. This analysis includes all controls from studies of abortions, CNS malformations, mongoloid infants and congenital heart disease. There was a rapid increase from approximately 1 percent of the patients with antibody among women with one pregnancy to 24 to 33 percent with antibody when the gravidity was four or more. These findings are in general agreement with previous reports.[4, 5] The figures are somewhat higher for most age groups than were observed when analyzing data for both white and black patients for cytotoxic antibodies using lymphocytes from white patients.[3] This points out the importance of controlling for race and ethnic groups when testing for cytotoxic antibodies.

TABLE-10-I

GRAVIDITY AND CYTOTOXIC ANTIBODIES*

Gravidity	Total Number of Women	No Antibodies	Possible Antibodies	Antibodies	% with Antibodies
1	97	91	5	1	1.0
2	69	58	3	8	11.6
3	53	43	3	7	13.2
4	37	27	1	9	24.3
5	46	30	4	12	26.1
6	37	25	3	9	24.3
7	15	10	1	4	26.6
≥8	27	17	1	9	33.3
Totals	381	301	21	59	

* Analysis includes all controls from studies of abortions, CNS malformations, Mongoloid infants, and congenital heart disease.

Women with Abnormal Pregnancy Outcomes

The frequency of cytotoxic antibodies among women whose pregnancies resulted in any one of five general categories of abnormal outcomes and antibodies in their controls is given in Table 10-II. In no category was there evidence of a significant increase in the frequency of cytotoxic antibodies for the study group when compared to the controls for either the presence of antibodies or "possible antibodies." For the category CNS malformations there was a slightly greater percentage of mothers with abnormal outcomes with antibodies than for the controls. The numbers of patients however were small and this distribution was due to the subgroups of hydrocephaly and anencephaly.

The analysis of cytotoxic antibodies among mothers of children with specific types of congenital heart diseases and matched controls is given in Table 10-III. Here again there was no evidence of a significant increase in cytotoxic antibodies for any of these specific groups of defects. However, in almost all groups the number of patients was too small to be analyzed satisfactorily.

TABLE-10-II

FREQUENCY OF HL-A CYTOTOXIC ANTIBODIES AMONG MOTHERS
WITH ABNORMAL PREGNANCY OUTCOMES AND
MATCHED CONTROLS

	Total Women in Group	No Antibodies	Possible Antibodies	Antibodies	% with Antibodies
Abortion	28	24	0	4	14.3
controls	56	48	1	7	12.5
CNS Malformations					
Hydrocephaly	9	8	0	1	11.1
controls	18	10	7	1	5.6
Anencephaly	17	12	3	2	11.7
controls	33	29	1	3	9.1
Misc. CNS	3	3	0	0	0.0
controls	6	4	2	0	0.0
Total CNS	29	23	3	3	10.3
controls	57	43	10	4	7.0
Monogoloid infants	28	25	2	1	3.6
controls	56	45	2	9	16.1
Congenital heart					
disease	43	32	1	10	23.3
controls	84	61	2	21	25.0
Microcephaly	12	11	0	1	8.5
controls	24	16	1	7	29.2

TABLE 10-III

CYTOTOXIC ANTIBODIES AMONG MOTHERS OF CHILDREN WITH
SPECIFIC TYPES OF CONGENITAL HEART DISEASE
AND MATCHED CONTROLS

	Total Women in Group	No Antibodies	Possible Antibodies	Antibodies	% with Antibodies
Ventricular septal					
defect	7	6	0	1	14.3
controls	14	12	0	2	14.3
Pulmonic stenosis	3	2	0	1	33.3
controls	6	5	0	1	16.7
Endocardial cushion					
defect	4	2	0	2	50.0
controls	8	4	0	4	50.0
Endocardial					
fibroelastosis	2	1	0	1	50.0
controls	4	4	0	0	0.0
Endomyocardial					
fibrosis	1	1	0	0	0.0
controls	2	1	1	0	0.0
Atrial septal					
defect primum	1	1	0	0	0.0
controls	2	0	0	2	100.0
Atrial septal					
defect secundum	1	1	0	0	0.0
controls	2	0	0	2	100.0
Truncus	1	1	0	0	0.0
controls	2	0	0	2	100.0
Preductal coarctation					
of the aorta	5	3	0	2	40.0
controls	9	7	0	2	22.2
postductal coarctation					
of the aorta	1	1	0	0	0.0
controls	2	0	0	2	100.0
Preductal coarctation					
plus septal defect	3	2	1	0	0.0
controls	6	6	0	0	0.0
Tricuspid atresia	1	1	0	0	0.0
controls	2	2	0	0	0.0
Pulmonary atresia	1	1	0	0	0.0
controls	2	1	0	1	50.0
Transposition of					
the great vessels	3	3	0	0	0.0
controls	6	6	0	0	0.0
Complex transposition					
of the great vessel	1	1	0	0	0.0
controls	2	2	0	0	0.0
Vascular ring	2	2	0	0	0.0
controls	3	1	0	2	66.7
Abnormalities of the					
coronary arteries	1	0	0	1	100.0
controls	2	2	0	0	0.0
Misc. (only 1					
of a type	5	3	0	2	40.0
controls	10	8	1	1	10.0

DISCUSSION AND SUMMARY

In this study of cytotoxic antibodies in the sera of pregnant women we have confirmed the positive relationship between increasing gravidity and higher frequencies of HL-A antibodies. Since these antibodies are of the immunoglobulin G class and are known to cross the placenta, we are concerned that they may be responsible for fetal disease and damage. The present study failed to show any significant association with abortions, CNS malformations, mongoloid infants, congenital heart disease or microcephaly.

The lack of significant association between cytotoxic antibodies and abnormal pregnancy outcomes in this study should not be considered as excluding of the possible significance of these antibodies. Several factors may have contributed to these negative findings: First, the abnormal outcomes caused by these antibodies may be somewhat infrequent; the majority being due to other causes. Thus larger numbers of patients would have to be studied to detect these associations. Second, the abnormalities may be types not included in the present study. Investigations of many types of abnormalities will have to be conducted to analyze this problem in detail. Third, the abnormalities may represent a "syndrome" which is lost to detection when analysis is based on specific groupings of abnormal outcomes. In the future analysis of patients with antibodies we will have to consider not only individual outcomes but also outcome groups to detect associations of this type. Fourth, the development of increasing levels of cytotoxic antibodies during a pregnancy may be of greatest significance to that pregnancy outcome. Studies of paired sera taken early in pregnancy and during the postpartum period will be necessary for the investigation of this important possibility. Lastly, tests of other tissue antigens should be included along with HL-A before the question of fetal damage due to maternal-fetal incompatabilities can be considered to have been adequately explored.

PROSPECTS FOR THE FUTURE

The presence of cytotoxic antibodies against HL-A tissue antigens constitutes a tantalizing possible mechanism for the production of placental-fetal damage. In view of the conflicting data concerning the pathogenic activities of these antibodies, we have now initiated studies in four areas to explore this feto-maternal incompatability in greater detail. These studies include: 1) larger investigations involving the abnormal outcomes most likely to be associated with increasing development of anti-fetal antibodies. These outcomes include repeat abortions and/or repeat stillbirths as well as defects such as anencephaly and spina bifida which are known to be more frequent in women with several prior pregnancies. In addition, following Dr. Peter Gruenwald's suggestions we are including late developmental defects which are probably related to cell necrosis such as malformations of the eyes, limbs, gastrointestinal tract and cysts of the brain. 2) Analysis of multiple groups of abnormal outcomes for the possible presence of patterns of abnormalities or syndromes. 3) Studies of paired sera obtained early and late in pregnancy to detect antibody increases as well as particular cytotoxic HL-A antibody types and 4) studies of other tissue antigens for other cells in addition to lymphocytes.

Cytotoxic antibody to HL-A antigens in pregnant women is a potentially pathogenic process in search of a disease. With the approaches described we hope to be able to resolve the question of the possible teratogenic or other damaging effects of these antibodies.

REFERENCES

1. Brent, R. L.: The production of congenital malformations using tissue antisera. *Am J Anat, 119*:555-562, 1966.
2. Hitzig, W. H., and Gitzelmann: Transplacental transfer of leukocyte agglutinins. *Vox Sang, 4*:445-455, 1959.
3. Sever, J. L., and Terasaki, P. I.: Maternal-fetal incompatability III, Central nervous system and cardiac anomalies. *Histocompatability Testing* 1970, Copenhagen, Pub. Munksgaard, 1970, pp. 495-500.

4. Terasaki, P. I., and McClelland, J. D.: Microdroplet assay of human serum cytotoxins. *Nature* (Lond.), *204*:998-100, 1964.
5. Terasaki, P. I.; Mickey, M. R.; Ymazaki, J. N., and Vredevoc, D. L.: Maternal-fetal incompatability I. Incidence of HL-A antibodies and possible association with congenital anomalies. *Transplantatum,* 9:538-543, 1970.
6. Terasaki, P. I., and Singal, D. P.: Human histocompatability antigens of leukocytes. XXVI. *Ann Rev Med,* 2:175-193, 1969.
7. vanRood, J. J.; vanLeevwen, A., and Eernisse, J. G.: Leucocyte antibodies in sera of pregnant women. *Vox Sang,* 4:427-444, 1959.

Chapter 11

INTRAUTERINE DETECTION OF BIOCHEMICAL DISORDERS

H. L. NADLER

INTRODUCTION

PRENATAL STUDIES OF fetal diseases and malformations have been attempted, to a limited extent, since earliest times. It has only been in recent years that systematic studies utilizing a variety of techniques have been developed. Among the many recently proposed methods of investigation, including direct visualization of the fetus, maternal blood and urine analysis, and fetal tissue sampling, the most fruitful approach has been the analysis of amniotic fluid and its components. For many years, amniocentesis was used exclusively for the prenatal detection of erythroblastosis fetalis. With the development of reliable diagnostic methods, the detection of Down's syndrome and other chromosomal abnormalities as well as the determination of fetal sex in pregnancies at risk for severe X-linked recessive disorders have become a reality. Most recently, it has become clear that these techniques can be applied to the prenatal diagnosis of a number of inborn errors of metabolism (Table 11-I).

Amniotic fluid obtained during pregnancy by amniocentesis offers three possible sources for diagnostic analysis: amniotic fluid, amniotic fluid cells, and cultivated amniotic fluid cells. The first of these is the amniotic fluid itself, separated from the suspended cells by centrifugation. Among the components of the amniotic fluid that have been utilized in prenatal diagnosis are

TABLE 11-I

INBORN ERRORS OF METABOLISM DETECTABLE *IN UTERO**

Disease	Method of Detection	Reference
Lipid Metabolism Disorders		
GM₁ Gangliosidosis, Type 1	β-galactosidase deficiency	1, 2
GM₁ Gangliosidosis, Type 2	β-galactosidase deficiency	3
GM₂ Gangliosidosis, Type 1 (Tay-Sachs Disease)	Hexosaminidase A deficiency	4-7
GM₂ Gangliosidosis, Type 2 (Sandhoff's Disease)	Hexosaminidase A & B deficiency Ultrastructural examination	8, 9
GM₂ Gangliosidosis, Type 3	Hexosaminidase A deficiency	10
Fabry's Disease	α-galactosidase deficiency	8, 11
	Ceramide trihexoside accumulation	11
Gaucher's Disease	β-glucosidase deficiency	12
Krabbe's Disease	Galactocerebroside β-galactosidase deficiency	13
Lactosyl ceramidase deficiency	Lactosyl Ceramidosis**	
Metachromatic Leukodystrophy	Aryl sulfatase A deficiency	14
Niemann-Pick Disease	Sphingomyelinase deficiency	15
Refsum's Disease**	Phytanic acid ovidase deficiency	16
Carbohydrate Metabolism Disorders		
Glycogen Storage Diseases:		
Type 2: (Pompe's Disease)	α-1, 4-glucosidase deficiency	17-19
	Ultrastructural findings of abnormal lysosomes	20
Type 3: (Debrancher Deficiency)**	Amylo-1, 6-glucosidase deficiency	
Type 4: (Brancher Deficiency)**	Brancher enzyme deficiency	21
Galactosemia	Galactose-1-phosphate uridyl transferase deficiency	22
Fucosidosis**	α-fucosidase deficiency	23
Mucopolysaccharide Metabolism Disorders		
Mucopolysaccharidoses:	Metachromasia (not reliable alone)	24
	Accumulation of mucopolysaccharides in amniotic fluid (not reliable alone)	25, 26
	Serial assay of mucopolysaccharides in amniotic fluid	27
	³⁵SO₄ uptake	28, 29
Type 1: Hurler Syndrome	Mixing experiments**	30
	α-L-iduronidase deficiency**	31, 32
Type 2: Hunter Syndrome	Mixing experiments**	30
	Iduronic acid sulfatase deficiency**	33
Type 3A: Sanfilippo A Syndrome	Sulfamidase deficiency**	34
Type 3B: Sanfilippo B Syndrome	α-acetylglucosaminidase deficiency	35, 36
Type 5: Scheie Syndrome	α-L-iduronidase deficiency**	32
Type 7:	β-glucuronidase deficiency**	37
Amino Acid Metabolism Disorders		
Argininosuccinic Aciduria	Argininosuccinase deficiency Argininosuccinic acid accumulation	38
Citrullinemia	Ureido-¹⁴C-citrulline incorporation	39
Cystathionuria	Amino acid composition of amniotic fluid	40

Disease	Method of Detection	Reference
Cystinosis	Cystine accumulation	41
	Radioactive cystine accumulation	42
Cystinuria**	Amino acid composition of amniotic fluid	43
Hartnup's Disease**	Amino acid composition of amniotic fluid	43
Histidinemia**	Histidase deficiency	44
Homocystinuria	Cystathionine synthase deficiency in amniotic fluid fibroblasts	23, 45
Hyperammonemia, Type 2	Ornithine transcarbamylase deficiency	16
Hypervalinemia**	Valine transaminase deficiency	46
Maple Syrup Urine Disease	Branched chain ketoacid decarboxylase deficiency	47
Methylmalonic Acidemia	Methylmalonate accumulation	48
	Methylmalonyl CoA isomerase or mutase deficiency	49, 50
Methylmalonic Aciduria	Methylmalonyl CoA isomerase deficiency	49
	Elevated maternal urinary excretion of methylmalonic acid	48
Ornithine α-Ketoacid Transaminase Deficiency	Ornithine α-ketoacid transaminase deficiency	51
Phenylketonuria**	Maternal excretion of phenylalanine Loading tests	
Propionic Acidemia	Propionyl CoA carboxylase deficiency	52

Miscellaneous Disorders

Disease	Method of Detection	Reference
Adrenogenital Syndrome	Elevated 17-ketosteroids and pregnanetriol levels in amniotic fluid	53-55
	Elevated maternal urinary excretion of estriol	56, 57
Combined Immunodeficiency Disease**	Adenosine deaminase deficiency	58
Congenital Erythropoietic Porphyria**	Uroporphyrinogen III cosynthetase deficiency	
Congenital Hypothyroidism**	Decreased PBI or T₄ in amniotic fluid	
Cystic Fibrosis**	"ciliary inhibitory factor"	59
Hemoglobinopathies**	Fetal blood sampling	60
I-Cell Disease	Decreased lysosomal hydrolases in amniotic fluid cells	61
	Elevated hydrolases in amniotic fluid	
Lesch-Nyhan Syndrome	HGPRT deficiency Autoradiography	62-64
Lysosomal Acid Phosphatase Deficiency	Acid phosphatase deficiency	65
Neonatal Grave's Disease	Elevated PBI in amniotic fluid	66
Sickle Cell Anemia and Thalassemia**	Globin chain synthesis in mixed placental blood	67
Xeroderma Pigmentosum**	5-Bromodeoxyuridine uptake	

* Detected in cultivated amniotic fluid cells unless specified otherwise.
** Detection has been postulated.

enzymes, amino acids, hormones, and abnormal metabolic products. Although a number of metabolic disorders have been diagnosed on the basis of a deficiency of enzyme activity in the cell-free amniotic fluid, the origin of these enzymes is, at present, largely unknown. It is obvious that further studies of the origin and characteristics of the enzymes present will be essential if analysis of the amniotic fluid is to be of value in the prenatal diagnosis of the inborn errors of metabolism. Recent studies indicate that at least some of the enzymes present in the fluid originate in the amnion and thus are fetal in origin.[68] Other authors have suggested that certain enzymes may originate in the decidua and enter the amniotic fluid by diffusion through the amniotic membrane.[69] An alternative route by which enzymes may reach the amniotic fluid is by way of the fetal urine. There is some indication that the a-glucosidase present in the amniotic fluid may enter by this mechanism.[70]

Current data indicate that high-speed centrifugation and fractionation of the amniotic fluid may be of some value in determining the origin of enzymes in the amniotic fluid.[71] After the initial centrifugation, the fluid still contains some cells, cell fragments, and organelles. It has been demonstrated that individual enzymes may be present in specific fractions of the amniotic fluid and that this may be determined by their degree of binding to lysosomes, mitochondria, and other membranous structures. It is likely that the presence of the organelles is the result of lysis of intact amniotic fluid cells, and thus the enzymes present in the amniotic fluid may actually represent enzymes that have been released from amniotic fluid cells.

Tay-Sachs disease[4, 5] and Pompe's disease[17] have been diagnosed on the basis of a deficiency of enzyme activity in the amniotic fluid. It has since been established, however, that the determination of a-1, 4-glucosidase activity in the amniotic fluid is not reliable in the prenatal diagnosis of Pompe's disease.[18, 70] In general, enzyme activity in the amniotic fluid should not be used as the sole criterion for the intrauterine diagnosis of an inborn error of metabolism. Further knowledge of the nature and origin of the enzymes present and further experience with the prenatal diagnosis of each disorder will be necessary to determine the reliability of enzyme assays of the cell-free amniotic fluid.

The amino acid composition of normal amniotic fluid has recently been quantitated from the ninth week of gestation to term.[43, 72] This information may prove to be of great value in the intrauterine diagnosis of a number of disorders of amino acid transport or metabolism characterized by excess urinary excretion of various amino acids. Indeed, the analysis of the amino acid composition of the amniotic fluid has been used in the evaluation of pregnancies at risk for a number of these disorders (Table 11-I).

Recently, quantitative amino acid analysis of amniotic fluid has been carried out at various stages of gestation in thirty-three cases of central nervous system malformations.[73] In a large number of these cases, abnormal elevations of many amino acids, particularly the neutral amino acids, were observed. In most instances, the amniotic fluid for thees studies was obtained during the third trimester of pregnancy although fluid samples with abnormal amino acid profiles were obtained from a case of spina bifida at twelve weeks' gestation and from a case of anencephaly at twenty weeks' gestation. There is, as yet, no explanation for these findings since the amino acid composition of fetal cerebrospinal fluid is not grossly different from that of normal amniotic fluid.[73]

Large numbers of steroid and non-steroid hormones have been detected in the amniotic fluid, and the presence of a number of these may be relevant to the intrauterine diagnosis of certain genetic disorders. Determination of 17-ketosteroid and pregnanetriol levels in the amniotic fluid have been used in the third trimester of pregnancy in the intrauterine diagnosis of the adrenogenital syndrome.[53, 55] This approach has been shown to be unreliable, however, during the mid-trimester of pregnancy.[74] Normal levels of PBI and thyroxine in the amniotic fluid have recently been established[66, 75] and, in one instance, elevated PBI was detected in the amniotic fluid of an infant who subsequently developed neonatal Graves' disease.[66] It is conceivable that congenital hypothyroidism secondary either to an enzymatic defect in thyroxine synthesis or to the absence of the thyroid gland might be reflected in decreased levels of amniotic fluid PBI or T_4.

A number of normal and abnormal metabolic products detectable in the amniotic fluid have proven to be of value in the prenatal diagnosis of genetic disorders. Hurler's snydrome has been diagnoses *in utero* at fourteen and twenty weeks' gestation on the basis of elevated levels of mucopolysaccharides in the amniotic fluid.[25] In this same case, heparitin sulfate, a compound not found in normal amniotic fluid, was found to comprise 63 percent of the mucopolysaccharides in the abnormal sample. Another amniotic fluid sample obtained at twenty weeks' gestation from a pregnancy at risk for Hurler's syndrome contained only slightly elevated levels of total mucopolysaccharides but exhibited a markedly abnormal mucopolysaccharide profile with striking elevations of both heparitin sulfate and dermatan sulfate.[26] The fetus was found to be affected with the Hurler syndrome.

Methylmalonic aciduria has been diagnosed prenatally on the basis of the detection of methylmalonic acid in amniotic fluid obtained during the third trimester of pregnancy.[48] Normal amniotic fluid contains no detectable methylmalonic acid. Elevated levels of ceramide trihexoside, a substance excreted in large quantities in the urine of patients with Fabry's disease, have been detected in the amniotic fluid obtained during the mid-trimester of pregnancy from a fetus affected with this disorder.[8]

It has recently been suggested that the estimation of fetoprotein in amniotic fluid might be of value in the prenatal diagnosis of anencephaly and meningomyelocele during the second trimester of pregnancy.[76] Numerous reports have demonstrated the potential usefulness of determining α-fetoprotein levels in amniotic fluid. A number of cases of anencephaly have been detected on the basis of increased levels of α-fetoprotein in amniotic fluid. More recently, Brock, *et al.*[77] have detected anencephaly on the basis of increased α-fetoprotein in maternal serum at sixteen and twenty-one weeks of pregnancy. This approach is extremely promising; however, confirmation of reliability is required before it can be recommended for routine use.

It has also been demonstrated that an absorption peak at 450 mμ, once thought to be a specific finding in Rh-immunized pregnancies, may be present in the amniotic fluid of at least some infants with anencephaly.[78, 79] Although this may be a valid finding in late pregnancy, it is unlikely that spectrophotometric analysis of amniotic fluid would be of value in the mid-trimester prenatal diagnosis of this disorder.

A second source of material for diagnostic analysis, derived from the amniotic fluid, is the uncultivated amniotic fluid cells. Amniotic fluid cells have been shown to originate primarily from the amnion or from desquamation of the fetal skin, buccal mucosa, vaginal epithelium, umbilical cord, and fetal urine. These cells have been used in a number of cases in the prenatal diagnosis of genetic disorders. Perhaps their greatest use to date has been in the detection of male fetuses at risk for sex-linked disorders by sex chromatin analysis and Y-chromosome fluorescence. The uncultivated cells have also been used for biochemical studies in a number of metabolic disorders, but their reliability for this purpose is questionable. It has been demonstrated that a large percentage of these cells are nonviable and have essentially no enzymatic activity,[80] thus making biochemical analyses impossible or uninterpretable. In addition, maternal white blood cells may contaminate the sample of uncultivated cells and lead to erroneous results. Pompe's disease[17] and Tay-Sachs disease[4] have been diagnosed *in utero* on the basis of an enzyme deficiency in the uncultivated amniotic fluid cells. Hexosaminidase A has been shown to be unstable in uncultivated amniotic fluid cells, however, so that this may not be a reliable method for the prenatal diagnosis of Tay-Sachs disease.[6] Certainly the biochemical analysis of the uncultivated amniotic fluid cells should not, at this point, be the sole determinant for the prenatal diagnosis of an inborn error of metabolism.

Histochemical and ultrastructural studies of the uncultivated amniotic fluid cells have been of some value in the prenatal diagnosis of certain genetic disorders. Abnormal lysosomes, characteristic of Pompe's disease, have been detected in uncultivated amniotic fluid cells and have been used as a clue to the prenatal diagnosis of this disorder.[18, 20] Histochemical techniques might conceivably be used to determine the presence of abnormal components or the accumulation of normal components in the uncultivated amniotic fluid cells. The viability of the cells used, however, is again an important consideration in the interpretation of the results of such studies.

Cultivated amniotic fluid cells represent the third and most significant source of material for analysis in the prenatal diagnosis of genetic disorders. The techniques of cell cultivation have been described in great detail elsewhere.[81-87] The cultivated cells have been used extensively for cytogenetic studies in the prenatal diagnosis of chromosome abnormalities. Amniotic fluid cell karyotyping is also utilized for fetal sex determination in sex-linked disorders, either alone or in combination with sex-chromatin analysis and/or Y-chromosome fluorescence of the uncultivated cells.

The cultivated amniotic fluid cells recently have been used a great deal in the study of the inborn errors of metabolism characterized by a known enzyme deficiency, or by some other specific biochemical abnormality. With cultivation, a number of factors are introduced that may alter the biochemical properties of the cells. These include the type of growth medium used, the length of cultivation, the degree of confluency of cultures, and a number of other parameters.[88] It is essential in the study of these cells that the effect of such factors be recognized and that conditions be standardized before any reliable diagnoses can be made on the basis of biochemical analyses.

To be of value in the prenatal diagnosis of metabolic disorders, it is essential that normal levels of enzyme activity be established in cultivated amniotic fluid cells obtained at specific stages of gestation. It has been demonstrated that there are significant changes in the levels of glucose-6-phosphate dehydrogenase activity in amniotic fluid cells obtained between the tenth and sixteenth weeks of gestation, as well as qualitative changes in the glucose-6-phosphate dehydrogenase and lactate dehydrogenase detectable.[86] In addition, aryl sulfatase A and β-galactosidase activities have been shown to increase with increasing gestational age.[89]

Although most enzymes present in cultivated skin fibroblasts are also found to be present in cultivated amniotic fluid cells, the levels of activity obtained from skin fibroblasts cannot be used as an index of normal activity in amniotic fluid cells. A number of enzymes, including cystathionine synthase[45] and β-galactosidase,[89] are present in higher levels in skin fibroblasts than in amniotic fluid cells. Other enzymes, including argininosuccinase,[90] ornithine ketoacid transaminase,[51] and aryl sulfatase A[89] exhibit substantially lower levels of activity in the cultivated amniotic fluid cells.

There is an additional factor that must be considered in the study of enzymes in cultivated amniotic fluid cells. For some time, it has been observed that amniotic fluid cells in short-term tissue culture may segregate into two distinct populations based on morphological criteria, epithelial-like cells and fibroblasts. In the past, enzyme studies have been performed on mixed cell populations without regard to the ratio of the two cell types present. Recently, however, it has been demonstrated that there are basic biochemical, as well as morphological, differences between the two cell types.[91] It has been shown that the enzyme histidase is absent in amniotic fluid fibroblasts from normal controls but present in high levels in epithelial cells from the same amniotic fluid samples.[44] Mixed-cell cultures exhibit intermediate levels of activity. This enzyme had been demonstrated previously in epidermal outgrowths of human skin explants in culture, whereas it could not be detected in fibroblasts derived from the original explants.[92] These data seem to indicate that some cells in culture retain tissue-specific properties. Recently, similar discrepancies in activity between the epithelial and fibroblast-like cells of amniotic fluid have been demonstrated for the enzyme cystathionine synthase.[23] In this case, however, the activity of the enzyme was significantly higher in fibroblasts than in the epithelial cells. Certain enzymes, including hexosaminidase, β-galactosidase, and aryl sulfatase exhibit no differences in activity in cultures that are predominantly epithelial, fibroblast-like or mixed.[93] It is clear from these data that the normal biochemical properties of cultivated amniotic fluid cells must be studied differentially in the individual cell types.

Despite the delay and technical difficulty involved in cell

cultivation, cultivated amniotic fluid cells have been the most reliable index for prenatal diagnosis of both chromosomal and biochemical disorders. The techniques of chromosome analysis, enzyme analysis, histochemistry, autoradiography, electron microscopy and electrophoresis have all been applied to these cells in the *in utero* diagnosis of various disorders. In the future, new and improved techniques will undoubtedly lead to more effective analysis of the cultivated cells.

CONCLUSION

Genetic counseling has rapidly changed from a simple presentation of Mendelian probability to the identification of high risk marriages and *in utero* diagnosis of specific genetic defects, both chromosomal and biochemical.

Techniques for more rapid, safe, and accurate intrauterine diagnosis of an increasing number of genetic defects are being integrated into the practice of medicine almost as fast as they are being developed. Continued carefully controlled studies of the precise risks to the mother and fetus are essential. Centralization of facilities and the formation of a central registry will prove to be of great value in identifying patients at risk, eliminating duplication of services particularly for rare disorders, and evaluating present and future techniques.

This chapter briefly presents the current state of knowledge of prenatal detection of genetic disorders, specifically as pertains to familial metabolic disorders. These techniques provide some parents with methods for having children without fear of producing a child with a specific deformity. In addition, the development of approaches which will increase the number of disorders detectable *in utero,* is essential if intrauterine treatment of genetic disorders becomes a reality.

REFERENCES

1. Lowden, J. A.; Cutz, E.; Conen, P. E.; Rudd, N., and Doran, T .A.: Prenatal diagnosis of GM$_1$ gangliosidosis. *N Engl J Med, 288*:225, 1973.
2. Kaback, M. M.; Sloan, H. R.; Sonneborn, M.; Herndon, R. M., and

Percy, A. K.: GM$_1$ gangliosidosis, type I: *in utero* detection and fetal manifestations. *J Pediatr, 82*:1037, 1973.

3. Booth, C. W.; Gerbie, A. B., and Nadler, H. L.: Intrauterine detection of GM$_1$ gangliosidosis, type 2. *Pediatrics, 52*:521, 1973.

4. Schneck, L.; Friedland, J.; Valenti, C.; Adachi, M.; Amsterdam, D., and Volk, B. W.: Prenatal diagnosis of Tay-Sachs disease. *Lancet, I*:582, 1970.

5. Friedland, J.; Perle, G.; Saifer, A.; Schneck, L., and Volk, B. W.: Screening for Tay-Sachs disease *in utero* using amniotic fluid. *Proc Soc Exp Biol Med, 136*:1297, 1971.

6. Rattazzi, M. C., and Davidson, R. G.: Prenatal detection of Tay-Sachs disease. In Dorfman, A. (Ed.): *Antenatal Diagnosis*. Chicago, U of Chicago Pr, 1971, p. 207.

7. O'Brien, J. S.; Okada, S.; Fillerup, D. L.; Veath, M. L.; Adornato, B.; Brenner, P. H., and Leroy, J. G.: Tay-Sachs disease: prenatal diagnosis. *Science, 172*:61, 1971.

8. Desnick, R. J.; Raman, M. K.; Bendel, R. P.; Kersey, J.; Lee. J. C.; Krivit, W., and Sharp, H. L.: Prenatal diagnosis of glycosphingo-lipidoses: Sandhoff's and Fabry's diseases. Presented at the Midwest Society for Pediatric Research, Chicago, Illinois, November 1-2, 1972.

9. Okada, S.; Veath, M. L.; Leroy, J., and O'Brien, J. S.: Ganglioside GM$_2$ storage disease: hexosaminidase deficiencies in cultured fibroblasts. *Am J Hum Genet, 23*:55, 1971.

10. O'Brien, J. S.: Ganglioside storage diseases. *N Engl J Med, 284*:893, 1971.

11. Brady, R. O.; Uhlendorf, B. W., and Jacobson, C. B.: Fabry's disease: antenatal detection. *Science, 172*:174, 1971.

12. Nadler, H. L.: Unpublished data.

13. Suzuki, K.; Schneider, E. L., and Epstein, C. J.: *In utero* diagnosis of globoid cell leukodystrophy (Krabbe's disease). *Biochem Biophys Res Commun, 45*:1363, 1971.

14. Nadler, H. L., and Gerbie, A. B.: Role of amniocentesis in the intrauterine detection of genetic disorders. *N Engl J Med, 282*:596, 1970.

15. Epstein, C. J.; Brady, R. O.; Schneider,, E. L.; Bradley, R. M., and Shapiro, D.: *In utero* diagnosis of Niemann-Pick disease. *Am J Hum Genet, 23*:533, 1971.

16. Nadler, H. L., and Gerbie, A. B.: Enzymes in non-cultured amniotic fluid cells. *Am J Obstet Gynecol, 103*:710, 1969.

17. Nadler, H. L., and Messina, A.: *In utero* detection of Type II glycogenosis (Pompe's disease). *Lancet, II*:1277, 1969.

18. Nadler, H. L., Bigley, R. H., and Hug, G.:' Prenatal detection of Pompe's disease. *Lancet, II*:369, 1970.

19. Cox, R. P.; Douglas, G.; Hutzler, J.; Lynfield, J., and Dancis, J.: *In utero* detection of Pompe's disease. *Lancet, II*:893, 1970.
20. Hug, G.; Schubert, W. K., and Soukup. S.: Prenatal diagnosis of Type II glycogenosis. *Lancet, I*:1002, 1970.
21. Howell, R. R.; Kaback, M. M., and Brown, B. I.: Type IV glycogen storage disease: branching enzyme deficiency in skin fibroblasts and possible heterozygote detection. Presented at the annual meeting of the American Pediatric Society and Society for Pediatric Research, Atlantic City, April 29-May 2, 1970.
22. Nadler, H. L.: Antenatal detection of hereditary disorders. *Pediatrics, 42*:912, 1968.
23. Melancon, S. B., and Nadler. H. L.: Unpublished data.
24. Danes, B. S., and Bearn, A. G.: Hurler's syndrome: demonstration of an inherited disorder of connective tissue in cell culture. *Science, 149*:987, 1965.
25. Matalon, R.; Dorfman, A.; Nadler, H. L., and Jacobson, C. B.: A chemical method for the antenatal diagnosis of mucopolysaccharides. *Lancet, I*:83, 1970.
26. Omura, K.; Higami, S.; Issiki, G.; Nishizawa, K., and Tada, K.: Prenatal diagnosis of the Hurler syndrome: mucoploysaccharide pattern in amniotic fluid. Submitted for publication.
27. Danes, B. S.; Queenan, J. T.; Gadow, E. C., and Cederquist, L. L.: Antenatal diagnosis of mucopolysaccharidosis. *Lancet, I*:946, 1970.
28. Fratantoni, J. C.; Hall, C. W., and Neufeld, E. F.: The defect in Hurler's and Hunter's syndrome: faulty degradation of mucopolysaccharide. *Proc Natl Acad Sci, 60*:699, 1968.
29. Fratantoni, J. C.; Neufeld, E. F.; Uhlendorf, B. W., and Jacobson, C. B.: Intrauterine diagnosis of the Hurler and Hunter syndromes. *N Engl J Med, 280*:686, 1969.
30. Fratantoni, J. C.; Hall, C. W., and Neufeld, E. F.: Hurler and Hunter syndromes: mutual correction of the defect in cultured fibroblasts. *Science, 162*:570, 1968.
31. Matalon, R., and Dorfman, A.: Hurler's syndrome, an α-L-iduronidase deficiency. *Biochem Biophys Res Commun, 47*:959, 1972.
32. Bach, G.; Friedman, R.; Weissman, B., and Neufeld, E. F.: The defect in the Hurler and Scheie syndromes: deficiency of α-L-iduronidase. *Proc Natl Acad Sci, 69*:2048, 1972.
33. Bach, G.; Cantz, M.; Okada, S., and Neufeld, E. F.: Enzymatic defect in the Hunter syndrome (mucopolysaccharidosis III). *Fed Proc, 32*:483/1471, 1973.
34. Matalon, R., and Dorfman, A.: The Sanfilippo A syndrome: a sulfamidase deficiency. *Pediatr Res, 7*:384/156, 1973.
35. O'Brien, J. S.: Sanfilippo syndrome: profound deficiency of alpha-

acetylglucosaminidase activity in organs and skin fibroblasts from Type B patients. *Proc Natl Acad Sci,* 69:1720, 1972.

36. von Figura, K., and Kresse, H.: The Sanfilippo B corrective factor: a N-acetyl-α-D-glucosaminidase. *Biochem Biophys Res Commun,* 48:262, 1972.

37. Sly, W. S.; Quinton, B. A.; McAlister, W. H., and Rimoin, D. L.: Beta-glucuronidase deficiency: report of clinical, radiologic, and biochemical features of a new mucopolysaccharidosis. *J Pediatr,* 82:249, 1973.

38. Goodman, S. I.; Mace, J. W.; Turner, B., and Garrett, W. J.: Antenatal diagnosis of argininosuccinic aciduria. *Clin Res,* XXI:295, 1973.

39. Roerdink, F. H.; Gouw. W. L. M.; Okken, A.; van der Blij, J. F.; Luit-de Haan, G., and Hommes, F. A.: Citrullinemia, report of a case, with studies on antenatal diagnosis. *Pediatr Res,* 7:863, 1973.

40. Frimpter, G. W.; Greenberg, A. J.; Hilgartner, M., and Fuchs, F.: Cystathionuria: management. *Am J Dis Child,* 113:115, 1967.

41. Schulman, J. D.; Fujimoto, W. Y.; Bradley, K. H., and Seegmiller, J. E.: Identification of heterozygous genotype for cystinosis *in utero* by a new pulse-labeling technique: preliminary report. *J Pediatr,* 77:468, 1970.

42. Schneider, J. A.; Verroust, F. M.; Garvin, A. J.; Horger, III, E. O., and Jacobson, C.: The prenatal diagnosis of cystinosis. *Pediatr Res,* 7:291/63, 1973.

43. Emery, A. E. H.; Burt, D.; Scrimgeour, J. B., and Nelson, M. M.: Antenatal diagnosis and amino acid composition of amniotic fluid. *Lancet, I*:307, 1970.

44. Melancon, S.; Lee, S., and Nadler, H. L.: Histidase activity in cultivated human amniotic fluid cells. *Science,* 173:627, 1971.

45. Uhlendorf, B. W., and Mudd, S. H.: Cystathionine synthase in tissue culture derived from human skin: enzyme defect in homocystinuria. *Science,* 160:1007, 1968.

46. Dancis, J.: Personal communication.

47. Dancis, J.: Maple syrup urine disease. In Dorfman, A. (Ed.): Chicago, U of Chicago Pr, 1972, p. 123.

48. Morrow, G., III; Schwarz, R. H.; Hallock, J. A., and Barness, L. A.: Prenatal detection of methylmalonic acidemia. *J Pediatr,* 77:120, 1970.

49. Mahoney, M.; Hsia, Y. E., and Rosenberg. L.: Abnormalities of vitamin B$_{12}$ metabolism. In Dorfman, A. (Ed.): *Antenatal Diagnosis.* Chicago, U of Chicago Pr, 1972, p. 95.

50. Mahoney, M.; Rosenberg, L. E.; Waldenstrom, J.; Lindblad, B., and Zetterstrom, R.: Prenatal diagnosis of methylmalonic aciduria. *Pediatr Res,* 7:342/114, 1973.

51. Shih, V. E., and Schulman, J. D.: Ornithine-ketoacid transaminase activity in human skin and amniotic fluid cell culture. *Clin Chim Acta, 27*:73, 1970.
52. Gompertz, D.; Goodey, P. A.; Thom, H.; Russell, G.; MacLean, M. W.; Ferguson-Smith, M. E., and Ferguson-Smith, M. A.: Antenatal diagnosis of propionic acidaemia. *Lancet, I*:1009, 1973.
53. Jeffcoate, T. N. A.; Fliegner, J. R. H.; Russell, S. H.; Davis, J. C., and Wade, A. P.: Diagnosis of the adrenogenital syndrome before birth. *Lancet, II*:553, 1965.
54. Fuchs, F.: Discussion of paper by Jacobson and Barter. *Am J Obstet Gynecol, 99*:806, 1967.
55. Nichols, J.: Antenatal diagnosis and treatment of the adrenogenital syndrome. *Lancet, I*:83, 1970.
56. Cathro, D. M.; Bertrand, J., and Coyle, M. G.: Antenatal diagnosis of adrenogenital hyperplasia. *Lancet, I*:732, 1969.
57. Nichols, J., and Gibson, G. G.: Antenatal diagnosis of the adreno-genital syndrome. *Lancet. II*:1068, 1967.
58. Chen, S-H., and Scott, C. R.: Adenosine deaminase in cultured skin fibroblasts and amniotic fluid cells: potential use for prenatal diagnosis of combined immunodeficiency disease. *Am Soc Hum Genet.* 25th Anniversary Meeting—Program and Abstracts, 1973, p. 21a.
59. Conover, J. H.; Beratis, N. G.; Conod, E. J.; Hathaway, P., and Hirsch-horn, K.: Ciliary dyskinesia factor produced in tissue culture from cystic fibrosis. *Clin Res, XXI*:531, 1973.
60. Valenti, C.: Antenatal detection of hemoglobinopathies. *Am J Obstet Gynecol, 115*:851, 1973.
61. Warren, R. J.; Condron, C. J.; Hollister, D.; Huijing, F.; Neufeld, E. F.; Hall, C. W.; McLeod, A. G. W., and Lorincz, A. E.: Antenatal diagnosis of mucolipidosis II (I-cell disease). *Pediatr Res, 7*:343-115, 1973.
62. Fujimoto, W. Y.; Seegmiller, J. E.; Uhlendorf, B. W., and Jacobson, C. B.: Biochemical diagnosis of an X-linked disease. *in utero. Lancet, II*:511, 1968.
63. DeMars, R.; Sarto, G.; Felix, J. S., and Benke, P.: Lesch-Nyhan mutation: prenatal detection with amniotic fluid cells. *Science, 164*:1303, 1969.
64. Boyle, J. A.; Raivio, K. O.; Astrin, K. H.; Schulman, J. D.; Seegmiller, J. E.; Graf, M. L., and Jacobson. C. B.: Lesch-Nyhan syndrome: preventive control by prenatal diagnosis. *Science, 169*:688, 1970.
65. Nadler, H. L., and Egan, T. J.: Deficiency of lysosomal acid phos-phatase: a new familial metabolic disorder. *N Engl J Med, 282*:302, 1970.

66. Hollingsworth, D. R., and Austin, E.: Thyroxine derivatives in amniotic fluid. *J Pediatr, 79*:923, 1971.

67. Kan, Y. W.; Dozy, A. M.; Alter, B. P.; Frigoletto, F. D., and Nathan, D. G.: Detection of the sickle gene in the human fetus. *N Engl J Med, 287*:1, 1972.

68. Geyer, V. H.: Die herkunft der fruchtwasser-enzyme. *Z Klin Chem, 8*:145, 1970.

69. Tornqvist, A.; Jonassen, F.; Johnson, P., and Fredholm, A. M.: Studies on diamine oxidase activity during pregnancy.*Acta Obstet Gynecol Scand, 50*:79, 1971.

70. Salafsky. I., and Nadler, H. L.: α-1,4-glucosidase activity in Pompe's disease. *J Pediatr, 79*:794, 1971.

71. Salafsky, I. S., and Nadler, H. L.: Intracellular organelles and enzymes in cell-free amniotic fluid. *Am J Obstet Gynecol, 111*:1046, 1971.

72. Scott, C. R.; Teng, C. C.; Sagerson, R. N., and Nelson, T.: Amino acids in amniotic fluid: changes in concentrations during the first half of pregnancy. *Pediatr Res, 6*:659, 1972.

73. Emery, A. E. H., and Burt, D.: Amino acid composition of amniotic fluid in central nervous system malformations. *Lancet, 1*:970, 1973.

74. Merkatz, I. R.; New, M. I.; Peterson, R. E., and Seaman, M. P.: Prenatal diagnosis of adrenogenital syndrome by aminocentesis. *J Pediatr, 75*:977, 1969.

75. Kaufman, S.: Protein-bound iodine (PBI) in human amniotic fluid. *J Pediatr, 68*:990, 1966.

76. Brock, D. J. H., and Sutcliffe, R. G.: Alpha-fetoprotein in the antenatal diagnosis of anencephaly and spina bifida. *Lancet, II*:197, 1972.

77. Brock, D. J. H.; Bolton, A. E., and Monoghan, J. M.: Prenatal diagnosis of anencephaly through maternal serum-alphafetoprotein measurement. *Lancet, II*:7835, 1973.

78. Lee, T. Y., and Wei, P. Y.: Spectrophotometric analysis of amniotic fluid in anencephalic pregnancies. *Am J Obstet Gynecol, 107*:917. 1970.

79. Cassady, G., and Caillitetau, J.: The amniotic fluid in anencephaly. *Am J Obstet Gynecol, 97*:395, 1967.

80. Nadler, H. L.: Prenatal detection of genetic defects. *J Pediatr, 74*:132, 1969.

81. Uhlendorf, B. W.; Jacobson, C. B.; Sloan, H. R.; Mudd, S. H.; Herndon, J. H.; Brady, R. O.; Seegmiller, J. E., and Fuqimoto, W.: Cell cultures derived from human amniotic fluid: their possible application in the intrauterine diagnosis of heritable metabolic disease. Nineteenth Annual Meeting of the Tissue Culture Association, Schedule and Abstracts. San Juan, Puerto Rico, 1968, *In Vitro*, p. 158.

82. Gregson, N. M.: A technique for culturing cells from amniotic fluid. *Lancet, I*:84, 1970.
83. Valenti, C., and Kehaty, T.: Culture of cells obtained by aminocentesis. *J Lab Clin Med, 73*:355, 1969.
84. Nelson, M. M., and Emery, A. E. H.: Amniotic fluid cells: prenatal sex prediction and culture. *Br Med J, 1*:523, 1970.
85. Nadler, H. L.; Gerbie, A. B.; Jacobson, C. B.; Valenti, C., and Macintyre, M. N.: Personal communication.
86. Nadler, H. L.: Patterns of enzyme development using cultivated human fetal cells from amniotic fluid. *Biochem Genet, 2*:119, 1968.
87. Nadler, H. L., and Ryan, C. A.: Amniotic cell culture. In Yunis, J. (Ed.): *Human Chromosome Methodology.* New York, Academic Press, Inc., in press.
88. Ryan, C. A.; Lee, S. Y., and Nadler, H. L.: Effect of culture conditions on enzyme activities in cultivated human fibroblasts. *Exp Cell Res, 71*:388, 1972.
89. Kaback, M. M.; Leonard, C. O., and Parmley, T. H.: Intrauterine diagnosis: comparative enzymology of cells cultivated from maternal skin, fetal skin, and amniotic fluid cells. *Pediatr, Res, 5*:366, 1971.
90. Shih, V. E., and Littlefield, J. W.: Arginosuccinase activity in amniotic fluid cells. *Lancet, II*:45, 1970.
91. Gerbie, A. B.; Nadler, H. L.; Melancon, S. B., and Ryan, C.: Cultivated epithelial-like cells and fibroblasts from amniotic fluid: their relationship to enzymatic and cytologic analysis. *Am J Obstet Gynecol, 114*:314, 1972.
92. Barnhisel, M. L.; Priest, R. E., and Priest, J. H.: Histidase activity in human epidermal cells. *J Cell Physiol, 76*:7, 1970.
93. Kaback, M. M., and Leonard, C.: Morphological and enzymological considerations in antenatal diagnosis. In Dorfman, A. (Ed.): *Antenatal Diagnosis.* Chicago, U of Chicago Pr, 1972, p. 81.

Chapter 12

INTRAUTERINE DETECTION OF FETAL MALNUTRITION*

J. Metcoff, M. Mameesh, Gail Jacobson,
P. Costiloe, and Warren Crosby

Background

WHETHER FETAL MALNUTRITION results from fetal, placental or maternal factors or various combinations of these, is not known. We hypothesize that idiopathic fetal malnutrition is essentially maternal in origin. Thus, maternal cells, particularly rapidly replicating cells, should illustrate phenomena which also characterize replicating fetal cells. Further, if alterations in cell function are present in maternal cells, the changes should be concurrent with the time of rapid fetal cell replication during the last ten to twelve weeks of pregnancy in the human. Such changes, if characteristic of the mother bearing an infant with fetal malnutrition, should serve as biochemical markers of fetal malnutrition. Whether such markers are intrinsic characteristics of the mothers or of events during that particular pregnancy is not known. If the cellular changes are a characteristic of the mother, not of the pregnancy, they should persist after delivery and should be present in some nonpregnant women. Biochemical markers, indicating fetal malnutrition, have not been reliably identified as yet in pregnant women.

Various chemical substances have been found in urine,

* Supported by a program project grant IPOI-HD-06915 from the National Institute of Child Health and Human Development, NIH, USPHS.

213

amniotic fluid or serum of pregnant women which have provided helpful indices of fetal or placental status with regard to successful outcome of the pregnancy. The items measured have not, however, contributed significantly to a prenatal diagnosis of fetal malnutrition.

The prevalent view of fetal malnutrition holds that cell replication is impaired *in utero*. Cell replication, of course, depends on protein synthesis. Protein synthesis requires energy as well as sufficient substrate and essential enzymes. Winick and Ross[1] first reported a reduced content of DNA, indicating a reduced number of cells, in brain of infants with severe protein-calorie malnutrition and later in those who had characteristics of fetal malnutrition.[2] In experimental animals, the myelin-related phospholipids in brain were reduced per cell.[3, 4] Dobbing[5] has shown that during the critical period of intrauterine growth, when cell replication or hyperplasia is occurring most rapidly, the brain is most vulnerable to insults, including malnutrition.[5] In the human fetus, about two-thirds of the brain cells are formed during the last trimester of pregnancy. The remaining one-third of the brain cells are acquired during the first year of postnatal life. Although there has been some correlation between learning performance of experimental animals and the DNA content (or number of cells) in their brains[6, 7] there appears to be no solid evidence that the number of brain cells is closely correlated with either intellectual potential or performance in the human being.

Gruenwald[8] suggested long ago that the spotty areas of maturational defects observed in the brains of small-for-dates infants dying at birth might be associated with abnormalities in the inter-relationships of integrated brain functions had the infants survived. A prospective study of the neurological and intellectual sequelae of being born small-for-dates recently was reported by Fitzhardinge and Steven.[9] Although there was a low incidence of major neurological defects in their series, 25 percent of the children had minimal cerebral dysfunction and EEG abnormalities. Frequently, these infants also had speech defects. Although the average full scale intelligence score was not remarkably reduced in these children, 50 percent of the boys and 36 percent of the girls did poorly in school. In fact, one-third of the children with IQ results over 100 were failing consistently. Drillien[10] in a smaller series previously observed that the small-for-dates infants were likely to show poor intellectual functioning. The present evidence therefore, indicates that the infant who is born small-for-dates with characteristics of fetal malnutrition might not reach the intellectual potential achieved by other infants of equivalent birth weight but shorter gestational age (prematures) or equivalent gestational age but normal birth weight. If, indeed, there is some correlation between neuronal and synaptosome cell number in the cerebral cortex and subsequent integrative performance of the child, if brain cell numbers are achieved largely before birth, and if brain cell hyperplasia does not "catch-up" postnatally, then prevention of fetal malnutrition will be the only effective treatment.

Gruenwald,[8] Naeye,[11] and Scott and Usher[12] have estimated that between one-third to one-half of low birth weight babies are not true prematures, but are small for their gestational age and suffer from fetal malnutrition. Using a median figure derived from their estimates and our national vital statistics, I have estimated that about 114,000 babies are born with fetal malnutrition annually in this country. If, as Usher reports, about one-third of fetal deaths may be attributed to fetal malnutrition,[13] perhaps 16,000 to 17,000 fetal deaths may be attributed to this cause. Together these figures suggest that the annual incidence of fetal malnutrition in the United States could approximate 130,000 annually (Table 12-I). This estimate is based largely on birth weight for gestational age. Miller and Hassanein[14, 15] have emphasized the use of Rhorer's "Ponderal Index" ($100 \times$ weight$_G \div$ length$^3{}_{CM}$) to define fetal malnutrition.[14, 15] If that index is used, the estimated figure would be increased. The enormity of the problem might be appreciated if, as Fitz-hardinge's work suggests, 25 percent of those live born infants will show minimal cerebral dysfunction, about one-third of them will have speech defects and between 35 percent and 50 percent of children born with fetal malnutrition will do poorly in school. In some series, as many as 50 percent of fetally malnourished neonates who survive, are estimated to have congenital anomalies.[10]

TABLE 12-I

ESTIMATED ANNUAL INCIDENCE OF SMALL-FOR-GESTATIONAL
AGE BIRTHS (FETAL MALNUTRITION) IN THE
UNITED STATES, 1968[1]

Actual:

Live births	3,501,564
Births under 2500g (LBW)	286,528
Fetal deaths	55,293

Estimated:

% LBW $\cong$ F.M.[2-4] = 33-50 (40)

LBW = F.M.	114,611
% Fetal deaths $\cong$ F.M.[5] = 30	
Fetal deaths = F.M.	16,588
Annual Incidence F.M.	131,199

[1] U.S. Demographic Survey—Date from National Vital Statistics System.
[2] Gruenwald, P.: *Pediatrics, 34*:157, 1964.
[3] Naeye, R. L.: *Arch Path, 79*:284, 1965.
[4] Scott, K. E., and Usher, R.: *Am J Obstet Gynec, 94*:951, 1966.
[5] Usher:*Ped Clin N Amer, 17*:169, 1970.

The relationship between maternal nutrition and fetal malnutrition is not clear. In several large studies, there appears to be a positive correlation between weight gain during pregnancy and birth weight of the baby.[16, 17] Poor weight gain in pregnancy has been related to fetal malnutrition as well as to inadequate nutrition of the pregnant women. Provision of supplemental calories during the last half of pregnancy will increase the birth weight of the child.[18] However, in the study of Habicht, *et al.*[18] the babies of nonsupplemented mothers usually had normal birthweights, while the babies of the supplemented mothers were bigger. Although nutritional deprivation during pregnancy may account for poor fetal growth,[19] there is also some suggestion from animal investigations[20] and from demographic data (U.S. Vital Statistics) that certain women may have intrinsic predisposition to produce babies with fetal malnutrition even though their nutritional state during pregnancy was not significantly impaired. If nutritional factors in the pregnant women are determinants of fetal malnutrition, then it is essential to identify these factors as early as possible in pregnancy. Presumably, malnutrition not only influences replication of fetal cells, but finds equivalent expression in rapidly replicating nucleated maternal cells.

The peripheral blood leukocyte is a rapidly replicating maternal cell, whose metabolism resembles that of other nucleated cells, although glycolysis is the principal energy pathway. In human beings, the polymorphonuclear neutrophil is the principal leukocyte cell type in the peripheral blood. It has a short life span which probably does not exceed fourteen days.[21] The hexose monophosphate shunt, Krebs cycle, aerobic mitochondrial oxidative metabolism, and protein synthesis also are present in the leukocyte (Table 12-II). Peripheral blood leukocyte levels increase during pregnancy, reaching a plateau during the second trimester.[22] Recently, Mitchell, *et al.*[23] reported that activities of the hexose monophosphate shunt and of the enzyme myeloperoxidase are increased during human pregnancy.[23] These usually constitute the biochemical drive for phagocytosis by the

TABLE 12-II

SOME CHARACTERISTICS OF THE HUMAN BLOOD LEUKOCYTE

Short Half Life ⌐ 14 days
Glycolysis predominates
Hexose monophosphate shunt
Krebs cycle
Aerobic mitochondrial oxidative metabolism
Protein synthesis
Reflects genetic defects, e.g.:
  Gangliosidosis
  Phosphorylase-deficient glycogen storage
  Fructose 6-diphosphatase
  Ataxia telangiectasia
  chronic granulomatous disease
Reflects nutritional cell biochemical changes, e.g.:
  Protein-calorie malnutrition
  Vitamin C deficiency
  Lysine deficiency

leukocyte; however, phagocytic capacity was not increased during pregnancy. Other studies have shown that specific enzyme defects or altered metabolite levels found in the liver cells of some genetically determined diseases, such as gangliosidosis[24] and phosphorylase-deficient glycogen storage disease,[25] are also present in the leukocyte. Some amino acid deficiencies,[26] vitamin C deficiency,[27] and altered protein synthesis[28] are reflected by the leukocyte. Leukocyte pyruvate kinase has kinetic properties similar to that of the enzyme in muscle.[29] The activity of the muscle enzyme is impaired by protein-calorie malnutrition.[30] These, and other observations, lend support to the thesis that metabolic changes in the leukocyte may be an index of similar changes in the cells of other organs[31] hence we have used it as a model, easily accessible cell.

Leukocyte Characteristics in Mothers and Babies with FM, at Term

Our method for leukocyte isolation requires about 20 ml of blood.[32] The isolated leukocyte extract contains 10^6 to 10^7 leukocytes/mm³ with over 95 percent being polymorphonuclear leukocytes. Some years ago, changes in the energy metabolism of leukocytes were related to the degree of protein-calorie malnutrition in young children.[33] More recently, we have extended these observations to neonates who are appropriately grown for their gestational age or to those who showed impaired fetal growth with characteristics of fetal malnutrition. Certain metabolic features of the peripheral blood leukocyte at term were noted to characterize mothers who delivered babies with fetal malnutrition. Metabolic changes found in maternal leukocytes at term included reduced levels of the adenine nucleotides and lowered activities of the enzymes pyruvic and adrenylate kinase.[34] Activities of these enzymes tend to increase during the last ten to twelve weeks of pregnancy.[35] Activities of the enzyme RNA polymerase also were noted to increase during the last part of normal gestation. A particularly interesting feature was the observation that activity of RNA polymerase in maternal leukocytes seemed to correlate with birth weight of the baby.[36] Most of these studies were obtained at term. Only a few observations were sequential during pregnancy.

Prospective Study of Maternal Leukocytes in Pregnancy

Recently a multidisciplinary project entitled "Maternal Malnutrition and Fetal Development" (MMFD) has been initiated at the University of Oklahoma Health Sciences Center. Several collaborating institutions include the Centro Medico Nacional of the Seguro Social in Mexico City, the Human Nutrition Research Laboratories (Grand Forks, North Dakota) and the Protein

Research Laboraties (Beltsville, Maryland) of the U.S. Department of Agriculture. Some of the preliminary results obtained by our MMFD group* are presented here. Since our study has been underway for less than a year, and our sample size is still small, conclusions are not warranted, but the preliminary results support the hypothesis that studies of leukocyte metabolism during pregnancy may indicate patterns of fetal development.

Design of Study

Monthly status reports provide raw data tables, summary data tables and various biostatistical outputs, which are reviewed by our biostatistician and other members of the group. Pregnant women are entered into the study at sixteen weeks of gestation, with the first blood and urine samples being obtained at twenty-four weeks of pregnancy. Subsequent samples are obtained at thirty-two weeks and at the time of delivery. Follow-up studies occur at three days postpartum, six weeks, six months and one year postnatally. Of course, the baby is entered into the study at the time of delivery and is followed for the first year of life.

Items Studied

In addition to the demographic and medical information obtained at each study time, some of the items assayed in leukocytes, blood, plasma, urine and hair are listed in Table 12-III.

Preliminary Results of Leukocyte Studies

Some of the leukocyte results at twenty-four and thirty-two weeks of gestation, at delivery and in cord blood are summarized in Tables 12-IV and 12-V. Enzyme activities and cell size shown in Table 12-IV vary considerably in different women, hence the group mean values have rather large deviations above or below the mean. The energy indices of Table 12-V are variations based

---

* MMFD group includes: Warren Crosby, M.D.; Mostafa Mameesh, Ph.D.; Gail Jacobson, Ph.D.; David Vore, Ph.D.; Gayle Burns; Katherine Fowler; Judy Page; Sherri Beck, M.S.; Sherri Cook; Irene Smith; Robert Theimer, M.S.; Paul Costiloe, M.S.; Paul Anderson, Ph.D.; William Reid; Ardith Wilson; Ray Kling, Ph.D.; Kim Murphy; Bonnie Bradshaw; Joyce Mesoner; and Jack Metcoff, Principal Investigator, Program Director.

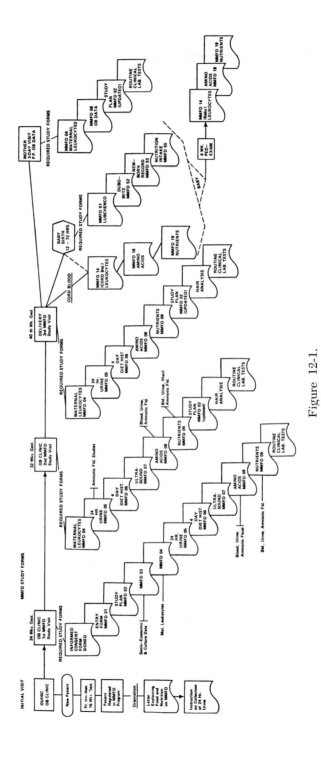

Figure 12-1.

TABLE 12-III

PARTIAL LIST OF ITEMS MEASURED IN WOMEN AT 24 AND 32
WEEKS OF GESTATION, AT TERM AND POSTNATALLY
(MMFD PROJECT)

A. BLOOD

1. *Leukocytes*	2. *Erythrocytes*	3. *Plasma*
DNA	Transketolase activity	22 free amino acids
Protein	Coefficient	Total Protein
	(Thiamin)	
Pyruvic Kinase	Glutathione reductase	Albumin
Adenylic Kinase	activity coefficient	Plasma Electro-
		phoresis
Phosphofructokinase	(Riboflavin)	Cholesterol
Glucose-6-phosphate	Transaminase activity	Iron & Iron binding
dehydrogenase	coefficient (Vit. B_6)	capacity
ATP	Folate activity	Zn
ADP		Copper
AMP		Selenium
Pyruvate		Creatinine
Glucose-6-phosphate		Vitamin A
protein Synthesis		Carotene
(^{3}H-Leucine incorporation)		Vitamin C
RNA Synthesis (^{3}H-Uridine		
incorporation)		

B. URINE

Estrogens
Creatinine
21 free amino acids

C. HAIR

Shaft—Zinc, chromium, copper, manganese, nickel
Roots—protein, DNA

D. OTHER

Ultrasound encephalography of fetal head
Sociocultural information
3 day diet record + 24 hour diet recall
weight, OB observations, etc.
Aminocentesis (for OB indication)

on the "energy charge" model of Atkinson.[37] Each relates to the
essential balance between ATP utilization and regeneration.

Correlations Between Leukocyte Metabolism and Other Items During Pregnancy

Figure 12-2 is an example of some correlations between
maternal leukocyte enzymes and metabolities, and maternal diet
protein and calorie intakes. The correlations refer to paired
observations in the same leukocyte extract of the women and
represent a plot of an asymetrical matrix in which any one

TABLE 12-IV

ENZYME ACTIVITIES IN LEUKOCYTES DURING PREGNANCY

	Week of Gestation			
	24 ± 1	32 ± 1	40 or delivery	Baby at birth*
PROT/DNA	16.2 ± 9.5† (64)**	17.7 ± 8.1 (48)	17.5 ± 5.3 (33)	13.3 ± 5.3 (28)
PK μmoles/ gDNA/min	9149 ± 3681 (62)	12116 ± 5101 (47)	11578 ± 4794 (32)	9048 ± 4638 (28)
AK μmoles/ gDNA/min	454 ± 184 (65)	557 ± 287 (48)	481 ± 211 (32)	547 ± 226 (27)
PFK μmoles/ gDNA/min	22 ± 18 (60)	31 ± 37 (48)	33 ± 40 (32)	29 ± 30 (26)
G6PDH μmoles/ gDNA/min	2527 ± 1050 (56)	2498 ± 1626 (48)	2856 ± 1329 (32)	2333 ± 1942 (27)

    * Cord blood.
    † mean ± S.D.
    ( ) indicates number of women sampled at each sequential study period.
    ** study sample size to 11/73.

TABLE 12-V

ENERGY INDICES IN LEUKOCYTES DURING PREGNANCY

	Week of Gestation			
	24 ± 1	32 ± 1	40 delivery	Baby cord blood
E charge[1]	0.85 ± 0.68* (58)	0.85 ± 0.74 (44)	0.86 ± 0.56 (30)	0.83 ± 0.09 (28)
E capacity[2]	1.57 (58)	1.99 (44)	2.19 (29)	2.1 (27)
E Metab[3]	19.52 ± 8.57 (53)	23.06 ± 11.98 (42)	31.95 ± 49.30 (28)	

[1] $\text{E Charge} = \dfrac{\text{ATP} + \frac{1}{2}\,\text{ADP}}{\text{ATP} + \text{ADP} + \text{AMP}}$

[2] $\text{E Capacity} = \text{ATP} + \frac{1}{2}\,\text{ADP (AK)}$

[3] $\text{E Metab} = \text{Ech} \times \dfrac{\text{PK}}{\text{AK}}$

( ) refers to number of women sampled at each sequential study period.
* mean ± S.D.

TABLE 12-VI

PROTEIN SYNTHESIS BY LEUKOCYTES DURING PREGNANCY

	Week of Gestation			
	24 ± 1	32 ± 1	40 delivery	Baby cord blood
Protein Synthesis nmole leucine/ hr/g DNA	1573 ± 226* (11)	1572 ± 327 (14)	1485 ± 664 (14)	931 ± 501 (4)
RNA Synthesis nmole uridine/ hr/g DNA	27 ± 13 (6)	31 ± 7 (7)		

( ) refers to number of women at each sequential study period.
* mean ± S.D.

TABLE 12-VII

SOME ESTIMATES OF NUTRITIONAL STATUS

	Week of Gestation		
	24 ± 1	32 ± 1	40 delivery
Diet Prot. g/kg	1.1 ± 0.5* (47)	1.1 ± 0.3 (23)	
Diet Calories Kcol/kg	30.0 ± 11.7 (47)	29.7 ± 7.8 (23)	
Hair Root Prot. μg/hair		10.4 ± 7.0 (25)	8.70 ± 5.8 (21)
Hair Root DNA μg/hair		0.089 ± 0.048 (21)	0.072 ± 0.06 (21)
Weight kg	66.94 ± 15.64 (30)	70.66 ± 15.31 (30)	71.20 ± 13.99 (28)

( ) refers to number of subjects.
* mean ± S.D.

measured item may be correlated with each of the other items. Since the number of women in our sample is still quite small, the results, although statistically significant, should be considered to be tentative. The correlations may change as the study progresses. The solid circles indicate statistically significant correlations made at twenty-four weeks of gestation in the accumulated group of fifty-two women. The open circles indicate statistically significant correlations obtained at thirty-two weeks of gestation in thirty-two of these same pregnant women. The negative signs indicate a negative correlation. For example, in these preliminary data, activity of adenylate kinase in the lekuo-

TIME-TRENDS DURING GESTATION IN MATERNAL LEUKOCYTES

(POOLED REGRESSION ANALYSIS FOR ALL SUBJECTS WITH AT LEAST 2 STUDIES BETWEEN 23-41 WKS. OF GESTATION)

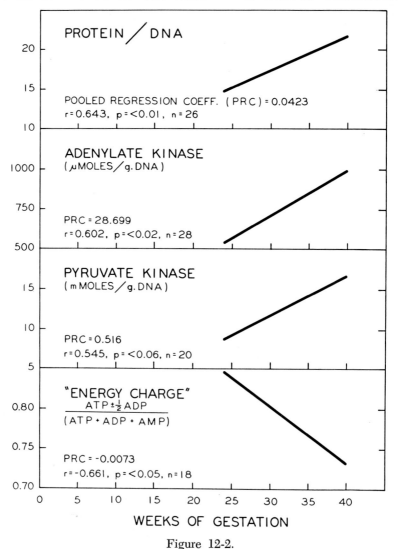

Figure 12-2.

cytes is correlated with those of pyruvic kinase at twenty-four and thirty-two weeks. Phosphofructokinase activity at thirty-two weeks correlate with those of pyruvic kinase and adenylate kinase. Dietary protein intake of the pregnant women at twenty-four weeks appears to be correlated with leukocyte protein synthesis.

Gestational Trends in Leukocyte Metabolism

Time-trends may be partially assessed by determination of pooled regression coefficients for various aspects of metabolism in the maternal leukocytes where at least two sequential determinations are available during gestation. Some of these are illustrated in Figures 12-3a & 3b. Between twenty-four and forty weeks of gestation the leukocyte cell size, reflected by the protein/DNA ratio, appears to increase as do the activities of the enzymes adenylate and pyruvate kinase. The energy charge seems to decrease.

Recently we have determined some of the kinetic properties of pyruvate kinase in leukocytes of mothers at parturition in Mexico City.[†] A preliminary assessment of the Michaelis-Menten constant (K_M) was calculated from the measured enzyme-substrate complex changes. The points for each curve were the mean values for initial velocities found at each substrate concentration in each group of women: Mothers who delivered fetally malnourished infants (FM=6) and mothers who delivered normal full term infants (N=6). Lines were calculated and the Lineweaver-Burk plots were made (Fig. 12-4a & 4b). Reported values for the Michaelis-Menton constant (K_M) for pyruvate kinase range from 0.35 to 0.06 M x 10^{-3}.[38] In human leukocytes $PK_{KM\ PEP\&ADP}$ were found to be 0.1 and 0.18 x 10^{-3} M.[39] These values are closely approximated by the values we observed in leukocytes from women at term. There is a distinct difference in the slopes of the curves for the FM mothers in comparison with

[†] These studies were carried out in the Departamento de Investigaciones Cientifica, Seccion Bioquimica de Reproduccion, Centro Medico Nacional, Instituto Mexicano de Seguro Social, with the assistance of Katherine Fowler, B.A. and in collaboration with Alfonso Bernal, M.D., Susanna Chew, M.S., Myriam Morales, M.S., Pablo Yoshida, M.D. and Adolfo Rosado, M.D., Ph.D. These studies were supported by grants from the Ross Laboratories and Abbott International (de Mexico).

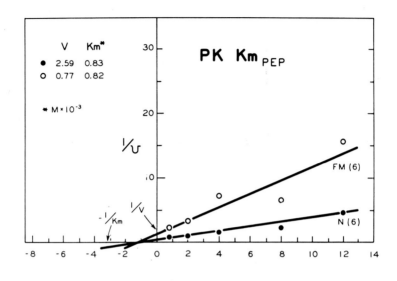

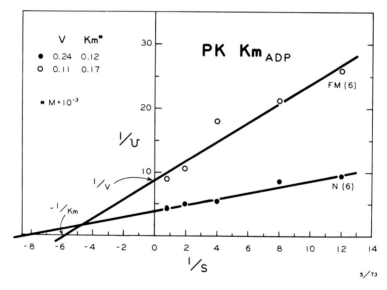

Figure 12-3.

PRENATAL MATERNAL LEUKOCYTES AND

BABY SIZE AT BIRTH

(ASYMETRICAL CORRELATIONS)
24 - 30 PAIRED VALUES

MATERNAL LEUKOCYTES

BABY	PROT/DNA	PYRUVATE KINASE	PHOSPHO-FRUCTOKINASE	GLUCOSE-6-P DEHYDROG.	ADP	ENERGY CHARGE
WEIGHT	●					
PERCENTILE WEIGHT	○					
C - H LENGTH		○				
PERCENTILE CHL						
PONDERAL INDEX*		●		●	●	-○
PERCENTILE PI			●	●		
HEAD CIRCUMF.						
PERCENTILE FOC	(-)●					

* P.I. = $100X \ WT_g \div C - H \ LENGTH^3_{cm}$

● = MATERNAL LEUKOCYTES AT 24 WEEKS

○ = MATERNAL LEUKOCYTES AT 32 WEEKS

11/73

Figure 12-4.

PRENATAL MATERNAL LEUKOCYTES AND

BABY SIZE AT BIRTH

(ASYMETRICAL CORRELATIONS)
24 - 30 PAIRED VALUES

MATERNAL LEUKOCYTES

BABY	PROT/DNA	PYRUVATE KINASE	PHOSPHO-FRUCTOKINASE	GLUCOSE-6-P DEHYDROG.	ADP	ENERGY CHARGE
WEIGHT	●					
PERCENTILE WEIGHT		○				
C - H LENGTH			○			
PERCENTILE CHL						
PONDERAL INDEX*		●		●	●	-○
PERCENTILE PI				●	●	
HEAD CIRCUMF.						
PERCENTILE FOC	(-)●					

$$* \quad \text{P.I.} = 100X \ WT_g \div C - H \ LENGTH^3_{cm}$$

● = MATERNAL LEUKOCYTES AT 24 WEEKS

○ = MATERNAL LEUKOCYTES AT 32 WEEKS

11/73

N mothers for both substrates. The difference is attributable largely to the lower V_{MAX} value for the enzyme in FM mothers. This suggests either the presence of some inhibitor or a reduction of enzyme protein and/or allosteric change in binding sites. These preliminary data do not warrant firm conclusions, particularly since purified enzyme was not used for these kinetic studies.

Tentative Correlation Between Maternal Leukocytes and Fetal Development

Although these particular interpretations are subject to changes as more data are accumulated, the analyses indicate that characteristic patterns of metabolism might be expected in the maternal leukocyte during pregnancy. It is still too early in the course of our studies to determine whether metabolism of the maternal leukocyte during pregnancy will predict fetal outcome. Some preliminary correlations and covariance analyses suggest that it might. Tentative correlations between some items in the maternal leukocyte at twenty-four and thirty-two weeks with anthropometric measures of the baby at birth are illustrated in Figure 12-4. Items measured in the maternal leukocytes are shown on the upper border and the baby measures are shown on the left ordinate. We consider the correlations tentative, although they are statistically significant. The ponderal index is used here as an index of fetal malnutrition.‡[14] A low ponderal index indicates that the baby would be underweight for length at any specific gestational age. Pyruvate kinase, glucose-6-phosphate dehydrogenase, ADP and the energy charge of the maternal leukocytes are correlated with either the ponderal index or the ponderal index percentile of the baby at birth. Similarly the cell size, that is the protein/DNA ratio, of the maternal leukocyte at twenty-four weeks correlates with the birth weight of the baby. These preliminary observations are subject to the qualification noted above, but do support the thesis that some patterns of leukocyte metabolism during pregnancy indicate

---

‡ If both weight and crown-heel length are reduced proportionately, the Ponderal Index may be within the normal range. In fetal malnutrition of long duration, both weight and crown-heel length may be proportionately reduced.[40, 41]

MATERNAL LEUKOCYTE METABOLISM
TRENDS DURING PREGNANCY & FETAL GROWTH

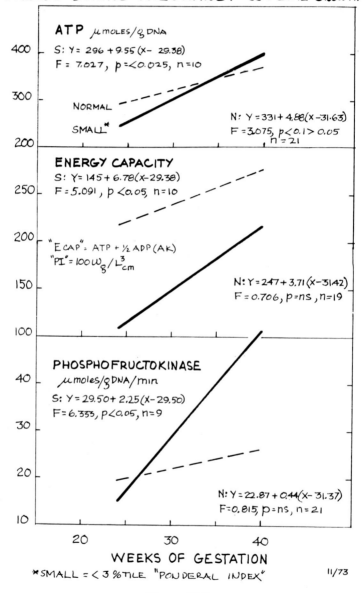

ATP μ moles/g DNA

S: $Y = 296 + 9.55(x - 29.38)$
F = 7.027, $p = <0.025$, n = 10

NORMAL

SMALL*

N: $Y = 331 + 4.88(x - 31.63)$
F = 3.075, $p < 0.1 > 0.05$
n = 21

ENERGY CAPACITY
S: $Y = 145 + 6.78(x - 29.38)$
F = 5.091, $p < 0.05$, n = 10

"E CAP" = ATP + ½ ADP (AK)
"PI" = $100 W_g / L^3_{cm}$

N: $Y = 247 + 3.71(x - 31.42)$
F = 0.706, p = ns, n = 19

PHOSPHOFRUCTOKINASE
μ moles/g DNA/min
S: $Y = 29.50 + 2.25(x - 29.50)$
F = 6.333, $p < 0.05$, n = 9

N: $Y = 22.87 + 0.44(x - 31.37)$
F = 0.815, p = ns, n = 21

WEEKS OF GESTATION

*SMALL = < 3 %TILE "PONDERAL INDEX"   11/73

Figure 12-5.

fetal growth. Trends for weight gain and ultrasound measures of fetal headsize in the pregnant women who later delivered normal babies are shown by the broken lines; whereas those who later delivered small babies are illustrated by the solid line. In the upper portion of Figure 12-5, the trend for weight gain of the women who delivered small babies was similar to that of women who later delivered normal babies. The absolute weights were slightly less in the latter group. In the lower portion of the diagram, there appears to be little or no difference between the growth of the fetal head as determined by ultrasound encephalography during pregnancy between babies who are later born with low ponderal indices versus those having normal fetal growth.

At this early stage of our study, it seems that neither weight gain during pregnancy nor growth of the fetal head hold much promise for differentiating those women who are likely to deliver small babies. For normal or large size babies, recent reports suggest that weight gain during pregnancy does correlate with size of the baby at birth. Recently, Miller indicated that mothers of FM babies (based on low ponderal indices) gained less weight during pregnancy than those who delivered babies with normal PIs.[15]

Gestation Trends in Leukocyte Metabolism as Predictors of Fetal Growth

Our preliminary observations suggest that trends of maternal leukocyte metabolism during pregnancy may serve as a predictor of fetal growth. For example, Figure 12-5 illustrates trends in ATP, energy capacity and phosphofructokinase activities. The solid lines illustrate trends in mothers who delivered babies whose ponderal indices were below the three percentile. The broken line illustrates maternal leukocyte trends in mothers who delivered normal sized babies. In each instance the pooled regression analysis for the few mothers of small babies was statistically significant, whereas the trend lines in the leukocytes in mothers who later delivered normal babies did not differ significantly from zero, and the trend was not statistically significant.

Relation of Maternal Nutrition to Fetal Development Being Studied

As yet, we do not know what role the mother's nutritional status plays in fetal development. The evidence that maternal malnutrition inhibits or alters development of the human fetus to produce a malnourished infant is largely circumstantial. In another aspect of our study, evaluation of dietary intakes by three-day diet records as well as the twenty-four hour recall history obtained by a nutritionist on at least three occasions during pregnancy should provide a reasonable assessment of recent dietary intake associated with the pregnancy. Quantitative assessments of vitamins, free amino acid levels, proteins and trace minerals in blood and urine will provide an objective estimate of nutrient status of the mothers. Assay of hair root protein and DNA contents obtained at thirty-two weeks of gestation and at delivery should provide evidence of protein nutrition. When coupled with studies of leukocyte metabolism it should be possible to determine whether nutritional status of the mother during pregnancy modifies the trends of fetal development and is related to outcome of the pregnancy.

CONCLUSIONS

As our study sample size increases, it is possible that the trends noted so far will either be confirmed or changed, or that other trends will emerge. The particular items noted in these figures illustrate only a few of the many variables being studied. We do not yet know whether the enzymes referred to are the most pertinent ones to measure, whether ATP or some more comprehensive index of cell metabolism will prove to be the most useful measurements, or whether protein synthesis or one of the other variables now being studied will be a better predictor of fetal growth. However, studies of the metabolism of the maternal leukocyte during pregnancy seem to offer promise as a predictor of fetal development and especially of fetal malnutrition.

REFERENCES

1. Winick, M., and Ross, P.: The effect of severe early malnutrition on cellular growth of human brain. *Pediatr Res, 3*:181, 1969.
2. Winick, M.: Cellular growth of fetus and placenta. In Waisman, H. A., and Kerr, G. (Eds.): *Fetal Growth and Development.* New York, McGraw-Hill, 1970, Chap. 3.
3. Winick, M.: Nutrition and nerve cell growth. *Fed Proc, 29*:1510, 1970.
4. Chase, H. P.; Dabrere, C. S.; Welch, N. N., and O'Brien, D.: Intrauterine undernutrition and brain development. *Pediatrics, 47*:491, 1971.
5. Dobbing, J.: Vulnerable periods in developing brain. In Davidson, A. N., and Dobbing, J. (Eds.): *Applied Neurochemistry,* Oxford, Blackwell Scientific Publications, Ltd., 1968.
6. Simonson ,M., and Chow, B. F.: Maze study on progeny of underfed mother rats. *J Nutr, 100*:685, 1970.
7. Hanson, H. M., and Simonson, M.: Effect of fetal undernourishment on experimental anxiety. *Nutr Reports Int'l, 4*:307, 1971.
8. Gruenwald, P.: Chronic fetal distress and placental insufficiency. *Biol Neonat, 5*:215, 1963.
9. Fitzhardinge, P. M., and Steven, E. M.: The small-for-date infant. II. Neurological and intellectual sequelae. *Pediatrics, 50*:50, 1972.
10. Drillien, C. M.: The small for date infant: etiology and prognosis. *Pediatr Clin North Am, 17*:9, 1970.
11. Naeye, R. L.: Malnutrition, a probable cause of fetal growth retardation. *Arch Pathol, 79*:284, 1965.
12. Scott, K. E., and Usher, R.: Fetal malnutrition: its incidence, causes and effects. *Am J Obstet Gynec, 94*:951, 1966.
13. Usher, R. H.: Clinical and therapeutic aspects of fetal malnutrition. *Pediatr Clin North Am, 17*:169, 1970.
14. Miller, H. C., and Hassaein, K.: Diagnosis of impaired fetal growth in newborn infants. *Pediatrics, 48*:511, 1971.
15. Miller, H. C., and Hassanein, K.: Fetal malnutrition in white newborn infants: maternal factors. *Pediatrics, 52*:504, 1973.
16. Inger, J. E.; Westphal, M., and Nisevander, K.: Relatonship of weight gain during pregnancy to birth weight and infant growth and development in the first year of life. Report from Collaborative Study of Cerebral Palsy. *Obstet Gynecol, 3*:417, 1968.
17. Bergner, L., and Susser, M. W.: Low birth weight and prenatal nutriton. An interpretive review. *Pediatrics, 46*:946, 1970.
18. Habicht, J-P; Yarborough, C.; Lechtig, A., and Klein, R. E.: Relation of maternal supplementary feeding during pregnancy to birth-

weight and other socio-biological factors. In Winick, Myron (Ed.):
Nutrition and Fetal Development, John Wiley, New York, 1974,
p. 127.

19. Naeye, R. L.; Blanc, W., and Paul, C.: Effects of maternal nutrition
on the human fetus. *Pediatrics, 52*:494, 1973.

20. Zamenhof, S.; Van Marthens, E., and Gruel, L.: DNA (cell number)
in neonatal brain: second generation (F_2) alteration by maternal
(F_0) dietary protein restriction. *Science, 172*:850, 1969.

21. Galbraith, P. R.; Chickkappa, G., and Abu-Zahra, H. T.: Patterns of
granulocyte kinetics in acute myelogenous and myelomonocytic
leukemia. *Blood, 37*:371, 1970.

22. Mitchell, G. W., Jr.; McRipley, R. J.; Selvaraj, R. J., and Sbarra, A. J.:
The role of the phagocyte in host-parasite interactions. IV. The
phagocytic activity of leukocytes in pregnancy and its relationship
to urinary tract infections. *J Obstet Gynecol, 96*:687, 1966.

23. Mitchell, G. W., Jr.; Jacobs, A. A.; Haddad, V.; Paul. B. B.; Strauss,
R. R., and Sbarra, A. J.: The role of the phagocyte in host-parasite
interactions. XXV. Metabolic and bacteriacidal activities of leukocytes from pregnant women. *Am J Obstet Gynecol, 108*:805, 1970.

24. Holmes, B.; Page, A. R., and Good, R. A.: Studies of the metabolic
activity of leukocytes from patients with a genetic abnormality of
phagocytic function. *J Clin Invest, 46*:1422, 1967.

25. Williams, H. E., and Field, J. B.: Low leukocyte phosphorylase in
hepatic phosphorylase-deficient glycogen storage disease. *J Clin
Invest, 40*:1841, 1961.

26. Leise, E. M.; Monta, T. N.; Gray, I.; LeSane, F., and Rodriquez, M.:
Leukocyte enzymes as indicators of nutritional deficiency. *Biochem
Med, 4*:347, 1970.

27. Loh, J. S., *et al.*: Relationship between leukocyte and plasma ascorbic
acid concentrations. *Br Med J, 3*:733, 1971.

28. Gordon, R. O.; Oppenheim, J. J.; Souther, S. G., and Spinson, E. B.:
Immediate in vitro leukocyte DNA synthesis: an early indicator of
heart allograft rejection. *Surg Forum, 22*:258, 1971.

29. Koler, R. D., and Van Bellinghen, P.: The mechanism of precursor
modulation of human pyruvate kinase I by fructose diphosphate.
In Weber. E. (Ed.): *Advances in Enzyme Regulation, 6*:127,
Oxford, England, Pergamon, 1968.

30. Metcoff, J.; Frenk, S.; Yoshida, T.; Torres-Pinedo, R.; Kaiser, E., and
Hansen, J. D. L.: Cell composition and metabolism in Kwashiorkor
(severe protein-calorie malnutrition in children). *Medicine, 45*:
365, 1966.

31. Jemelin, M., and Frei, J.: Leukocyte energy metabolism: III. Anaerobic
and aerobic ATP production and related enzymes. *Enzym Biol
Clin, 11*:289, 1970.

32. Yoshida, T.; Metcoff, J.; Frenk, S., and de la Pena, C.: Intermediary metabolism and adenine nucleotides in leukocytes of children with protein-calorie malnutrition. *Nature, 214*:5087, 1967.
33. Yoshida, T.; Metcoff, J., and Frenk, S.: Reduced pyruvic kinase activity, altered growth patterns of ATP in leukocytes and protein-calorie malnutrition. *Am J Clin Nutr, 21*:162, 1968.
34. Metcoff, J.; Yoshida, T.; Morales, M.; Rosado, A.; Urristi, J.; Sosa, A.; Yoshida, P.; Frenk, S.; Velasco, L.; Ward, A., and Al-Ubaidi, Y.: Biomolecular studies of fetal malnutrition in maternal leukocytes. *Pediatrics, 47*:180, 1971.
35. Yoshida, T.; Metcoff, J.; Morales, M.; Rosado, A.; Sosa, A.; Yoshida, P.; Urristi, J.; Frenk, S., and Velasco, L.: Human fetal growth retardation. II. Energy metabolism in leukocytes. *Pediatrics, 50*:559, 1972.
36. Metcoff, J.; Wikman-Coffelt, J.; Yoshida, T.; Bernal, A.; Rosado, A.; Yoshida, P.; Urristi, J.; Frenk, S.; Madrazo, R., and Velasco, L.: Energy metabolism and protein synthesis in human leukocytes during pregnancy and in placenta related to fetal growth. *Pediatrics, 51*:866, 1973.
37. Atkinson, D. E.: The energy charge of the adenylate pool as a regulatory parameter. Interaction with feedback modifiers. *Biochemistry, 7*:4030, 1968.
38. Taylor, C. V.; Morris, H. P., and Wever, G.: A comparison of the properties of pyruvate kinase from hepatoma 3924-A, normal liver and muscle. *Life Sciences, 8* (Part II):635, Pergamon, 1965.
39. Campos, J. O.; Koler, R. D., and Bigley, R. H.: Kinetic differences between human red cell and leukocyte pyruvate kinase. *Nature, 208*:194, 1965.
40. Urrusti, J., et al.: Human Fetal Growth Retardation. I. Clinical features of sample with intrauterine growth retardation. *Pediatrics, 50*:547, 1972.
41. Metcoff, J.: Biochemical markers of intrauterine malnutrition. In Winick, M. (Ed.): *Nutrition and Fetal Development*. John Wiley, 1974, p. 27.

Chapter 13

ROLE OF ALPHA$_1$-FETOPROTEIN AS A MARKER IN FETAL DISTRESS

M. Seppälä and E. Ruoslahti

INTRODUCTION

ALPHA$_1$-FETOPROTEIN (AFP) is a major plasma protein of early human fetuses.[1] Evidence has accumulated indicating the fetal liver as a major site of AFP origin.[2] During the embryonal period, the highest AFP concentrations in fetal serum occur around weeks twelve to fifteen of gestation, while the total amount of AFP in the fetus increases until about the twenty-second week. Between the twenty-second and thirty-second weeks the concentration is constant, and decreases thereafter.[3]

In our studies, human AFP was immunochemically isolated and purified.[4] A highly sensitive radioimmunoassay was developed[5] enabling demonstration of AFP in various types of neoplastic and non-neoplastic liver diseases,[6] during pregnancy[7] and in normal human serum.[5]

Circulating maternal AFP levels increase during the course of normal pregnancy with the highest AFP levels occurring during the mid-third trimester.[7] Abnormally high maternal AFP levels were first demonstrated in pregnancies associated with intrauterine fetal death.[8] Recently AFP levels have been introduced to the detection of antenatal fetal complications, which are frequently associated with elevated AFP levels in maternal serum[9, 10] and amniotic fluid.[11-13]

The mechanisms leading to increased maternal AFP levels in

236

fetal disorders are poorly understood, the AFP levels in various types of high risk pregnancies have not been documented. In order to clarify these phenomena and the significance of maternal AFP levels in the assessment of fetoplacental function, we have extended our studies to include various types of high risk pregnancies.

METHODS AND MATERIALS

A detailed description of the double antibody radioimmunoassay for AFP has been presented previously.[5]

AFP concentrations of 204 pregnant women were measured to establish the 95 percent confidence limits.[14] Six hundred and sixteen serum samples from 296 women with various types of high risk pregnancies were studied for AFP concentrations. Included in these were 140 samples from seventy-four women with hypertension, 130 sera from eighty-two women with toxemia, ninety-two samples from fifty-seven women with a liver disorder, 164 sera from thirty-eight women with diabetes, forty-four sera from twenty-four Rh-immunized women,[15] and forty-six samples from twenty-one women with multiple pregnancies.[16] Forty-four serum samples from thirty women whose fetuses had died or were later to die *in utero* were considered separately. All samples were taken while the fetus was *in utero*.

The criteria used to classify pregnancies according to the fetoplacental function are listed in Table 13-I. Two criteria had

TABLE 13-I

CRITERIA FOR THE CLASSIFICATION OF FETOPLACENTAL FUNCTION

Normal fetoplacental function	*Severe fetoplacental dysfunction*
1. Normal fetal heart action	1. Abnormal fetal heart action —late deceleration —variation greater than 110-170 beats/min.
2. Normal fetal blood gas analysis	2. Fetal acidosis below pH 7.25
3. Normal colored amniotic fluid	3. Green amniotic fluid
4. Normal intrauterine growth	4. Intrauterine growth retardation (fetal weight below the normal 10 percentile)
5. Normal placenta	5. Marked placental infarction
6. Apgar score of seven or more	6. Apgar score of six or less
	7. Intrauterine fetal death

to be fulfilled before the case was classified as severe fetoplacental dysfunction, while all criteria had to be normal to be considered as normal fetoplacental function. Thus, the two clearly defined categories did not contain any questionable cases.

RESULTS

The occurrence of severe fetoplacental dysfunction in high risk pregnancies varied according to the type of the complication (Table 13-II). The lowest frequency of fetal distress occurred

TABLE 13-II

OCCURRENCE OF SEVERE FETOPLACENTAL DYSFUNCTION
IN HIGH RISK PREGNANCIES

Complication	*Frequency of Fetal Distress*
Hypertension	11/74 (15)
Toxemia	22/82 (27)
Liver disorder	9/57 (16)
Diabetes	14/38 (37)

( ) Denotes percent.

in hypertensive pregnancies and the highest frequency in diabetic pregnancies.

In high risk pregnancies, the AFP levels also varied (Table 13-III). In hypertonic and toxemic pregnancies the AFP levels tended to be lower than normal, whereas in diabetic and Rh-immunized mothers the AFP levels were higher than normal.

The individual AFP levels in seventy-four *hypertensive pregnancies* are presented in Figure 13-1. Among pregnancies with normal fetoplacental function, the highest individual AFP concentrations exceeded the normal 97.5 percentile in one out of forty-eight cases, while this level was more frequently exceeded in cases with fetal distress (2 out of 11 cases). Consequently, when the maternal AFP level was higher than the normal 97.5 percentile in hypertensive pregnancies, fetal distress was associated with two of three cases (Table 13-IV). When examining AFP levels to establish normal fetoplacental function versus severe dysfunction, the levels exceeding 250 ng/ml coincided

TABLE 13-III

MATERNAL AFP LEVELS IN HIGH RISK PREGNANCIES (SAMPLES).
N.S. = NOT SIGNIFICANT

Complication	AFP Concentration		
	Below the Normal Median	Above the Normal Median	Significance of Difference from X^2 normal P
Hypertension	81/140 (58)	59/140 (42)	1.76 N.S.
Toxemia	73/130 (56)	57/130 (44)	0.97 N.S.
Liver disorder	42/92 (46)	50/92 (54)	0.32 N.S.
Diabetes	58/164 (35)	106/164 (65)	7.34 <0.01
Rh-immunization[15]	8/44 (18)	36/44 (82)	13.58 <0.001
Fetal death			
—before	2/14 (14)	12/14 (86)	5.34 <0.05
—after	4/30 (13)	26/30 (87)	12.75 <0.001
Multiple pregnancy[16]	1/46	45/46 (98)	33.49 <0.001

( ) Denotes percent.

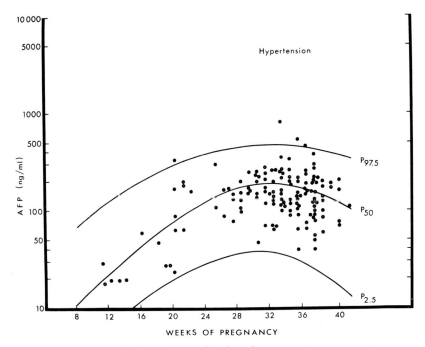

Figure 13-1.   Maternal AFP levels in hypertensive pregnancies.

TABLE 13-IV

HIGHEST INDIVIDUAL MATERNAL AFP LEVELS AND
FETOPLACENTAL FUNCTION IN PREGNANT WOMEN
WITH HYPERTENSION

AFP Level	Fetoplacental Function Normal	Severe Dysfunction	Association with Fetal Distress of a Given AFP Level
>97.5 percentile	1/48 (2)	2/11 (18)	2/3 (67)
>250 ng/ml	6/48 (12)	9/11 (82)	9/15 (60)

( ) Denotes percent.

with normal fetoplacental function in six out of forty-eight cases and with fetal distress in nine out of eleven cases (p<0.01). Thus, a given value exceeding 250 ng/ml in hypertensive pregnancies is associated with fetal distress in about 60 percent of the cases. The frequency of incorrect classifications is 16.9 percent if the normal 97.5 percentile is applied, and 13.6 percent if the level of 250 ng/ml is used.

In toxemia, the AFP levels were also somewhat lower than in normal pregnancies (Fig. 13-2). Among the twenty-two toxemic women with severe fetoplacental dysfunction, abnormally high AFP levels were found in nine cases (41%), while similar levels occurred less frequently (1 out of 54 cases, p<0.001) in pregnancies with normal fetoplacental function. Thus, abnormally high maternal AFP levels were associated with fetal distress in nine out of ten cases, compared to twenty-two out of eighty-two cases of fetal distress in all toxemic pregnancies (p<0.001), (Tables 13-II and 13-V).

The AFP concentrations of 300 ng/ml or higher occurred in fourteen out of twenty-two cases with fetal distress and in eight out of fifty-four individuals with a normal fetoplacental function (p<0.01). This means that a given AFP level exceeding 300 ng/ml in toxemia is associated with fetal distress in 64 percent of the cases, compared to the 27 percent occurrence of fetal distress in all toxemic pregnancies (p<0.01).

AFP levels in *maternal liver disorder* were above the normal median in fifty out of ninety-two samples (Fig. 13-3). Two out of nine pregnancies with severe fetoplacental dysfunction were associated with abnormally high AFP levels while two out of

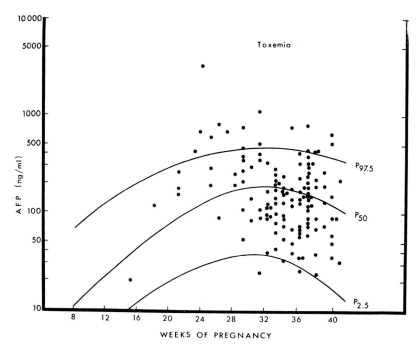

Figure 13-2.   Maternal AFP levels in toxemic pregnancies.

TABLE 13-V

HIGHEST INDIVIDUAL AFP LEVELS AND FETOPLACENTAL FUNCTION
IN PREGNANT WOMEN WITH TOXEMIA

| *AFP Level* | *Fetoplacental Function* | | *Association with* |
	Normal	*Severe Dysfunction*	*Fetal Distress of a Given AFP Level*
⩾97.5 percentile	1/54 (2)	9/22 (41)	9/10 (90)
>300 ng/ml	8/54 (15)	14/22 (64)	14/22 (64)

( ) Denotes percent.

thirty-six pregnancies with normal fetoplacental function had similar levels. An AFP concentration of 350 ng/ml or higher occurred in five out of nine pregnancies with fetal distress and in six out of thirty-six cases with normal fetoplacental function ($p > 0.05$) (Table 13-VI).

In diabetic pregnancies, of 164 samples, 106 were above the normal median (Fig. 13-4). Abnormally high AFP concentra-

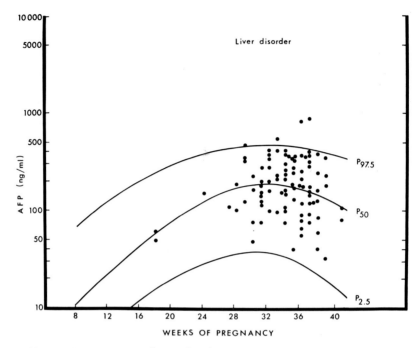

Figure 13-3. Maternal AFP levels in pregnancies with a maternal liver disorder.

TABLE 13-VI

HIGHEST INDIVIDUAL AFP LEVELS AND FETOPLACENTAL FUNCTION
IN PREGNANT WOMEN WITH LIVER DISORDER

AFP Level	Fetoplacental Function Normal	Severe Dysfunction	Association with Fetal Distress of a Given AFP Level
>97.5 percentile	2/36 (6)	2/9 (22)	2/4 (50)
>350 ng/ml	6/36 (17)	5/9 (56)	5/11 (45)

( ) Denotes percent.

TABLE 13-VII

HIGHEST INDIVIDUAL AFP LEVELS AND FETOPLACENTAL FUNCTION
IN PREGNANT WOMEN WITH DIABETES

AFP Level	Fetoplacental Function Normal	Severe Dysfunction	Association with Fetal Distress of a Given AFP Level
>97.5 percentile	0/20 (0)	4/14 (29)	4/4 (100)
>350 ng/ml	3/20 (15)	8/14 (57)	8/11 (73)

( ) Denotes percent.

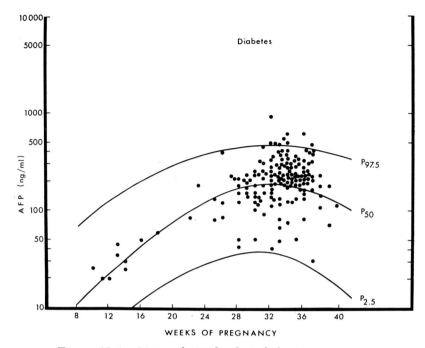

Figure 13-4.   Maternal AFP levels in diabetic pregnancies.

tions were present in four patients. All of these pregnancies were associated with severe fetoplacental dysfunction (Table 13-VII). The AFP concentration of 350 ng/ml or higher was associated with fetal distress in eight out of fourteen pregnancies and with normal fetoplacental function in three out of twenty pregnancies ($p < 0.05$). Consequently, a given value of 350 ng/ml or higher in diabetic pregnancies was associated with fetal distress in 73 percent of the cases, compared to the 37 percent occurrence of fetal distress in all diabetic pregnancies ($p < 0.05$).

Intrauterine fetal death was frequently associated with high maternal AFP concentrations (Fig. 13-5). Out of thirty pregnancies, the highest individual AFP levels exceeded the normal median in twenty-six and the levels were above the normal 97.5 percentile in eighteen individuals (60%). In most cases, the highest AFP concentrations were found after the fetus had died. In six pregnancies in which AFP was measured before the fetal death, abnormally high levels were present in four.

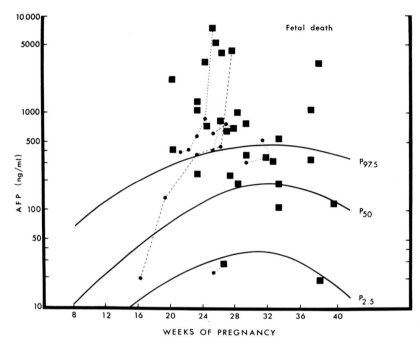

Figure 13-5. Maternal AFP levels in pregnancies associated with intra-uterine fetal death.

DISCUSSION

The mechanisms involved in the regulation of maternal AFP concentrations are not thoroughly understood. Since the fetal AFP levels even at term are still 300 to 600 times higher than the maternal levels,[7] all factors increasing the fetomaternal transfer of proteins are likely to increase the maternal AFP level. These include placental disorders and increased trans-amniotic passage of fetal elements to the mother. The latter mechanism may play a role especially during the second trimester, where the amniotic fluid AFP levels are high.[17]

An important question arising from the present results is whether there is variation in the fetal AFP levels in high risk pregnancies, and whether this can affect the maternal levels. Retarded maturation of the fetal liver is associated with high fetal AFP levels in mice.[18] In the case of the fetal lung, retarded maturation has been indicated in group A-C diabetes by the lecithin/sphingomyelin ratio. Whether the high maternal AFP levels in diabetic pregnancies indicate an ananlogous situation in the maturation of the fetal lung has been suggested to occur in hypertensive and toxemic pregnancies.[19] Our results showing low AFP levels in association with these complications may indicate that a similar condition occurs in the fetal liver. While more trivial mechanisms can be proposed to explain high AFP levels in diabetic pregnancies and low levels in hypertensive and toxemic pregnancies, variation of the biological timetable regarding differentiation of the fetal liver remains a possibility that merits attention.

Our results show that maternal AFP levels can be clinically important in identifying pregnancies at greater risk. A simple guess would point out fetal distress in 27 percent of toxemic pregnancies, while AFP levels exceeding the normal 97.5 percentile indicate pregnancies 90 percent of which are associated with fetal distress ($p < 0.001$). Calculated from the present data, the frequency in toxemia of incorrect classifications is 18.4 percent if the normal 97.5 percentile is used, and 21.1 percent if the level of 300 ng/ml is used.

As in the case of other biochemical parameters, AFP levels can indicate only certain types of fetoplacental disorders. Therefore, cumulative information of various parameters can serve as a more meaningful guide for obstetric decisions. Our recent findings[16] indicate that a combination of several parameters (e.g. maternal AFP and HPL levels) provides a better index for the assessment of fetoplacental function than either determination alone.

SUMMARY

Abnormally high maternal serum alpha₁-fetoprotein (AFP) levels were previously found in association with fetal distress and intrauterine fetal death. In a continuing analysis of high risk pregnancies, the maternal AFP levels appeared to be lower in hypertensive and toxemic pregnancies than if the maternal complication was diabetes or Rh-immunization. Irrespective of the type of maternal complication, high AFP levels were frequently associated with fetal distress.

The factors regulating maternal AFP levels include those affecting transplacental and transamniotic passage of fetal elements to the mother, while the role of fetal AFP levels in this regulation remains to be established. AFP is becoming increasingly important in the study of fetal differentiation.

Our results indicate that in certain cases maternal AFP levels may increase the cumulative efficacy of other biochemical methods available for antenatal fetal monitoring. However, the elevation of AFP in fetal distress is a late phenomenon and indicates that fetal life is severely jeopardized, while normal AFP levels cannot be relied upon to indicate that the fetus is doing well. These results also suggest the necessity of simultaneous analysis of both fetal and maternal AFP levels in various types of high risk pregnancies in order to achieve better understanding of the mechanisms regulating the synthesis and fetomaternal distribution of AFP.

REFERENCES

1. Bergstrand, C. G., and Czar, B.: Demonstration of a new protein fraction in serum from the human fetus. Scand J Clin Lab Invest, 8:174, 1956.
2. Gitlin, D., and Boesman, M.: Sites of serum α-fetoprotein synthesis in the human and in the rat. J Clin Invest, 46:1010, 1967.
3. Gitlin, D., and Boseman, M.: Serum α-fetoprotein, albumin and δG-globulin in the human conceptus. J Clin Invest, 45:1826, 1966.
4. Ruoslahti, E., and Seppälä, M.: Studies on carcino-fetal proteins: Physical and chemical properties of human α-fetoprotein. Int J Cancer, 7:218, 1971.
5. Ruoslahti, E., and Seppälä, M.: Studies on carcino-fetal proteins. III. Development of a radioimmunoassay for α-fetoprotein. Demonstration of α-fetoprotein in serum of healthy human adults. Int J Cancer, 8:374, 1971.
6. Ruoslahti, E., and Seppälä, M.: Normal and increased alpha-fetoprotein in neoplastic and non-neoplastic liver disease. Lancet, 2:278, 1972.
7. Seppälä, M., and Ruoslahti, E.: Radioimmunoassay of maternal serum alpha fetoprotein during pregnancy and delivery. Am J Obstet Gynecol, 112:208, 1972.

8. Seppälä, M., and Ruoslahti, E.: α-fetoprotein in normal and pregnancy sera. *Lancet, 1*:375, 1972.
9. Seppälä, M., and Ruoslahti, E.: Alpha fetoprotein in maternal serum: A new marker for detection of fetal distress and intrauterine death. *Am J Obstet Gynecol, 115*:48, 1973.
10. Cohen, H.; Graham, H., and Lau, H. L.: Alpha-1 fetoprotein in pregnancy. *Am J Obstet Gynecol, 115*:881, 1973.
11. Brock, D. J. H., and Sutcliffe, R. G.: Alpha-fetoprotein in antenatal diagnosis of anencephaly and spina bifida. *Lancet, 2*:197, 1972.
12. Seppälä, M., and Ruoslahti, E.: Alpha-fetoprotein in antenatal diagnosis. *Lancet, 1*:155, 1973.
13. Seppälä, M.: Increased alpha fetoprotein in amniotic fluid associated with a congenital esophageal atresia of the fetus. *Obstet Gynecol, 42*:613, 1973.
14. Seppälä, M., and Ruoslahti, E.: Alpha fetoprotein: Physiology and pathology during pregnancy and application to antenatal diagnosis. *J Perinatal Med, 1*:104, 1973.
15. Seppälä, M., and Ruoslahti, E.: Alpha fetoprotein in Rh-immunized pregnancies. *Obstet Gynecol, 42*:701, 1973.
16. Garoff, L., and Seppälä, M.: Alpha fetoprotein and placental lactogen levels in multiple pregnancies. *J Obstet Gynaec Br Commonw, 80*:695, 1973.
    press, 1973.
17. Seppälä, M., and Ruoslahti. E.: Alpha fetoprotein in amniotic fluid: An index of gestational age. *Am J Obstet Gynecol, 114*:595, 1979.
18. Coid, C. R., and Ramsden, D. B.: Retardation of foetal growth and plasma protein development in foetuses from mice injected with Coxackie B3 virus. *Nature* (Lond.), *241*:460, 1973.
19. Gluck, L., and Kulovich, M. V.: Lecithin/sphingomyelin ratios in amniotic fluid in normal and abnormal pregnancy. *Am J Obstet Gynecol, 115*:539, 1973.

SECTION IV

ANOMALIES OF
FETAL DEVELOPMENT

Chapter 14

EMBRYOLOGICAL BASIS OF ABNORMAL DEVELOPMENT WITH SPECIAL REFERENCE TO CELL DEATH

P. Gruenwald

INTRODUCTION

In its early days teratology was an armchair science: embryologists determined the time and manner of development of malformations based on their knowledge of normal stages of an organ.

One assumption was that during organogenesis some developmental step altered from its normal direction or intensity to produce a structural abnormality seen much later, usually at birth. A few instances have been known in which degeneration altered a part of the body which had developed normally during organogenesis, but it was not realized until fairly recently that this is one of the most common mechanisms in teratogenesis. There are many instances in which abnormal organogenesis as postulated in the early days must have occurred. Either truncus arteriosus communis or transposition of the great vessels must arise at the time when the early truncus arteriosus would normally divide into the aorta and the pulmonary artery. Other examples could readily be adduced. However, examination of actual embryonic stages of hereditary or experimental malformations in animals has shown that in many instances degenerative changes, usually cell death, alter the structure of parts which originally had been formed normally. These secondary changes

251

can occur at any time, from early embryonic stages to late fetal life, or to degenerative diseases in later life. The present account will deal with this manner of pathogenesis of abnormalities up to and including the neonatal period.

CAUSES OF MALDEVELOPMENT

Circumstances which trigger development of malformations are basically the same for primary aberrations of organogenesis as well as secondary, degenerative ones. In both forms, genetic and environmental causes are recognized. Genetic factors occur in man spontaneously by mutation, and the environmental ones inadvertently by radiation, chemicals, drugs, pollutants, or other poisons. In experimental animals, genetic traits may be pinpointed by breeding or environmental agents which are administered under controlled conditions. In such animals, series of embryonic stages can be examined, or the interaction of synergistic and antagonistic factors investigated. Differences between species and even strains are considerable, and the applicability of details of experimental results to man is limited even though the principles are the same.

Genetic Causes

An increasing number of gene mutations have been subjected to embryologic study. In many instances degeneration of previously well-formed parts has been documented. The embryology of chromosomal abnormalities of vertebrates is not known, but it is likely that they lead to secondary degeneration. This could be true of those chromosome imbalances which are found with considerable frequency among spontaneous early abortions.[18, 64]

In genetically as well as environmentally mediated abnormalities, development may not be visibly abnormal until long after the particular structures are well-formed, then, a "time bomb" effect of tissue destruction sets in at a specific stage. Genetic and environmental factors may influence each other, one enhancing or reducing the effect of the other. This was demonstrated by the effect of chemical teratogens on mouse embryos heterozygous for the defect of the caudal end of the body due to the *brachyury* gene, enhancing the effect of the gene under circumstances which they would otherwise not be teratogenic.[127] Excessive cell death occurred in these experiments.

Environmental Agents

Any conceivable kind of environmental influence may be teratogenic, and many cause degenerative changes. In some instances the mode of action is quite mysterious, for instance, the abnormalities in the offspring of "stressed" mice.[52] Best known are the visible effects of ionizing radiation and of chemicals, particularly cytotoxic agents such as those used in cancer chemotherapy. Infectious diseases, particularly viruses affect the embryo; however, many potent teratogens do not produce recognizable disease in the mother. More and more "sporadic" abnormalities manifested by degeneration before or after birth, have been recognized as caused by drugs, pollutants or viruses.

PATHOGENESIS

Various proven or postulated mechanisms of teratogenesis are shown diagrammatically in Figure 14-1. We are concerned here with the mechanism indicated by the last line as it applies to prenatal life and the neonatal period.

Many investigators have addressed themselves to the question, "What determines the kind of malformation produced by an environmental agent: time of action vs. nature of the agent?" At one time it was suggested that the embryo is not capable of specific reaction, and that only the pattern of sensitivity existing at the time, and perhaps the intensity of the insult determines the result. It is now clear that considerable specificity exists as to the effect of one agent or another. Yet the timing of teratogenic action along with the nature of the agent is of paramount importance. The effects of the reacting agent change very rapidly, by day or hour, during early development.

Cell death is a normal morphogenetic process. Its widespread distribution in normal embryos has been reviewed by Ernst[29] and Glücksmann.[34] Källen[65] studied cell death in the brains of nine to fifteen-day rabbit embryos, and Saunders[101] discussed in

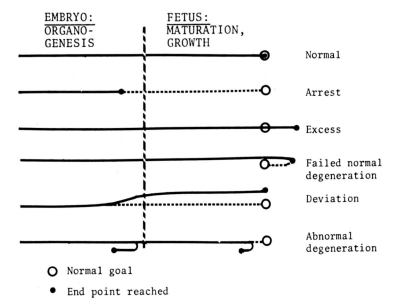

Figure 14-1.   Diagram of various mechanisms in the pathogenesis of malformations. The one dealt with in this review is indicated on the bottom
line. Contrary to others, this mechanism, or at least its visible manifestation, can be initiated at any time.

depth the problems involved, largely on the basis of the avian
wing bud which he had investigated by a variety of methods.
Schweichel and Merker[108] studied normal and teratogen-induced
embryonic cell death by electron microscopy. Its role in over-all
teratogenesis has been discussed by Zwilling,[131] Beck and Lloyd[6]
and Saxén and Rapola.[103] A review by Menkes, *et al.*[85] deals in
great detail with embryonic stages, but does not consider later
(fetal) occurrence of the process. Goerttler[36] reviewed disease
processes in the embryo and fetus, including necrosis, as basic
mechanisms from the point of view of the pathologist.

   Blebs, clear or hemorrhagic. In some instances regressive
changes are ushered in, or become apparent by blebs filled with
clear fluid or blood. This is followed by defects in the same
areas. This mechanism acquired some notoriety when Bonnevie
stated in 1934,[11] after studying the embryogenesis of defects in

the limbs and other parts of Little and Bagg's mutant mouse strain, that the blebs at first had clear contents and consisted of cerebrospinal fluid which had left the myelencephalon in abnormal amounts via the foramen anterius. Plagens had previously[94] described these blebs and considered them as local occurrences, and their origin from cerebrospinal fluid was discredited by Jost[62] and Carter.[20] However, the pediatrician Ullrich had theorized in 1938[122] that many malformations are due to Bonnevie's myelencephalic blebs, and this gave rise to the "status Bonnevie-Ullrich." The concept was used rather indiscriminately by Ullrich and others to explain, without knowledge of developmental stages, a staggering variety of malformations. It is hoped that this monstrous concept is no longer perpetuated.

The existence of clear or hemorrhagic blebs in the early phases of degeneration has been documented in many instances. Greene and Saxton[41] described the sequence of vascular dilatation, hemorrhage, necrosis and sloughing in a mutant strain of rabbits with defects of the feet, outer ears, nose and eyes, similar to Little and Bagg's mice. Radio-cobalt treatment of pregnant hamsters produces blisters in the embryos which lead to defects.[55] Vascular changes with hemorrhagic necrosis were produced in mouse embryos by salycylates[75] and in chick embryos by lead compounds.[69] Deficiency of linoleic acid[83] and of pantothenic acid[32] has similar effects. Mitomycin C causes oligodactyly by necrosis and hematomas of the limb primordia in mice.[119]

During the last twenty years Jost[63] experimented with the effect of vasopressor substances transmitted transplacentally to rat and rabbit embryos. He came to the conclusion that vascular changes leading to hemorrhagic blebs and eventual defects, are caused by these substances which change the partition of the blood volume between fetus and placenta. The ensuing congestion leads to changes in areas of predilection (Fig. 14-2). This challenging concept does not exclude the possibility of the reverse sequence, namely, necrosis followed by hemorrhage, in other circumstances.

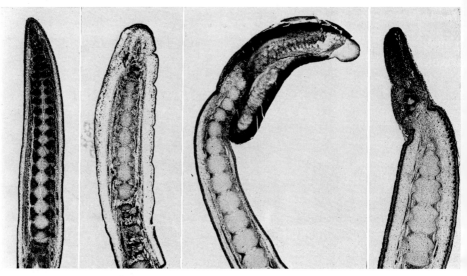

Figure 14-2.   Changes in the tail of rat fetuses after treatment with a vasopressor. From left to right: control; edema six hours after injection; hemorrhagic blister and necrosis twenty-two hours after injection; demarcation four days after injection. From Jost, with permission of author and The International Medical Congress Ltd., 1964.)

Early Embryonic Stages; Defects of the Caudal Parts of the Body

Degeneration in early stages of development occurs particularly in those hereditary abnormalities which are dominant for a viable malformation in heterozygous form, but lethal in the homozygous state. Best studied with regard to embryonic stages are mutations producing tail defects in the mouse (at the t locus), rumplessness in the chick, and their teratogen-induced phenocopies. Bennett[3] reviewed a large volume of research on the embryonic stages of mouse embryos homozygous for various t alleles. Necrosis occurring in the neural tube, somites and mesenchmye are described in detail in some of the reports mentioned in that review. The mechanisms involved in the morphogenesis may not all involve cell death. Differences in the morphogenesis of these and other mutants affecting the tail cannot be deduced from the appearance of late stages seen at birth. The lethal homozygous condition varies according to the allele involved; some die as early as the morula stage; while others never develop the caudal portion of the body, perhaps because of degeneration of part of the primitive streak. Actinomycin D produces phenocopies of some of the features of homozygotes, including cell death, when given to heterozygotes in doses not teratogenic in normal mice.[127]

The role of cell death has been clearly demonstrated in two mutations causing rumplessness (tail defects) in chick embryos. In dominant rumplessness the presumptive tail tissue degenerates before differentiating, by exaggeration of cell death normally going on in the region of the cloaca. Zwilling's[129] diagrams are shown here in Figure 14-3. In recessive rumplessness, on the other hand, the tissues first differentiate and then degenerate, at later stages than in the dominant form.[130] Here again, phenocopies can be produced by actinomycin D; degeneration occurs in the undifferentiated mesoderm or trunk-tail node, and the level of the ensuing defect depends on the timing of treatment.[93]

Grüneberg[46] compiled a list of forty-two mutants in the mouse which affect early development up to day fourteen. Experimentally, selective necrosis of somites follows administration of high doses of vitamin A to pregnant hamsters on the eighth day.[81]

Regarding the early stages of sporadic malformations, particularly those in man, we are almost completely in the dark. An accidental observation by Politzer and Sternberg[95] concerns a very well-preserved 6-mm human embryo which had numerous malformations and was irregularly arrested in development so that various primordia were judged to correspond to normal stages at 0 to 30 pairs of somites. The mesenchyme contained many necrotic cells, including large numbers in the trunk-tail-node. This may have been the result of a lethal mutation; the same may be suggested for the many misshapen small embryos in "blighted" ova. These are not sufficiently well-preserved when expelled to allow satisfactory examination. Prolonged survival of the placenta may make chromosome analysis possible after death of the embryo.

Extra-embryonic structures regularly undergo degeneration as part of normal development. Part of the primary yolk sac of the human embryo degenerates, leaving a much smaller,

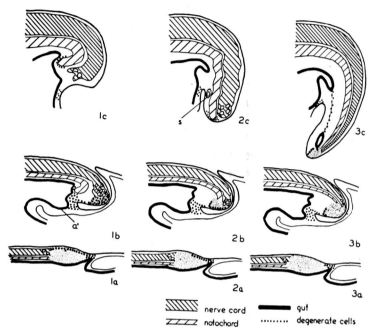

Figure 14-3. Diagrammatic sagittal sections illustrating the important morphological events in the development of rumpless embryos. 1, extreme rumplessness; 2, intermediate rumplessness; 3, normal; a, latter part of second day incubation; b, latter part of third day; c, latter part of fourth day; s, abortive somite; a, allantoic diverticulum. Fine stippling indicates the indifferent tail mass. Small circles in distal portion of the nerve cords represent multiple canals. (From Zwilling, by permission of *Genetics*, 1942.)

definitive yolk sac.[59] The inverted yolk sac placenta of rodents owes its existence to disappearance of the parietal wall of the yolk sac. In man, chorionic villi degenerate over the greater part of the chorionic surface, leaving the chorion laeve, except in the area of the definitive placental disc.

The Nervous System

The intricacies of structure and function of the nervous system pose numerous problems regarding development and disease that do not exist in other organs. The seriousness of relatively small defects is due to the inability of parts to compensate for loss of others, as might occur, for instance, in the liver. Part of the complexity of development is an intricate pattern of cell death, partly predetermined and partly influenced by the internal environment. Amputation in the embryo of a part such as a limb[51] or eye primordium[23] is followed by excessive cell death in related nuclei and ganglia; whereas, implantation of an additional limb causes more cells to persist. In normal development, necrosis of scattered cells is seen,[9, 34, 65] as well as the formation of cavities.[43] Postnatally, cell loss as determined by counts continues into old age.[15] A tremendous volume of information on teratology of the nervous system has been collected by Innes and Saunders[61] and Kalter.[66]

Genetic traits. Some traits affecting the neural tube in early stages were mentioned in the preceding section. Hereditary cerebellar atrophy with death of Purkinje cells occurs in lambs.[123] Interestingly, cerebellar ataxia of kittens which had been thought to be hereditary, is now known to be of viral origin. Degeneration of ganglion cells in the anterior horns of the spinal cord of dogs, presumably beginning shortly after birth, was described by Stockard[116] as a genetic trait. Hereditary demyelination, usually in the first few weeks after birth, occurs in several mutants of mice.[40, 71] Sidman *et al.*[112] compared similar end results in one strain with deficient myelin formation and one in which there was also destruction of myelin. Another comparison of a mouse strain with faulty myelination and one in the rabbit with degeneration was made by Anderson and Harman.[2]

Radiation and chemical agents. Necrosis caused by ionizing radiation has been documented in many studies as reviewed by D'Agostino and Brizzee[24] and Hicks and D'Amato.[60] A variety of malformations following irradiation are seen in late stages, but the pathogenesis of many of these is not known. This is also true of human malformations following therapeutic doses of x-rays during pregnancy.[37] Attempted restitution after cell loss leads to abnormal shape and architecture including formation of rosettes. Very similar effects follow the treatment of pregnant animals with toxic chemicals, including cancer-therapeutic drugs; 6-AN,[21] hydroxyurea,[109] monosodium glutamate,[89] or in vitamin

deficiency.[16, 111]   In chick embryos, hypoxia[39] or administration
of lead compounds[69, 82] cause degenerative changes in the brain.
In man and animals, fetal and neonatal asphyxia presumably
cause similar changes, but characteristic early stages are not
readily observed except in experiments.[126] At necropsy, some
time after the insult, one sees opaque areas of necrosis, usually
in the paraventricular white matter of the hemispheres, or cavities
in various parts of the telencephalon and mesencephalon. In
addition, degeneration in the fetal brain is caused by methyl-
mercury (fetal Minamata disease),[54, 84] lead poisoning,[53] carbon
monoxide poisoning in the attempted suicide of the mother,[50, 77]
or hypoglycemia.[4] In the neonatal period Kernicterus caused by
hyperbilirubinemia destroys ganglion cells.

Infectious agents. While infectious diseases such as syphilis
or toxoplasmosis are known to affect the fetal brain, sometimes
very seriously, viral infections pose further problems. Those
involving the cerebellum will be discussed separately. Early
stages with necrosis followed inocculation of Newcastle disease
virus at thirty-six to eighty-four hours of incubation. Microscopic
examination one day later[97] involved, in addition to lesions in
other organs, the dorsal portion of the neural tube. Later stages
with necrosis and rarefaction resulting in porencephaly or hydranencephaly at birth, were produced in fetal lambs by bluetongue
vaccine virus.[92] Fetal or neonatal inocculation of several species
of rodents with rat virus resulted in hemorrhagic encephalopathy.[79] In man, intrauterine infection with cytomegalovirus
results in tissue destruction. One example of severe damage was
described by Haymaker, *et al.*[56]

Pathologic manifestations. Hemorrhages and hemorrhagic
blebs as discussed above, are seen in early stages of cerebral
degeneration in some instances quoted here. Generally, the
appearance of necrosis is similar in both genetic and environmental instances. It can be recognized only when nuclear debris
is present, either free or within macrophages. If necrosis occurs
adjacent to a ventricle or the central canal, debris may be seen
in the lumen. This occurs in chick embryos containing selenium
compounds from the laying hen's diet.[44] Figure 14-4 shows
examples of necrosis caused by selenium compounds in the brain,

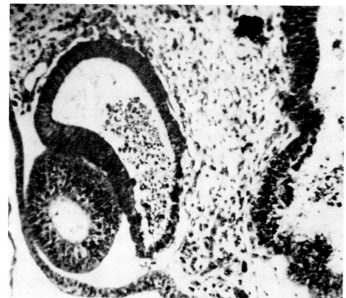

Figure 14-4.   Necrosis caused by selenium compounds transmitted to the egg by the laying hen. *a*, 3½-day embryo: note extensive destruction in the diencephalon (right) and the optic cup (left), with necrotic debris in the lumen. *b*, 4-day embryo: cell loss in the mid-lateral portions of the spinal cord, with some remnants of necrotic material. Mesenchymal cells growing across the central canal, partially obliterating it.

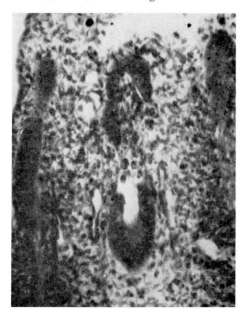

spinal cord, and optic cup. The section of spinal cord shows a late stage in which cells from the eroded surfaces grow across the central canal. The same process produces stenosis or obliteration of the aqueduct resulting in hydrocephalus, a hereditary form in the mouse,[22] a virus-induced form in rodents[78] and sporadically in man.[33]

In many species of mammals, the cerebellum has a peculiar sensitivity to noxious agents. Numerous viruses produce cerebellar degeneration[80] (Figure 14-5). In human neonates degeneration of Purkinje cells in the cerebellar cortex is, perhaps, the most readily ascertained effect of asphyxia. Some of these changes, particularly those induced by viruses, are phenocopies of hereditary traits. Ataxia of kittens, once thought to be hereditary, is now recognized as viral.[80]

If loss of tissue is very extensive, the entire hemispheres may

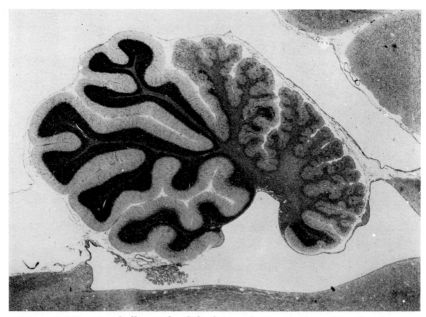

Figure 14-5. Cerebellum of adult ferret demonstrating abruptly demarcated anterior zone of the hypoplastic cortex (right) and contrasting posterior zone of spared cortex (left) following neonatal infection with feline panleukopenia virus. From Margolis, *et al.* (1971) with permission of authors and Grune and Stratton.

be reduced to barely visible remnants attached to the meninges (Fig. 14-6). This porencephaly, schizencephaly, or hydranencephaly cannot be a primary failure of development as shown by the shape of the hemispheres and the cranium.

A peculiar form of secondary change which affects a previously normal feature is the re-opening of the lumen of the central nervous system to the body surface. This was first described as a "brain catastrophe," an hereditary trait in mice,[12] and more recently in vincristine-treated rat fetuses.[88] In human anencephaly and open myelocele of whatever origin, the nervous tissue is completely, or nearly absent from the exposed areas at birth. It is generally accepted, and supported by examination of embryonic stages, that the neural plate is present at first and, according to some, even abnormally large and degenerates later, presumably under the macerating influence of amniotic fluid.

The Eyes

Two components of the eyes, the retina and the lens, are frequently sites of degenerative changes during development. Normally cell death occurs in the optic cup and lens placode of rat embryos;[34] seven specific sites were recently distinguished.[113]

The retina. The optic cup develops from the diencephalon, and both may be affected by noxious agents in early stages (Fig. 14-4).

In rodents and rabbits several genetic traits produce a rodless retina. This arises in some forms by failure of the rod cells to develop, and in others by degeneration of these cells after they have differentiated more or less fully. A phenocopy has been producd in rabbits with sodium iodoacetate. The entire subject has been reviewed by Karli.[68]

X-rays have a deleterious effect on the retina of embryos, fetuses and neonates. In the newborn rat necrosis is followed by the formation of rosettes.[35] Hall[49] found similar changes in rat fetuses after x-ray, as well as urethane treatment. Rosettes are also present in the eyes of human fetuses accidentally given therapeutic doses of x-rays.[38]

A variety of infectious agents, particularly viruses, affect the

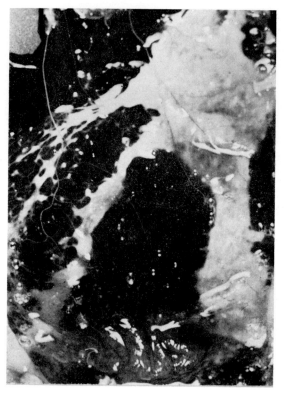

Figure 14-6. Part of a cerebral hemisphere of a newborn infant with nearly normal head size. The tissue consists of meninges with thin remnants of nervous tissue attached. *a,* gross appearance of a portion spread out; *b,* microscopic section of a similar area: at one point no nervous tissue is left along the meninges.

fetal retina. Silverstein, *et al.*[114] produced retinal dystrophy in lamb fetuses by bluetongue virus. In man, cytomegalovirus infection acquired *in utero* is known to result in chorioretinitis.[7] In this respect and others, toxoplasmosis may have similar effects on the human fetus.

The lens. Hereditary cataract has been found in many mammals such as the mouse,[25] dog[1] and cattle.[42]

The literature on radiation-induced cataract has been reviewed by Rugh, *et al.*;[97] a detailed morphologic study in man and several mammalian species was undertaken by Geeraets.[31]

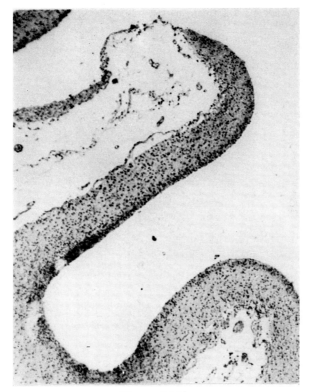

Figure 14-6b.

That viruses can cause prenatal cataract, is now well known through the effect of rubella in human pregnancy.[10, 120] Two studies involving the experimental induction of cataract by viruses include that of Scheidegger[105] who used ectromelia, psittacosis and rabies virus in chick embryos, and Levitt, *et al.*[76] who infected monkey fetuses at 97 to 104 days *in utero* with Venezuelan equine encephalitis virus, obtaining cataracts as well as hydro-cephalus.

Chemical disturbances producing fetal cataracts include excessive galactose feeding[5] and urethane administration[49] to pregnant mice, and hypoxia in the rat.[124]

The Inner Ears

Two areas have been explored in depth: genetic changes in the mouse leading to disturbed vestibular function, and viral effects in man resulting in deafness. Examples of the former are the "shaker—1",[47] "spinner"[28] and "waltzer"[27] mutants of the mouse. Kocher[72] compared the pathologic changes in eight mutants, and concluded that degeneration occurs from the suckling period to old age, depending on the mutation involved.

Rubella of the human fetus has long been known to cause deafness. Töndury and Smith[120] demonstrated degeneration in the inner ear; this was subsequently confirmed by Schall, *et al.*,[104] Kelemen and Gotlib[70] and others.

Teeth

The tooth germ, particularly the enamel epithelium while it forms enamel, is exquisitely sensitive to extrinsic influences, so much so that the normal birth process leaves a mark of slight enamel hypoplasia, the neonatal line, in every infant. Many agents cause reversible or irreversible degeneration of the enamel epithelium, leading either to interruption or cessation of enamel formation, or to the production of abnormal masses of enamel instead of normal rods. If interruption of enamel formation is reversible, a line is produced within the enamel which is visible on section (Fig. 14-7). If no further enamel is formed, a hypoplastic band encircles the crowns of the deciduous teeth, followed, in apical direction, by new formation from undamaged enamel epithelium. It may be possible to estimate the time of insult from the thickness of subsequently formed enamel. In the continuously erupting teeth of rodents, similar changes may be produced later in life as well. A variety of agents produce similar effects in man[45, 73] and in experimental animals.[74] This is one of the few examples where a variety of noxious agents such as fetal and perinatal distress,[45] infection with rubella in man[120] or experimental animals,[74] or chemical agents,[107, 125] produce qualitatively similar results, with only localization depending on the time of action.

Digestive Tract

The digestive canal is formed in the earliest embryonic stages. In the process of formation of the body from the flat germinal disc, it separates from the yolk sac, first as the fore- and hind-gut

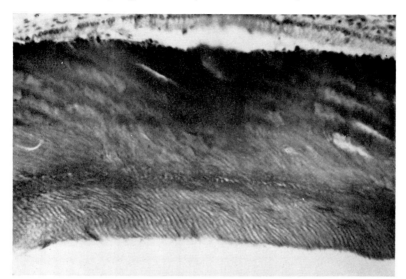

Figure 14-7. Enamel of a tooth germ from the mandible of a newborn infant with multiple areas of old tissue destruction in the brain, kidneys, and spleen. The space at the bottom is an artifact separating enamel from dentine. At the top is the enamel epithelium. At the lower third of the enamel is a double line. The thickness of the enamel above that line, formed after the injury, allows timing at about two months before birth.

connecting with the yolk sac lumen by the anterior and posterior intestinal portals. Eventually, as the portals approach each other, only a narrow duct connects the completed canal briefly with the yolk sac. Thus, since a patent digestive tube must exist in early stages, any atresia is a secondary change. In the esophagus, atresias may be related to the separation from the respiratory tract; in the stomach they are very rare.

Duodenum. Atresia is relatively common, its explanation complicated by the fact that it is the only part of the intestine which is occluded for a time by epithelial proliferation. Among others, Boyden, *et al.*[14] based their explanation of duodenal atresia on abnormal canalization of this occluding epithelium. If this explanation is at all valid, it does not apply to the rest of the intestine, even though similar atresias occur there as well.

Jejunum, ileum, colon. Atresias occur at any level, sometimes multiple, in the form of diaphragms across the lumen, or as a solid cord connecting the proximal and distal lumina, or complete interruption. Only a few among the vast number of papers dealing with this subject are mentioned here. Bernstein, et al.[8] examined the association with cystic fibrosis of the pancreas which was then well established, and suggested that secondary to meconium ileus, meconium infiltrates the intestinal wall from ulcerations and thus leads to scarring. As alternative explanations they suggested extrinsic scarring from meconium peritonitis, or necrosis caused by volvulus. Santulli and Blanc[100] thought that volvulus, pinching-off of the umbilical hernia, intussuspection, or other occlusion of mesenteric blood supply causes necrosis and complete disappearance of segments of bowel; this explains the reduced length of the intestine in some cases. The most extensive loss of bowel results when the entire umbilical loop, including part of the jejunum, the entire ileum, and part of the colon is cut off when the umbilical herina closes. This was described long ago by Misgeld,[87] and several similar cases have since been reported.

The stage at which the previously normal bowel may become atretic is attested to by the presence distal to the atresia, of cornified squames derived from vernix caseosa. These must have been swallowed, and moved past the level in question by peristalsis before the lumen was occluded.[30]

A mutation manifested by atresia of the colon in horses is on record but its pathogenesis is unknown.[128]

An unusual instance of complete loss of intestinal lumen and mucosa from the beginning of the jejunum to the ampulla of the rectum is known.[86] Only muscularis with a solid core of submucosa was present throughout the entire length. The ampulla of the rectum contained meconium (not histologically verified). What noxious agent could have caused nearly the entire intestinal mucosa to disappear is unknown.

Many attempts at producing intestinal atresia surgically in mammalian fetuses have been successful. Healing occurs with minimal scarring unless there is extravasation of meconium. As one example, experimental occlusion of mesenteric blood supply may be mentioned.[121]

Liver. Basically similar considerations apply to atresia of bile ducts as to intestinal atresia. While the development of intrahepatic bile ducts is more complex, it is true that the existence of hepatic parenchyma is predicated on the existence of a duct system in the early embryo; atresia, therefore, must be due to secondary obliteration. Liver cell necrosis occurs in the fetus, postnatally, under the influence of chemical and infectious agents. Gestational rubella in man may affect both liver cells and bile ducts, leading to giant cell hepatitis, focal liver cell necrosis, cholangitis, and fibrosis.[117]

Pancreas. In cystic fibrosis, prenatal changes are usually limited to distension of ducts with abnormal secretion. Whether mild fibrosis indicates past destruction of parenchyma, is not clear. Complete atrophy and disappearance of the exocrine portion takes years after birth.

Urogenital Tract

Gonads. Prenatal degeneration, rather than primary absence of germ cells in ovaries of XO females, has been suggested because of the presence of these cells in early stages.[19] Selective destruction of germ cells in the embryo is caused by certain drugs.[57, 58]

Genital ducts. Normal degeneration and its hormonal modification in the wolffian and müllerian ducts in the female and male, respectively, has been studied by many authors. Recently it has been discovered that sterility of males with cystic fibrosis of the pancreas is due to interruption of the ductus deferentes.[67] The presence of wolffian ducts in early stages is proven by the presence of kidneys; the atresia, therefore, must be due to secondary degeneration.

Kidneys. Oliver[90] examined cystic kidneys by microdissection, and concluded that in some (perhaps not all) forms there is "regressive dysplasia which results in atresias, atrophies and disruptions."

Skin

Two forms of lesions suggest secondary prenatal changes in previously normal skin; congenital skin defects or ulcers, and scars presumably associated with amniotic adhesions. Changes in underlying tissues occur particularly in the latter form. Hereditary hairlessness in the mouse develops long after birth.

Congenital skin defects occur particularly in the midline of the scalp and on the extremities. Since the surrounding and underlying tissues are normal, it is difficult to conceive that these lesions might be primary aplasias rather than secondary defects. Very severe epidermolysis bullosa, fatal shortly after birth, has been regarded as a lethal form of the hereditary disease.[26] Hereditary skin defects present at birth occur in cattle.[48] Ulcerated lesions of virus diseases such as smallpox can develop *in utero*, as reviewed by Schick.[106]

Defects that were demonstrated or assumed to be associated with amniotic adhesions have intrigued teratologists for a long time. Within a short period of time, scientists in three countries came to the conclusion that these adhesions occur at the site of pre-existing skin defects, and do not cause them.[91, 110, 118] In most instances, deep tissues are affected and sometimes extensive defects such as "congenital amputations" are present. Owing to a lack of specific tissue reaction in the fetus, and the time elapsed when changes are seen at birth, there is no factual information on the pathogenesis.

Limbs

Complex patterns of cell death in limb buds are among the processes responsible for normal development of the extremities, including the formation of distinct digits.[101, 102] The effects of excessive, abnormally located necrosis range from abnormal separation of digits to severe defects of large parts of the limbs.

Two forms of necrosis occur: (1) excessive numbers of necrotic cells depopulating the limb bud or, at later stages, portions of it, and (2) hemorrhage as described above under the heading of blebs. Prior to the appearance of mesenchymal condensations such as primordia of the skeleton, only the first of these forms has been observed. This occurs as a result of chemical insults such as those caused by selenium compounds[44] (Fig. 14-8) or nitrogen mustard[99] in chick embryos, or cytosine arabinoside in rat embryos.[96] In later stages, when the skeleton has begun

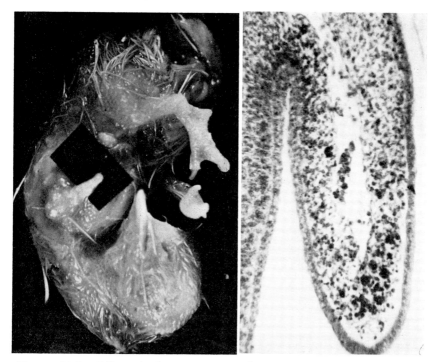

Figure 14-8.   Effect of selenium compounds transmitted to the egg by the laying hen, on the limbs of chick embryos. *a*, gross deformities in an embryo that failed to hatch; *b*, limb bud of a 4-day embryo with extensive necrosis appearing as loss of cells, and nuclear debris lying free or contained in macrophages.

to form as condensations of mesenchyme, hemorrhagic necrosis occurs in hereditary abnormalities with hemorrhagic blebs (see above). Jost's theory that extreme hyperemia resulting from maldistribution of blood between fetus and placenta produces these hemorrhages, may apply to hereditary forms as well.[63] Singh and Singh[115] found similar effects after amniocentesis, Giroud, *et al.*[32] in experimental pantothenic acid deficiency in the rat, and Takano[119] after treatment with mitomycin C in the mouse. In still later stages cell death occurs in the more or less well differentiated cartilaginous skelton, for instance after insulin administration to chick embryos;[132] or chlorambucil treatment,[17] or riboflavin deficiency accentuated by galactoflavin[111] in the rat.

Very late defects, once thought to be due to amputation by amniotic bands, occur in bizarre, sometimes familial forms. In the section on skin, mention was made of the possibility that amniotic adhesions associated with these defects, may be secondary to some other tissue damage.

CONCLUSION

This chapter has been limited to one mechanism in the pathogenesis of malformations, namely, secondary degeneration of previously well-formed parts. The causes are genetic, environmental, or unknown. The changes, usually in the form of cell death if the acute phase is observed, occur at a specific time in each form from the earliest embryonic stages on. While examples quoted here are limited to the embryonic, fetal, and neonatal period, similar changes are known to occur throughout the life span up to old age, including degenerative diseases and some aspects of the aging process itself.

In order to prevent these degenerative changes, one must learn their causes, and this is the principal challenge. Developmental genetics, epidemiology, toxicology (including the effects of drugs, pollutants and other poisons), and microbiology (particularly virology) all play a role in such endeavors. Within the last few years a viral etiology has been determined for degenerative diseases occurring at widely different points of the life span: ataxia of kittens and kuru.

Conditions generally considered as malformations are not necessarily caused by deviations of organogenesis, but may be closely related in their etiology and pathogenesis to mechanisms usually envisaged in pathology. It is time to drop the arbitrary borderline between teratology and pathology; yet the embryo and fetus need special consideration for several reasons: (1) basic developmental processes are interfered with in early life, (2) the reactions to extrinsic pathogens and to cell death itself differ from those of the older individual, and (3) the consequences tend to be more far-reaching the earlier an abnormality occurs.

REFERENCES

1. Anderson, A. C., and Shultz, F. T.: Inherited (congenital) cataract in the dog. *Am J Pathol, 34*:965, 1958.
2. Anderson, F. D., and Harman, P. J.: Neurohistology of two mammalian mutations. *Neurology, 11*:676, 1961.
3. Bennett, D.: Abnormalities associated with a chromosome region in the mouse. II. Embryological effects of letha lalleles in the t-region. *Science, 144*:263, 1964.
4. Banker, B. Q.: The neuropathological effects of anoxia and hypoglycemia in the newborn. *Develop Med Child Neurol, 9*:544, 1967.
5. Bannon, S. I.; Higginbottom, R. M.; McConnell, J. M., and Kaan, H. W.: Development of galactose cataract in the albino rat embryo. *Arch Ophthalmol, 33*:224, 1945.
6. Beck, F., and Lloyd, J. B.: Embryological principles of teratogenesis. In Robson, J. M., and Smith, R. L. (Eds.): *Embryopathic Activity of Drugs.* Boston, Little, 1965, p. 1.
7. Berenberg, W., and Nankervis, G.: Long-term follow-up of cytomegalic inclusion disease of infancy. *Pediatrics, 46*:403, 1970.
8. Bernstein, J.; Vawter, G.; Harris, G. B. C.; Young, V., and Hillman, L. S.: The occurrence of intestinal atresia in newborns with meconium ileus: the pathogenesis of an acquired anomaly. *Am J Dis Child, 99*:804, 1960.
9. Bodian, D.: Spontaneous degeneration in the spinal cord of monkey fetuses. *Bull Johns Hopkins Hosp, 119*:212, 1966.
10. Boniuk, M., and Zimmerman, L. E.: Ocular pathology in the rubella syndrome. *Arch Ophthalmol, 77*:455, 1967.
11. Bonnevie, K.: Embryological analysis of gene manifestation in Little and Bagg's abnormal mouse tribe. *J Exp Zool, 67*:443, 1934.
12. Bonnevie, K.: Pseudencephalie als spontane recessive (?) Mutation bei der Hausmaus. *Skr Norske Vidensk Akad Oslo, Math-nat Kl.9*, 39, 1936. (Quoted by Grüneberg, H.: *The Genetics of the Mouse.* Cambridge, University Press, 1943).
13. Bourne, M. C., and Grüneberg, H.: Degeneration of the retina and catract, a new recessive gene in the rat (*Rattus norvegicus*). *J Hered, 30*:131, 1939.
14. Boyden, E. A.; Cope, J. G., and Bill, Jr., A. H.: Anatomy and embryology of congenital intrinsic obstruction of the duodenum. *Am J Surg, 114*:190, 1967.
15. Brody, H.: Organization of the cerebral cortex. III. A study of aging in the human cerebral cortex. *J Comp Neurol, 102*:511, 1955.
16. Brown, E. E.; Fudge, J. F., and Richardson, L. R.: Diet of mother and brain hemorrhages in infant rats. *J Nutr, 34*:141, 1947.

17. Brummett, E. S.: Alterations in the developing fetal rat limb follow-
    ing administration of chlorambucil to the maternal animal. *Anat
    Rec, 172*:279, 1972.

18. Carr, D. H.: Chromosome studies in spontaneous abortions. *Obstet
    Gynecol, 26*:308, 1965.

19. Carr, D. H.; Haggar, R. A., and Hart, A. G.: Germ cells in the ovaries
    of XO female infants. *Am J Clin Pathol, 49*:521, 1968.

20. Carter, T. C.: Embryology of the Little & Bagg x-rayed mouse stock.
    J Genet, 56:401, 1959.

21. Chamberlain, J. C.: Early neurovascular abnormalities underlying
    6-aminonicotinamide (6-AN)-induced congenital hydrocephalus
    in rats. *Teratol, 3*:377, 1970.

22. Clark, F. H.: Anatomical basis of hereditary hydrocephalus in the
    house mouse. *Anat Rec, 58*:225, 1934.

23. Cowan, W. M., and Wenger, E.: Degeneration in the nucleus of
    origin of the preganglionic fibers of the chick ciliary ganglion
    following early removal of the optic vesicle. *J Exp Zool, 168*:105,
    1968.

24. D'Agostino, A. N., and Brizzee, K. R.: Radiation necrosis and repair
    in rat fetal cerebral hemisphere. *Arch Neurol, 15*:615, 1966.

25. Davidorf, F., and Eglitis, I.: A study of a hereditary catract in the
    mouse. *J Morphol, 119*:89, 1966.

26. Davidson, L. T.: Hereditary epidermolysis bullosa: report of a case
    with a résumé of the literature. *Am J Dis Child, 59*:371, 1940.

27. Deol, M. S., and Green, M. C.: Snell's waltzer, a new mutation
    affecting behaviour and the inner ear in the mouse. *Genet Res,
    8*:339, 1966.

28. Deol, M. S., and Robins, M. W.: The spinner mouse. *J Hered,
    53*:133, 1962.

29. Ernst, M.: Ueber den Untergang von Zellen während er normalen
    Entwicklung bei Wirbeltieren. *Zeitschr, f Anat Entwicklungsgesch,
    79*:228, 1926.

30. Fanconi, G.: Fünf Fälle von angeborenem Darmverschluss: Dünn-
    darmatresien, Duodenalstenose, Meconiumileus. *Virchows Arch,
    229*:207, 1921.

31. Geeraets, W. J.: Radiation cataract: biomicroscopic observations in
    rabbit, monkey and man. *Med Coll Virginia Quart, 8*:259, 1972.

32. Giroud, A.; Lefèbvres, J.; Prost, H., and Dupuis, R.: Malformations
    des membres dues à des lésions vasculaires chez le foetus de
    rat déficient en acide pantothénique. *J Embryol Exp Morphol,
    3*:1, 1955.

33. Globus, J. H., and Bergman, P.: Atresia and stenosis of the aqueduct
    of Sylvius. *J Neuropathol Exp Neurol, 5*:342, 1946.

34. Glücksmann, A.: Cell deaths in normal vertebrate ontogeny. *Biol Rev, 26*:59, 1951.
35. Glücksmann, A., and Tansley, K.: Some effects of gamma radiation on the developing rat retina. *Br J Ophthalmol, 20*:497, 1936.
36. Goerttler, K.: Die Aetiopathogenese angeborener Entwicklungsstörungen vom Standpunkt des Pathologen. *Anat Anz, 109*: suppl.: First European Congress of Anatomy: 35, 1962.
37. Goldstein, I., and Murphy, D. P.: Etilogy of ill-health in children born after maternal pelvic irradiation. Part II. Defective children born after postconception irradiation. *Am J Roentgenol, 22*:322, 1929.
38. Goldstein, I., and Wexler, D.: Rosette formation in the eyes of irradiated human embryos. *Arch Ophthalmol, 5*:591, 1931.
39. Grabowski, C.: The etiology of hypoxia-induced malformations in the chick embryo. *J Exp Zool, 157*:307, 1964.
40. Green, M. C.; Sidman, R. L., and Pivetta, O. H.: Cribriform degeneration (cri): a new recessive neurological mutation in the mouse. *Science, 176*:800, 1972.
41. Greene, H. S. N., and Saxton, Jr., J. A.: Hereditary brachydactylia and allied abnormalities in the rabbit. *J Exp Med, 69*:301, 1939.
42. Gregory, P. W.; Mead, S. W., and Reagan, W. M.: A congenital hereditary eye defect of cattle. *J Hered, 34*:125, 1943.
43. Gruenwald, P.: Studies on developmental pathology. III. Disintegration in the nervous system of normal and maldeveloped embryos. *J Neuropathol Exp Neurol, 4*:178, 1945.
44. Gruenwald, P.: Malformations caused by necrosis in the embryo, illustrated by the effect of selenium compounds on chick embryos. *Am J Pathol, 34*:77, 1958.
45. Gruenwald, P.: Disturbed enamel formation in deciduous tooth germs, and adjunct to the study of prenatal abnormality. *Arch Pathol, 95*:165, 1973.
46. Grüneberg, H.: Developmental genetics in the mouse, 1960. *J Cell Compar Physiol, 56, suppl. 1*:49, 1960.
47. Grüneberg, H.; Hallpike, C. S., and Ledoux, A.: Observations on the structure, development and electrical reactions of the internal ear of the shaker-1 mouse (*Mus musculus*). *Proc Roy Soc London, B: 129*:154, 1940.
48. Hadley, F. B.: Congenital epithelial defects of calves, epitheliogenesis imperfecta neonatorum bovis; recessive brought to light by inbreeding. *J Hered, 18*:487, 1927.
49. Hall, E. K.: Developmental anomalies in the eye of the rat after various experimental procedures. *Anat Rec, 116*:383, 1953.

50. Hallervorden, J.: Ueber eine Kohlenoxydvergiftung im Fetalleben mit Entwicklungsstörungen der Hirnrinde. *Allg Zeitschr Psychiat, 124:*289, 1949.

51. Hamburger, V.: The effects of wing bud extirpation on the development of the central nervous system in chick embryos. *J Exp Zool, 68:*449, 1934.

52. Hamburgh, M.; Lang, A.; Rader, M.; Silverstein, H.; Lynch, B.; Hoffman, K., and Miller, D.: Teratogenesis in offspring of stressed mice. *Teratology, 5:*256, 1972.

53. Hansmann, G. H., and Perry, M. C.: Lead absorption and intoxication in man unassociated with occupations or industrial hazards: absorption of lead from eleven weeks of intrauterine life to ninety-three years of age. *Arch Pathol, 30:*226, 1940.

54. Harada, Y.: Congenital Minamata disease. *Proc Cong Anom Res Assn Japan, 10-11:*2, 1971.

55. Harvey, E. B., and Chang, M. C.: Effects of radiocobalt irradiation of pregnant hamsters on the development of embryos. *J Cell Comp Physiol, 59:*293, 1962.

56. Haymaker, W.; Girdany, B. R.; Stephens, J.; Lillie, R. D., and Fetterman, G. H.: Cerebral involvement wth advanced periventricular calcification in generatized cytomegalic inclusion disease in the newborn. *J Neouropath, 13:*562, 1954.

57. Heller, R. H., and Jones, Jr., H. W.: Production of ovarian dysgenesis in the rat and human by busulfan. *Am J Obstet Gynecol, 89:*414, 1964.

58. Hemsworth, B. N., and Jackson, H.: Embryopathies induced by cytotoxic substances. In Sullivan, F. M., and Jackson, H. (Eds.): *Embryopathic Activity of Drugs.* Boston, Little, 1965, p. 116.

59. Heuser, C. H.; Rock, J., and Hertig, A. T.: Two human embryos showing early stages of the definitive yolk sac. *Contrib Embryol, 31:*85, 1945.

60. Hicks, S. P., and D'Amato, C. J.: Effects of ionizing radiations on mammalian development. *Adv Teratol, 1:*195, 1966.

61. Innes, J. R. M., and Saunders, L. Z.: *Comparative Neuropatholgy.* New York, Acad Pr, 1962.

62. Jost, A.: La dégénérescence des extremités du foetus de rat sous des actions hormonales (acroblapsie expérimentale) et la theorie des bulles myelencéphaliques de Bonnevie. *Arch Franc de Pediat, 10:*865, 1953.

63. Jost, A.: (Discussion of extrinsic factors in congenital malformations of man.) In *Congenital Malformations, Second International Congress.* New York, International Medical Congress Ltd, 1964, p. 290.

64. Kajii, T.; Ohama, K.; Niikawa, N.; Ferrier, A., and Avirachan, S.: Banding analysis of abnormal karyotypes in spontaneous abortion. *Am J Hum Genet, 25*:539, 1973.
65. Källén, B.: Cell degeneration during normal ontogenesis of the rabbit brain. *J Anat, 89*:153, 1955.
66. Kalter, H.: *Teratology of the central nervous system: induced and spontaneous malformations of laboratory, agricultural, and domestic mammals.* Chicago and London, U of Chicago Pr, 1968.
67. Kaplan, E.; Shwachman, H.; Perlmutter, A. D.; Rule, A.; Khaw, K. T., and Holsclaw, D. S.: Reproductive failure in males with cystic fibrosis. *N Eng J Med, 279*:65, 1968.
68. Karli, P.: Rétines sans cellules visuelles: recherches morphologiques, physiologiques et physiopathologiques chez les rongeurs. *Arch Anat Histol, Embryol, 35*:1, 1952.
69. Karnofsky, D. A., and Ridgway, L. P.: Production of injury to the central nervous system of the chick embryo by lead salts. *J Pharm Exper Therap, 104*:176, 1952.
70. Kelemen, G., and Gotlib, B. N.: Pathohistology of fetal ears after maternal rubella. *Laryngoscope, 69*:385, 1959.
71. Kelton, D. E., and Rauch, H.: Myelinaton and myelin degeneration in the central nervous system of dilute-lethal mice. *Exp Neurol, 6*:252, 1962.
72. Kocher, W.: Untersuchingen zur Genetik und Pathologie der Entwicklung von 8 Labyrinthmutanten (*Deaf- Waltzer- Shaker-Mutanten*) der Maus (*Mus musculus*). *Ztschr Vererbungsl, 91*:114, 1960.
73. Kreshover, S. J.; Clough, O. W., and Bear, D. M.: A study of prenatal influences on tooth development on humans. *J Am Dent Assoc, 56*:230, 1958.
74. Kreshover, S. J., and Hancock, Jr., J. A.: The effect of lymphocytic choriomeningitis on pregnancy and dental tissues in mice. *J Dent Des, 35*:467, 1956.
75. Larsson, K. S.; Boström, H., and Ericson, B.: Salicylate-induced malformations in mouse embryos. *Acta Paed, 52*:36, 1963.
76. Levitt, N. H.; London, W. T.; Kent, S. G., and Sever, J. L.: In utero induction of cataracts and hydrocephalus in rhesus monkeys using Venezuelan equine encephalitis virus. *Abst Ann Meet Am Soc Microbiol, 73*:226, 1973.
77. Maresch, R.: Ueber einen Fall von Kohlenoxydgasschädigung des Kindes in der Gebärmutter. *Wien med Wocherschr, 79*:454, 1929.
78. Margolis, G., and Kilham, L.: Hydrocephalus in hamsters, ferrets, rats and mice following inoculation with reovirus type I. II. Pathologic studies. *Lab Invest, 21*:189, 1969.
79. Margolis, G., and Kilham, L.: Parovirus infections, vascular endo-

thelium, and hemorrhagic encephalopathy. *Lab Invest,* 22:478, 1970.
80. Margolis, G.; Kilham, L., and Johnson, R. H.: The paroviruses and replicating cells: insights into the pathogenesis of cerebellar hypoplasia. *Prog Neuropath, 1*:168, 1971.
81. Marin-Padilla, M., and Ferm, V. H.: Somite necrosis and developmental malformations induced by vitamin A in the golden hamster. *J Embryol Exp Morphol, 13*:1, 1965.
82. Martin, A. H.; Chang, L. W., and Kreuhl, K.: The influence of heavy metals on the developing central nervous system in avian and mammalian embryos. *Anat Rec, 175*:384, 1973.
83. Martinet, M.: Hémorrhagies embryonnaires par deficience en acide linoléique. *Ann de Med, 53*:286, 1952.
84. Matsumoto, H.; Kola, G., and Takeuchi, T.: Fetal Minamata disease: a neuropathological study of two cases of intoxication by a methyl mercury compound. *J Neuropathol Exp Neurol, 24*:563, 1965.
85. Menkes, B.; Sandor, S., and Ilies, A.: Cell death in teratogenesis. *Adv Teratol. 4*:169, 1970.
86. Miller, M. M., and Amir-Jahed, A. K.: Total intestinal atresia. *Surgery, 55*:737, 1964.
87. Misgeld, G. C.: Ueber die Bedeutung des physiologischen Nabelbruchs bei der Entstehung von Atresien, Stenosen und Okklusionen im Bereich des Ileums. *Virchows Arch, 310*:697, 1943.
88. Murakami, U.; Hoshino, K., and Inouye, M.: An experimental observation of the morphogenesis of reopening of the cranium. *Proc Cong Anom Res Assn Japan, 12*:157, 1972.
89. Murakami, U., and Inouye, M.: Brain lesions in the mouse fetus caused by maternal administration of monosodium glutamate (preliminary report). *Proc Cong Anom Res Assn Japan, 11*:171, 1971.
90. Oliver, J.: Microcystic renal disease and its relation to "infantile nephrosis." *Am J Dis Child, 100*:312, 1960.
91. Ombrédanne, L., and Lacassie: La maladie ulcéreuse intra-utérine. *Arch Méd Enfants, 33*:199, 1930.
92. Osburn, B. I.; Silverstein, A. M.; Prendergast, R. A.; Johnson, R. T., and Parshall, Jr., C. J.: Experimental viral-induced encephalopathies, I. Pathology of hydranencephaly and porencephaly caused by bluetongue vaccine virus. *Lab Invest, 25*:197, 1971.
93. Pierro, L. J.: Teratogenic action of actinomycin D in the embryonic chick. II. Early development. *J Exp Zool, 148*:241, 1961.
94. Plagens, G. M.: An embryological study of a special strain of deformed x-rayed mice, with special reference to the etiology and morphogenesis of the abnormalities. *J Morphol, 55*:151, 1933.

95. Politzer, G., and Sternberg, H.: Ueber einen missbildeten menschlichen Embryo des ersten Monates. *Frankf Zeitschr Path, 37*:174, 1929.

96. Ritter, E. J.; Scott, W. J., ånd Wilson, J. G.: Relationship of temporal patterns of cell death and development to malformations in the rat limb. Possible mechanisms of teratogenesis with inhibitors of DNA synthesis. *Teratol, 7*:219, 1973.

97. Robertson, G. G.; Williamson,, A. P., and Blattner, R. J.: A study of abnormalities in early chick embryos inoculated with Newcastle disease virus. *J Exp Zool, 129*:5, 1955.

98. Rugh, R.; Duhamel, L.; Chandler, A., and Varma, A.: Cataract development after embryonic and fetal x-irratiation. *Radiol Res, 22*:519, 1964.

99. Salzgeber, B.: Production élective de la phocomélie sous l'influence d'yperite azotée, chez l'embryon de poulet. II. Étude histologique des bourgeons de membres aucours du développement. *J Embryol Exp Morpho, 16*:339, 1966.

100. Santulli, T. V., and Blanc, W. A.: Congenital atresia of the intestine: pathogenesis and treatment. *Ann Surg, 154*:939, 1961.

101. Sanders, Jr., J. W.: Death in embryonic systems. *Science, 154*:604, 1966.

102. Saunders, Jr., J. W.; Gasseling, M. T., and Saunders, L. C.: Cellular death in morphogenesis of the avian wing. *Develop Biol, 5*:147, 1962.

103. Saxén, L., and Rapola, J.: *Congenital Defects*. New York, Holt, Rinehart and Winston, 1969.

104. Schall, L. A.; Lurie, M. H., and Kelemen, G.: Embryonic hearing organs after maternal rubella. *Laryngoscope, 61*:99, 1951.

105. Scheidegger, S.: Entzündungen beim Embryo und Foetus bei experimenteller Virusinfektion des Muttertieres. *Bull Schweiz Ak Med Wiss, 8*:346, 1952.

106. Schick, B.: Diaplacental infection of the foetus with the virus of German measles despite immunity of the mother; analogous observations in smallpox. *Acta Paed, 38*:563, 1949.

107. Schour, I., and Poncher, H. G.: Rate of apposition of enamel and dentin, measured by the effect of acute flurorsis. *Am J Dis Child, 54*:757, 1937.

108. Schweichel, J. U., and Merker, H. J.: The morphology of various types of cell death in prenatal tissues. *Teratol, 7*:253, 1973.

109. Scott, W. J.; Ritter, E. J., and Wilson, J. G.: DNA synthesis inhibition and cell death associated with hydroxyurea teratogenesis in rat embryos. *Develop Biol, 26*:306, 1971.

110. Seizt, L.: Spontanamputationen durch amniotische Fäden künnen mit primärer Minderwertigkeit der Fruchtanale zusammenhängen. *Monatsschr Geburts, Gynäk, 94*:236, 1933.

111. Shepard, T. H.; Lemire, R. J.; Aksu, O., and Mackler, B.: Studies of the development of congenital anomalies in embryos of riboflavin-deficient, galactoflavin fed rats. I. Growth and embryologic pathology. *Teratol, 1*:75, 1968.
112. Sidman, R. L.; Dickie, M. M., and Appel, S. H.: Mutant mice (Quaking and Jimpy) with deficient myelination in the central nervous system. *Science, 144*:309, 1964.
113. Silver, J.: The role of cell degeneration in the developing rat eye. *Anat Rec, 172*:406, 1972.
114. Silverstein, A. M.; Parshall, Jr., C. J.; Osburn, B. I., and Prendergast, R. A.: An experimental, virus-induced retinal dysplasia in the fetal lamb. *Am J Ophthalmol, 72*:22, 1971.
115. Singh, S., and Singh, G.: Hemorrhages in the limbs of fetal rats after amniocentesis and their role in limb malformations. *Teratol, 8*:11, 1973.
116. Stockard, C. R.: An hereditary lethal for localized motor and preganglionic neurones with a resulting paralysis in the dog. *Am J Anat, 59*:1, 1936.
117. Strauss, L., and Bernstein, J.: Neonatal hepatitis in congenital rubella: a histopathological study. *Arch Path, 86*:317, 1968.
118. Streeter, G. L.: Focal deficiencies in fetal tissues and their relation to intrauterine amputation. *Contr Embryol, 22*:1, 1930.
119. Takano, M.: Experimental study on the development of congenital anomalies of the digits. *Proc Cong Anom Res Assn Japan, 10-11*:20, 1971.
120. Töndury, G., and Smith, D. W.: Fetal ribella pathology. *J Pediatr, 68*:867, 1966.
121. Tsujimoto, K.; Sherman, F. E., and Ravitch, M. M.: Experimental intestinal atresia in the rabbit fetus: sequential pathological studies. *Johns Hopkins Med J, 131*:287, 1972.
122. Ullrich, O.: Neue Einblicke in die Entwicklungsmechanik multipler Abartungen und Fehlbildungen. *Klin Wochenschr, 17*:185, 1938.
123. van Bogaert, L., and Innes, J. R. M.: Cerebellar disorders in lambs: a study in animal neuropathology with some comments on ovine neuroanatomy. *Arch Pathol, 50*:36, 1950.
124. Werthemann, A., and Reiniger, M.: Ueber Augenentwicklungsstörungen bei Rattenembryonen durch Sauerstoffmangel in der Frühschwangerschaft. *Acta Anat, 11*:329, 1950.
125. Wessinger, G. D., and Weinmann, J. P.: The effect of manganese and boron compounds on the rat incisor. *Am J Physiol, 133*:233, 1943.

126. Windle, W. F.; Becker, R. F., and Weil, A.: Alterations in brain structure after asphyxiation at birth; experimental study in guinea pig. *J Neuropath Exper Neurol, 3*:224, 1944.

127. Winfield, J. B., and Bennett, D.: Gene—teratogen interaction: potentiation of actinomycin D teratogenesis in the house mouse by the lethal gene brachyury. *Teratol, 4*:157, 1971.

128. Yamane, J.: Ueber die "Atresia coli," eine letale, erbliche Darmmissbildung beim Pferde, und ihre Kombination mit Gehirngliomen. *Zeitschr f indukt Abstamm Vererbungsl, 46*:188, 1927.

129. Zwilling, E.: The development of dominant rumplessness in chick embryos. *Genetics, 27*:641, 1942.

130. Zwilling, E.: The embryogeny of a recessive rumpless condition of chickens. *J Exp Zool, 99*:79, 1945.

131. Zwilling, E.: Teratogenesis. In Willier, B. H.; Weiss, P. A., and Hamburger, V. (Eds.): *Analysis of development.* Philadelphia and London, Saunders. 1955, p. 699.

132. Zwilling, E.: Micromelia as a direct effect of insulin; evidence from *in vitro* and *in vivo* experiments. *J Morphol, 104*:159, 1959.

Chapter 15

MULLERIAN DEFECTS

T. N. Evans

Since congential vaginal agenesis was first described in the sixteen century,[1] Müllerian defects have been of great interest to embryologists and gynecologists and more recently to those concerned with teratology. It has been estimated that Müllerian defects occur once in every 4,000 deliveries.[2] However, we suspect that this defect is much more frequent although our patient population which is refered from many areas makes true assessments of frequency difficult. If minor uterine defects detected by hysterosalpingography are included, Müllerian defects would be among the most common congenital anomalies.

Since the first recorded attempt to correct vaginal agenesis surgically in the early part of the last century,[3] numerous operations have been designed to correct vaginal agenesis. Segments of ileum, sigmoid and rectum have been used.[4] Simple pressure[5] has also been recommended, but many have abandoned this because of the long time required and the frequency of an unsatisfactory result. The most significant development in surgical technique occurred when utilization of a split-thickness skin graft was introduced.[6] A number of additional modifications will be detailed in this chapter which may represent significant improvements in operative technique.

EMBRYOGENESIS OF THE MÜLLERIAN SYSTEM

Fallopian tubes, uterus and upper vagina are derived from the Müllerian ducts. On or about the thirty-seventh day of human embryonic ovulation age a coelomic mesothelial groove develops parallel to the Wolffian ducts.[7] An enfolding occurs so that this groove is covered and the dorsal portion becomes thickened to form the uterus. The upper unfused Müllerian ducts develop into the fallopian tubes. The distal ducts fuse to form the vagina and descend to fuse with the sinovaginal bulbs which probably are derived from epithelium from both the Müllerian ducts and the urogenital sinus. These sinovaginal bulbs lose their core and form the locus of the hymen. Although it is still debated, the current consensus suggests that the definitive epithelium of the vagina for the most part is derived from the ectoderm of the cloacal membrane which reaches the vagina by way of the urogenital sinus.[8]

From this embryological sequence one can readily understand the clinical defects observed. Other than minor arcuate or bicornuate uterine deformities, the most common major congenital Müllerian defect involves complete vaginal agenesis and an absent or rudimentary uterus without functioning endometrium. Less frequently, one may encounter partial failure of fusion of the lower Müllerian ducts with occlusion of the upper and lower vagina and in some instances the development of transverse septa. Less than 5 percent of patients thus afflicted have a sufficiently normal upper Müllerian system to permit subsequent successful pregnancy after vaginal plastic surgery.[9, 10]

ETIOLOGY

There are a number of interrelated phenomena that may play a role in sexual organogenesis. These include (1) genetic substrate which determines male and female differentiation, (2) intrinsic epigenetic developmental factors (enzymes, inductive substances, hormones), and (3) extrinsic epigenetic factors (environment, trauma, teratogens).[11] The extent to which each of these is involved is speculative. However, we increasingly suspect a teratogen is implicated since (1) the same defect does not occur in siblings except in the case of male hermaphrodites, (2) there is a frequent occurrence of associated anomalies and (3) embryonic Müllerian defects have been observed in preg-

nant women exposed to known human teratogens, e.g. thalido-
mide. Although vaginal agenesis has been produced in monkeys
by the injection of androgens,[7] there is no other evidence that
virilizing factors play a role in the production of vaginal agenesis
in most patients with these defects.

IMPROVEMENTS IN SURGICAL TECHNIQUE

Utilization of segments of bowel have largely been abandoned
because of the associated morbidity and mortality and the
troublesome leukorrhea encountered by most who have performed these procedures. Dissection of a channel between the
bladder and rectum all the way to the peritoneum and insertion
of a split-thickness skin graft over a stent remains the procedure
of choice. Modifications of this technique which we have employed are illustrated in Figures 15-1 to 15-5. In order to achieve
better hemostasis and facilitate dissection, a vasopressor solution
consisting of 0.6 cc of 1 percent Neosynephrine® in 100 cc of
physiological saline is injected liberally into the area of the
vestibule and beyond. A small diamond-shaped piece of mucus
membrane is excised with a scalpel. It is generally unnecessary
to incise the perineal skin since the small opening where the
mucus membrane is excised is readily distensible. Blunt digital
dissection of this area has been abandoned in favor of the use of
Kelly clamps to initiate dissection of the channels on each side
of the midline. There is a vertical midline fibromuscular structure
which is readily identified after the channels have been dissected
on each side. This median raphe is cut with scissors and dissection of the entire channel completed up to the peritoneum. It
had been concluded previously that there was also a defect in the
distribution and location of the levator muscles in these patients
leading to the problem of contraction of the space for quite some
months after surgery unless it is held open with a stent. This
hypothesis was supported by the fact that total vaginectomy for
cancer followed by insertion of the same stent and split-thickness
skin graft is followed by little evidence of subsequent contraction of the vagina. Our supposition may have been erroneous
since the levator muscles had never really been separated pre-

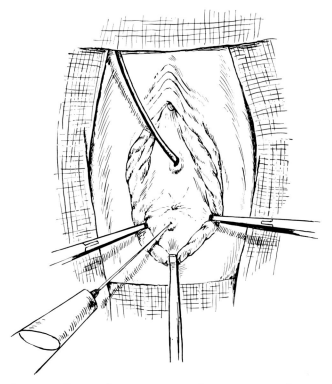

Figure 15-1. Instillation of a vasopressor solution (0.6 cc of 1% Neosyne-phrine in 100 cc of physiologic saline). About 10 or 15 cc of solution is injected to the full depth of the area of dissection.

viously in the vaginal agenesis patients. We now identify and resect the levator muscles on each side about halfway up the neovagina and believe that this has resulted in less of a problem with contraction subsequently. Although it is much easier to remove a skin graft of relatively uniform thickness from the thigh, we have in recent years utilized the hip primarily because of the type of clothing worn by most of these young patients. The greater difficulty in getting a graft of uniform thickness does not seem to compromise the end result. In an effort to reduce the frequency and the amount of granulation tissue which has proved to be a real problem postoperatively in these patients, in recent years we have filled the new vagina with a topical thrombin

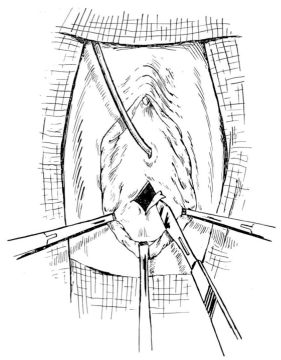

Figure 15-2.   Excision   of   a   small   diamond-shaped   piece   of   mucous
membrane.

solution leaving it in the vagina for several minutes before
insertion of the graft. The apparent beneficient effect of this
may well be due to the improved hemostasis rather than to any
direct suppression of granulation tissue. The graft-covered stent
is sutured deep into the vagina by No. 2 nylon sutures in the
vestibule which obscures the stent and produces less discomfort
than sutures placed in the more distal vulvar area. The graft-
covered stent is left in place for ten days during which time the
patient is confined to bed but may be turned from side to side.
Preoperatively, the patient is placed on a liquid diet for forty-
eight hours before surgery and the bowel thoroughly emptied
with enemas. She remains on a liquid diet throughout the ten
days before removal of the stent under anesthesia. During this
interval the patient receives tincture of opium, 4 cc four times

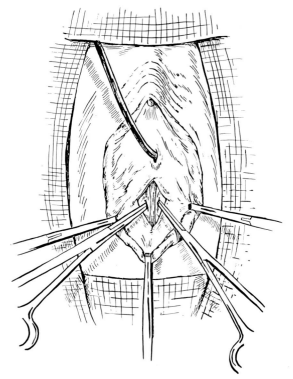

Figure 15-3.   Lateral dissection with Kelly clamps with a median raphe illustrated.

daily and 8 cc stat if there is any urge to defecate. The bladder is kept empty either with transurethral catheter or a suprapublic cystotomy. After the patient has been thoroughly instructed in removal of the stent and its reinsertion, she is discharged on or about the fourteenth postoperative day.

SURGICAL COMPLICATIONS

Postoperative complications seem to occur in direct proportion to the number of previous attempts at surgical construction of a vagina by inexperienced or unskilled operators.[9] With meticulous dissection, vesicovaginal and rectovaginal fistulas usually can be avoided. If there is extensive scarring in this area,

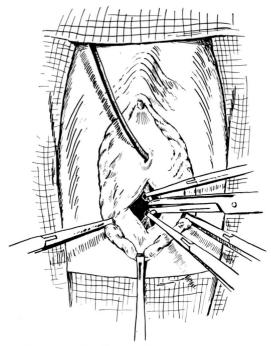

Figure 15-4.   The vertical pillar of fibrous tissue is incised progressively
to the apex of the vagina.

even the most meticulous dissection can still result in entering
the bladder and/or the rectum. Urinary tract infections are
common while a catheter is in place. Hemorrhage has not been
a problem in recent years with utilization of the technique
described. Occasionally, granulation tissue can grow so abund-
antly that it is necessary to do a curettage of the vagina under
anesthesia. Again, utilizing these changes in technique, this has
become less frequent.

ASSOCIATED ANOMALIES

Of the first 134 patients with partial or total vaginal atresia,
103 or 77 percent had only a rudimentary or totally absent uterus.[9]
There were six with an anomalous uterus with functioning endometrium, and five of these had crytomenorrhea at the time of

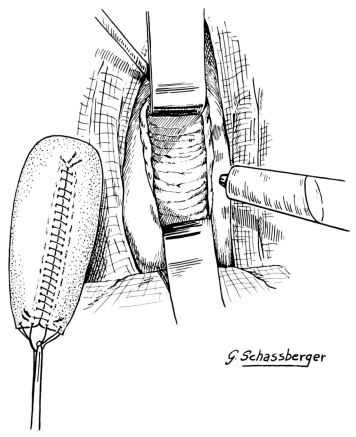

G. Schassberger

Figure 15-5.   After dissection has been carried all the way up to the full depth of the vagina, 15 to 20 cc of topical thrombin solution is instilled and left in place for several minutes before insertion of the stent covered with the split-thickness skin graft.

their initial examination. Two had associated pelvic endometriosis. There were only five in the entire series who had a sufficiently normal upper Müllerian tract to permit subsequent pregnancy.

There were twenty-seven (20%) with significant associated urinary tract defects. These included a single kidney in nine in a normal location and a single pelvic kidney in four. Another had two pelvic kidneys, one of which had been removed inadvertently suspecting it was a retroperitoneal neoplasm. There were thirteen with hydronephrosis, hydroureter and other lesser renal and ureteral anomalies.

Twenty-one or 16 percent had various associated musculoskeletal anomalies involving the spine, pelvis, extremities, ribs and abdominal wall. Most of these were comparatively minor and nondisabling anomalies except for one with partial absence of the rectus abdominis muscle.

There were ten hermaphrodites including three sets of siblings. Five had femoral or inguinal hernias, three congenital heart disease, and two had clubbed feet.

DISCUSSION

An apparent increase in the frequency of Müllerian defects may be attributable to the increased frequency of such patients seeking medical aid, a wider appreciation that such defects can be corrected surgically, and the increased utilization of hysterographic investigation of patients with infertility. Evidence presented of a possible teratogenic etiology is only presumptive. If in fact a teratogen is responsible, its identification may continue to be difficult since diagnosis of these defects is generally quite belated. Furthermore, teratogens can produce marked fetal defects when the mother is asymptomatic and unscathed.[12]

Great progress has been made in the treatment of these patients. Thorough psychiatric evaluation preoperatively and careful timing of surgery are critical. Because of the importance of her role in the postoperative care, the patient must be sufficiently mature to have a strong desire for sanative surgery and be emotionally stable to the extent that she will carry out explicit instructions postoperatively. Pre- and post-operative psychometrics and psychiatric evaluations have demonstrated some rather remarkable changes.[13] Virtually all of these patients become orgasmic, and many have been involved with successful marriages.

Fate of the skin graft has been of interest to many.[14] Exfoliative cytology not infrequently demonstrates anucleated cells, and in a few instances cyclic cytologic changes may be observed similar to those in patients without such defects. This suggests that over a period of time in some, the skin graft may be replaced in part by relatively normal mucosa.

Previous karyology has suggested that all of these patients except those in the hermaphrodite group have normal chromosomal patterns.[15] However, we are repeating these studies utilizing some of the newer karyological techniques in search of possible defects in the karyotype.

Although improvements in management have been great, further experience with the technical changes described here will be necessary to assess their effects in preventing or diminishing the two therapeutic enigmas involved—occasional prolonged periods of vaginal contraction and persistent granulation tissue in the neovagina.

REFERENCES

1. Steinmetz, E. P.: Formation of artificial vagina. *West J Surg,* 48:169, 1940.
2. Bryan, A. L.; Nigro, J. A., and Counseller, V. S.: One hundred cases of congenital absence of the vagina. *Surg Gynecol Obstet,* 88:79, 1949.
3. Dupuytren, cited by Whitacre, F. E., and Chen, C. Y.: Surgical treatment of the absence of the vagina. *Am J Obster Gynecol,* 49:789, 1945.
4. Counseller, V. S., and Flor, F. S.: Congenital absence of the vagina—further results of treatment and a new technic. *Surg Clin North Am,* 37:1107. 1957.
5. Frank, R. T.: The formation of an artificial vagina without operation. *Am J Obstet Gynecol,* 35:1053, 1938.
6. McIndoe, A. H., and Banister, J. B.: An operation for cure of congenital absence of the vagina. *J Obstet Gynaecol Br Commonw,* 45:490, 1938.
7. Wells, L. J.: Embryology and anatomy of the vagina. *Ann NY Acad Sci,* 83:80, 1959.
8. Politzer, G.: Zur normalen und abnormalen Enturcklung der menschlichen Scheide. *Anat Anz,* 102:271, 1955.
9. Evans. T. N.: The artificial vagina. *Am J Obstet Gynecol,* 99:944, 1967.
10. Miller, N. F., and Stout, W.: Congenital absence of the vagina. *Obstet Gynecol,* 9:48, 1957.

11. Gallien, L. G.: Genetic control of sexual differentiation in vertebrates. In DeHaan, R. L., and Ursprung, H. (Eds.): *Organogenesis.* New York, Holt, Rinehart, and Winston, 1965.

12. Evans, T. N.: Teratogenic agents. *Indust Med Surg, 32:*87, 1963.

13. Tourkow, L.: Psychic consequences of loss and replacement of body parts. *J Am Psychoanal Assoc,* In Press.

14. Ulfelder, H.: Agenesis of the vagina. A discussion of surgical management and morphologic comparison of end results with and without skin grafting. *Am J Obstet Gynecol, 100:*745, 1968.

15. Jones, H. W., Jr.; Ferguson-Smith, M. A., and Heller, R. H.: The pathology and cytogenetics of gonadal agenesis. *Am J Obstet Gynecol, 87:*578, 1963.

Chapter 16

MATERNAL HEALTH AND
FETAL DEVELOPMENT

H. W. Berendes

INTRODUCTION

Concern about the effect of maternal health on reproductive performance is part of modern obstetrics. Surely the call for early and optimal prenatal care of every pregnant woman is an expression of this concern. The feeling and experience of the profession is not only that of controlling maternal complications, but also reducing fetal risk in perinatal mortality, neonatal morbidity, as well as long range sequela. For obvious reasons, we can better understand the effects of maternal health on perinatal mortality than on postnatal long term sequelae. The difficulties involved in research into prenatal causes of developmental abnormalities in children are known to most of us. Obstetricians, have been rightly optimistic in what prenatal care can achieve with respect to fetal well-being and their successes prove this. Their optimism is reflected in the concern about high risk groups, their early identification, special care and provision of specialized services for them.

Eleven years ago in a national report[1] specific recommendations were made towards launching a national program, which would concentrate on high risk groups, whose prenatal care was frequently inadequate. This was an all out effort to reduce mental retardation. In response, as you well know, maternal infant care programs designed to serve the indigent high risk

groups, were developed. These trends are mentioned to emphasize the importance of our continuing concern about maternal
well-being and child development and to recognize the key role
played by the obstetrician in regard to this area of preventive
medicine.

Some liberties have been taken with the term "fetal development" for the purpose of this chapter, which deals with maternal
health factors and long-term sequelae. The implied assumption
here is that child development and performance is at least a
reflection of fetal development. Our ability to measure neurological integrity is extremely limited in the newborn. There
is at present no way to assess intelligence or other more complex
functions in the infant. It is necessary, therefore, to rely on
assessments of children during their first few years of life in
order to obtain information on neuropsychological disabilities.

Review of the Problem

Until recently our knowledge regarding maternal health
characteristics and fetal development was based largely upon
clinical experience and retrospective studies. These studies revealed associations between cerebral palsy, epilepsy, mental
deficiency, and several factors.[2-7] Among these were prenatal
hemorrhage, third trimester bleeding, toxemia of pregnancy,
placenta previa, abruptio placentae, cord prolapse, and breech
delivery. The association between diabetes and congenital malformation of the offspring was noted by several investigators.[8-11]
An increase in neurological disorders among the offspring of
diabetic women was also reported.[10]

Infections of the pregnant woman have long been recognized
as important hazards to fetal development. Known effects are
related to certain specific infections and to the particular time
in pregnancy when infections occurs. These range from congenital malformations to physical growth retardation; developmental delay, mental defects, sensory defects, convulsions and
the like.[12-17]

Furthermore, differences in incidence of certain malformations
and certain chromosomal aberrations according to maternal age
are a matter of record.[18-21]

Increases in some malformations and trisomies were seen among the offspring of older women.[18, 21] More recently, mental retardation has been reported among non-phenylketonuric children of phenylketonuric mothers.[22-24] PKU is an inborn error in the metabolism of phenylalanine associated with mental retardation. Untreated phenylketonuria during pregnancy exposes the fetus to an abnormal biochemical environment *in utero* resulting in mental retardation, even in the genetically normal offspring.

Highly suggestive data from a prospective study has recently been reported about the relationship between maternal subclinical hypothyroidism and developmental retardation in four and seven year olds.[25-27] The contention is that some of these cases are clinically unrecognized and are only reliably identified by laboratory means. The rate of mental retardation was increased among the offspring of untreated or inadequately treated hypothyroid women.

The importance of chronic alcoholism among pregnant women, affecting the development of their offspring, was only recently identified.[28, 29] Patterns of craniofacial, limb, and cardiovascular defects, together with stunted prenatal growth and mental retardation have been observed among children of chronically alcoholic mothers. If, as suggested, these developmental defects are found among one third of the children of such women, it is amazing that this has not been recognized and reported before. Whether these defects are the result of direct toxic effects of alcohol, or related to some nutritional deficit in the mother, is not known.

Intrauterine fetal growth results from a complex set of interactions of many factors. Maternal health characteristics are important contributors to fetal growth.[30-32] Several attempts have been made to construct a statistical model[33] explaining variances in birth weight. Important in these predictions are many maternal health variables, among them are: age of gravida, pre-pregnancy weight, height of gravida, diabetes, organic heart disease, smoking during pregnancy, history of hypertensive disease, number of specific diseases, toxemia, second trimester bleeding, various placental complications, maternal weight gain, incompetent cervix, various viral infections during pregnancy, and parity, to name only a few.

In turn, prematurity and low birth-weight are known to be important predictors of abnormal development and of long-term sequelae.[34] The consideration of specific effects of these factors on postnatal development is beyond the scope of this presentation.

The topic of maternal nutrition and fetal growth and development[35-38] is a most important research priority at this time, but will not be considered further in this chapter.

Recent results of several prospective investigations have become available. These begin with pregnant women and include a follow-up of their children during the first few years of life. These studies differ somewhat from each other in detail, sample size, population studies and, also, in the specific developmental characteristics of children ascertained. Some of these studies are still in progress, therefore, final information is not yet available. However, results from these projects and discussion of the incompletely analyzed information from the collaborative perinatal project[39] permits us to summarize certain current knowledge.

Buck and associates pursued the effect of prenatal complications upon the development of children of 2500 grams and above.[40] Among the characteristics of relevance to our discussion, the analysis considered toxemia, essential hypertension, inappropriate weight gain, hemorrhage during various stages of pregnancy (early stage, threatened abortion, after the 20th week). Comprehensive evaluation of offspring into the first year of school consisted of assessments of intelligence by Stanford-Binet, abnormal behavior score, Illinois psycholinguistic test, Graham Block sort, neurological abnormality score, copy form test and documentation of academic progress.

A significant difference was noted between children of women who had pre-eclampsia or toxemia and their controls. A small reduction in average intelligence of 4.5 IQ points was found among children of toxemic women as compared to their controls, with a very small variance in behavior. Furthermore, only 6.4 percent of the children of toxemic women were assigned to an advanced level of academic standing during their first year in school as compared to 18.8 percent of the controls.

Another prospective investigation of note was the follow-up of children from the Kauai Project which encompassed all births over a period of two years in the mid-fifties and their follow-up.[41, 42] The observed pre- and perinatal complications were scored by severity. Prenatal characteristics considered to be mild were mild pre-eclampsia, essential hypertension, renal insufficiency or anemia, controlled diabetes or hypothyroidism, positive Wasserman with no treatment, urinary tract infection in third trimester, treated asthma, second and third trimester bleeding. Among the moderate complications were marked pre-eclampsia, essential hypertension, renal insufficiency or anemia, diabetes in poor control, decompensated cardiovascular disease requiring therapy, untreated thyroid dysfunction, confirmed rubella, first trimester vaginal bleeding. Severe complications were eclampsia and renal or diabetic coma.

The children's psychological status were assessed at two years by the Cattell infant intelligence scale and the Doll Vineland social maturity scale. An association was found between the severity of pre- and perinatal complications and below normal mental and social development at two years of age. The children of women with severe complications showed the highest proportion of abnormalities. Further analysis, however, suggested an important interaction between abnormal performance at two years and various environmental factors such as socioeconomic status, family stability or mothers' intelligence. In fact, among children from families with high socioeconomic status, almost identical abnormality scores were observed at two years regardless of the severity of prenatal and perinatal complications. An increase in abnormality score at two years for severe perinatal complications was observed in children of families of intermediate socioeconomic status. Only children of low economic status showed consistent differences in developmental score by severity of pre- and perinatal complications. Quite clearly a favorable home environment can, to some extent, deal with and compensate for adverse pre- or perinatal influences.

A followup through ten years made use of available information about these children from their physicians, hospitals, schools, health and welfare departments, and their parents. Because of the stability of this island population more than 90 percent follow-up was obtainable at age ten. Associations were found between the severity of perinatal stress and mental retardation and IQ below 85, and also any significant physical handicap. Again, however, within the high and intermediate socioeconomic groups there were no differences in intelligence irrespective of severity of perinatal stress. Only the low socioeconomic group showed a decrease in intelligence because of the severity of perinatal score, which indicates the strong effect that postnatal environment has on subsequent child development. The authors concluded their report, that the continuum of reproductive casualties needs to be complemented with a greater concern of environmental casualties among the young.

As part of the follow-up of the Perinatal Mortality Survey in 1958 in Great Britain, all surviving children born in England, Scotland, and Wales during one week in March, 1958, were re-evaluated at seven years of age with measures made available within the school system.[43, 44] Among these were physical handicaps, reading attainment, and social adjustment in school. To evaluate the relationship of conditions during pregnancy, and events surrounding birth, complex statistical analyses of the composite effect on reading levels were undertaken. The variables included were: sex of child, social class, maternal height, maternal age, maternal smoking during pregnancy, length of pregnancy, child's birthweight, birth order, and number of younger children in household when index case was seven years old.

Aside from the expected marked effect of social class on reading ability, birth order had the next most sizable impact on this performance measure. Reading attainment of first-born children was sixteen months ahead of reading age compared to the fourth or later born children. Children of women aged twenty-five to thirty-four years were the best readers on the average; children of younger mothers the worst. Length of pregnancy and birthweight had a lesser effect on reading level. The reduction in birthweight by 1,000 gm. accounted for a reduction in reading attainment of four months. Smoking of ten cigarettes or more per day during pregnancy was associated with a decrease in reading level of four months.

To predict handicaps, two groups were arranged. Group A consisted of children with partial or severe hearing loss, visual loss, cerebral palsy, severe mental retardation and multiple defects. Group B consisted of children who received special schooling at age seven because of educational or mental backwardness. Predictor variables selected for study were: birth order, type of delivery, condition of baby during the first week, as well as social class, birth weight, and gestation.

For Group A, conditions of predictive value were: high birth order, that is, fifth birth or later, abnormal delivery, and abnormal signs of serious illness during the neonatal period. Social class and birth weight at gestation did not add much to the prediction when the three variables mentioned were included. For Group B, predictive usefulness in order of importance was established for factors of birth order, social class, birthweight-gestation and methods of delivery.

While few of the variables are directly relevant to our presentation, it is noteworthy that none of the conditions under study had a substantial effect on performance with the possible exception of young maternal age and high birth order on reading attainment.

It should be mentioned here that another detailed study of the effect of maternal smoking on long term development did not support this finding from the British study. Hardy and Mellits, based upon data collected at Johns Hopkins, as part of the collaborative perinatal project, reviewed maternal smoking in relation to postnatal physical growth, neurological status, intelligence, wide-range academic achievement, and visual motor perception of the offspring.[45] Height attainment during the first year was the only significant difference between matched pairs of children of smoking mothers and non-smoking mothers. No developmental differences in the measures observed were seen at one, four, and seven years in these children which could be attributed to maternal smoking.

A community wide study of mental retardation was conducted in the city of Aberdeen, Scotland, in the sixties.[46] This project ascertained all mentally abnormal children in that city in 1962, who were born in 1952, 1953 and 1954. Because of the well-known efforts in Aberdeen by the eminent obstetrician, Sir Dugald Baird, since 1948, excellent obstetrical records were available in these cases. Among the mentally retarded group, compared to a control group of children, there was an increase in moderate or severe pre-eclampsia, low birth weight, short gestation, and poor condition during the perinatal period, and also malpresentations during delivery. The association with obstetrical complications were stronger in children with retardation who had associated central nervous system damage. Among mildly subnormal children there was an excess of mothers with short stature and high pregnancy rate.

Overall, only a small effect could be attributed to clearly definable obstetric and perinatal conditions, but more to the presence of generally poor physical condition of the mother. The conclusion was that little could be attributed to a primary obstetric etiology for mental retardation in these cases. Instead, an interaction between social-environmental circumstances, familial factors, and ill-defined features of reproductive inadequacy were of etiological importance.

A sub-sample of the perinatal collaborative project studied at the University of Oregon concerned the relationship of selected perinatal variables to seven year intelligence.[47] Factors examined included, race, mother's occupation and education, neuro-psychiatric illness, family income, birth place, sex, toxemia, type of delivery, cord complications, birth weight, Apgar and sex of child. The multiple correlation of these variables to seven-year I.Q. was .34. This meant that only a small proportion of the variance, namely, 11.4 percent was explained by these factors. It is important to mention here that there were no significant correlations between birth weight, Apgar score, type of delivery, cord complications and toxemia and seven year IQ.

Prechll[48] also reviewed in a longitudinal investigation the impact of maternal complications on neurological sequelae and included a total of forty-two obstetric variables.[48] Severity of risk in abnormal neurological status seemed to relate to a number of abnormal conditions: women with the largest number of complications had the highest proportion of abnormal neurological children.

The topic pre- and perinatal etiological factors in children with epilepsy and other convulsive disorders was investigated in a prospective study from Denmark.[49] It showed some relationship to maternal and perinatal factors.

For children with febrile convulsions, and those with genuine and symptomatic epilepsy, maternal first trimester bleeding was increased. A tendency for toxemia and complicated deliveries was further noted among symptomatic epileptics. Furthermore, children with undefined convulsions revealed increases in maternal bleeding, pre-eclampsia, complicated delivery, asphysia, neonatal convulsions, and jaundice.

In summary, then, our introduction points out that while numerous studies have identified contributions of pre- and perinatal performance, the overall effect has been for the most part, rather small.

General Description and Methodology

A comprehensive evaluation of the relationship between maternal health during pregnancy and fetal development is possible within the framework of the Collaborative Perinatal Project.[50, 51] This is a prospective investigation of some 55,000 pregnancies with a follow-up of the children to age seven, to ascertain neurological, intellectual, physical and other developmental characteristics during the first seven years of life. While the data base is still not complete—some children are still awaiting the final seven to eight year examination this year—several comprehensive analyses have been undertaken, or are in progress. These deal with the relationship between pregnancy characteristics and complications, and developmental status, which include neurological deficits at one year and the intelligence level at four years.

In order to identify maternal characteristics, which appear to show an association with abnormal developmental findings at one year of age, a comprehensive set of cross tabulations was developed. The abnormalities in one-year-old children were classified into several mutually exclusive diagnostic categories:

specific disease states,* cerebral palsy, dyskinesia and ataxia, non-febrile seizures, hypotonia with deep tendon reflexes, delayed motor development, febrile seizures, cranial and peripheral nerve impairment, visual impairment, abnormalities of extraocular movements, nystagmus, and others.

The category, specific disease states, includes all neurological and developmental deficits obviously of a non-maternal and obstetric origin, which could be determined. The category, "others," is a catch-all of other conditions which could not be grouped conveniently under other headings.

Children whose abnormalities did not fall into any of these groups were classified as "normal." The sequence is arbitrary, based more upon a judgment of the severity of an affliction, rather than any other consideration. Certainly no insights into etiological considerations were available to guide this classification scheme. The scheme, as indicated, is mutually exclusive; thus, a child who had cerebral palsy and delayed motor development was classified as "cerebral palsy" but was not listed under "delayed motor development."

A vast set of pre- and perinatal variables were included in the tabulations. Many of these reflected maternal health status, such as: parity, gravidity, maternal age, sterility investigation, bleeding during the first, second, and third trimester, hypertension, albuminuria 2+ or more, hypertension and albuminuria, malformations of the gravida, history of seizures, motor defects, maternal mental retardation and mental illness, diabetes, low hemoglobin, anemia, organic heart disease, acute asthma, urinary tract infection, history of syphilis, convulsions in pregnancy, maternal height, weight gain during pregnancy, maternal weight, confining illnesses during the last twelve months, number of hospitalizations since last menstrual period, vomiting, fever, jaundice, and maternal smoking. The analysis was limited to blacks and whites and tabulations were produced separately for the two ethnic groups.

This chapter does not deal with all of the developmental

---

* Includes all malformations of the central nervous system, inborn errors of metabolism, and conditions which are obviously the result of catastrophic postnatal events, leading to neurological deficit.

abnormalities at one year. Several were omitted because they were infrequent, or were of traumatic origin. Therefore, dyskinesia and ataxia among blacks (only 5 cases), cranial and peripheral nerve abnormalities, visual impairment and nystagmus will not be considered further in this review.

Data was arranged for ease of comparison as in a retrospective analysis. Frequencies were tabulated for specific maternal characteristics in the various groups of abnormals at one year, and for normal children. Suggestive associations consisting of increases in these maternal characteristics among one or more groups of abnormals at one year as compared to normals, will be discussed.

Results

Maternal Health and Neurological Abnormalities at One Year

Observed increases in maternal characteristics among one or more abnormal groups were frequently not the same between whites and blacks. For discussion purposes, it may be easier to list for each specific abnormal group at one year those maternal characteristics which appear suspect.

Specific Disease States

Among blacks small increases were observed in first trimester bleeding, smoking for five years or more, parity five or more, gravidity six or more, as compared to normal (Table 16-I). For whites, there were more instances of second trimester bleeding, history of seizures, urinary tract infections, gravidity six or more, maternal age fifteen years or less, and maternal age thirty-five years or more (Table 16-II).

TABLE 16-I

(BLACKS)
PERCENT CASES AND CONTROLS WITH SELECTED
MATERNAL CHARACTERISTICS

Maternal Characteristics	Specific Disease States	Normal
	%	%
First Trimester Bleeding	14	10
Smoked 5 Years or oMre	34	26
Parity ± 5	23	19
Gravidity +6	20	16

TABLE 16-II

(WHITES)

PERCENT OF CASES AND CONTROLS WITH SELECTED
MATERNAL CHARACTERISTICS

Maternal Characteristics	*Specific Disease States* %	*Normal* %
Second Trimester Bleeding	10	4
History of Seizures	6	3
Kub Infections	11	8
Gravidity ± 6	14	10
Maternal Age — 15	4	.9
Maternal Age ± 35	11	7

Cerebral Palsy

An increased frequency of second trimester bleeding, third trimester bleeding, history of seizures, more than one illness, smoking five years or more and cigarettes smoked per day (11 or more) were found among black children with cerebral palsy as compared to controls (Table 16-III).

Among white cerebral palsy children, more frequently their mothers had smoked eleven or more cigarettes a day, had a parity of five or more, or a gravidity of six or more, than mothers of normal white children at one year (Table 16-IV). Dyskinesia and Ataxia (among white children only).

The mothers of these children had first trimester and third trimester bleeding more often, parity five or more, gravidity six or more, than mothers of normal white children (Table 16-V).

TABLE 16-III

(BLACKS)

PERCENT OF CASES AND CONTROLS WITH SELECTED
MATERNAL CHARACTERISTICS

Maternal Characteristics	*Cerebral Palsy* %	*Normal* %
Second Trimester Bleeding	10	5
Third Trimester Bleeding	17	11
History of Seizures	4	2
More Than One Illness	18	10
Smoking 5 Years or More	35	26
Cigarettes Smoked Per Day ± 11	19	9

TABLE 16-IV

(WHITES)

PERCENT OF CASES AND CONTROLS WITH SELECTED

MATERNAL CHARACTERISTICS

Maternal Characteristics	Cerebral Palsy %	Normal %
Cigarettes Smoked Per Day ± 11	33	29
Parity ± 5	19	11
Gravidity ± 6	22	10

TABLE 16-V

(WHITES)

PERCENT OF CASES AND CONTROLS WITH SELECTED

MATERNAL CHARACTERISTICS

Maternal Characteristics	Dyskinesia, Ataxia %	Normal %
First Trimester Bleeding	22	11
Third Trimester Bleeding	33	9
Parity ± 5	23	11
Gravidy ± 6	22	10

Non-Febrile Seizures

Among black chlidren with non-febrile seizure, higher rates of maternal anemia, urinary tract infections, low parity, and history of seizures were noted than among normals (Table 16-VI). Maternal history of seizures, anemia, more than one illness, and maternal age thirty-five years or more, were increased among whites with non-febrile seizures as compared to controls (Table 16-VII).

TABLE 16-VI

(BLACKS)

PERCENT OF CASES AND CONTROLS WITH SELECTED

MATERNAL CHARACTERISTICS

Maternal Characteristics	Non-Febrile Seizures %	Normal %
Anemia	36	24
Kub Infections	14	11
Parity — 1	42	32
History of Seizures	3	2

TABLE 16-VII

(WHITES)

PERCENT OF CASES AND CONTROLS WITH SELECTED
MATERNAL CHARACTERISTICS

Maternal Characteristics	Non-Febrile Seizures	Normal
	%	%
History of Seizures	10	3
Anemia	16	7
More Than One Illness	7	2
Maternal Age ± 35 Years	11	7

Hypotonia with Deep Tendon Reflexes

For blacks there were increases in second and third trimester bleeding, smoking five years or more, low parity, gravidity 6 or more, and maternal age fifteen years or younger (Table 16-VIII).

For whites, higher rates were noted in maternal first, second and third trimester bleeding, history of seizures, anemia, urinary tract infection, more than one illness, smoking five years or more, cigarettes smoked per day, eleven or more, parity five or more, gravidity six or more, and maternal age thirty-five years or older (Table 16-IX).

TABLE 16-VIII

(BLACKS)

PERCENT OF CASES AND CONTROLS WITH SELECTED
MATERNAL CHARACTERISTICS

Maternal Characteristics	Hypotonia with DTR	Normal
	%	%
Second Trimester Bleeding	10	5
Third Trimester Bleeding	24	11
Smoking 5 Years or More	30	26
Parity — 1	40	32
Gravidity ± 6	20	16
Maternal Age — 15	10	5

Delayed Motor Development

Mothers of black children with delayed motor development had more frequent first trimester bleeding, history of seizures, more than one illness, smoking five years or more, parity five or more, and gravidity six or more, than mothers of normal black children (Table 16-X).

For whites there were increases in second trimester bleeding, anemia, smoking five years or more, cigarette smoking, eleven or more per day, pariety five or more, gravidity six or more, and maternal age thirty-five or older (Table 16-XI).

TABLE 16-IX

(WHITES)

PERCENT OF CASES AND CONTROLS WITH SELECTED
MATERNAL CHARACTERISTICS

Maternal Characteristics	Hypotonia with DTR %	Normal %
First Trimester Bleeding	15	11
Second Trimester Bleeding	7	4
Third Trimester Bleeding	15	9
History of Seizures	7	3
Anemia	15	7
Kub Infections	10	8
More Than One Illness	5	2
Smoked 5 Years or More	55	41
Cigarettes Smoked Per Day + 11	34	29
Parity ± 5	15	11
Gravidity ± 6	21	10
Maternal Age ± 35	11	7

TABLE 16-X

(BLACKS)

PERCENT CASES AND CONTROLS WITH SELECTED
MATERNAL CHARACTERISTICS

Maternal Characteristics	Delayed Motor Development %	Normal %
First Trimester Bleeding	15	10
History of Seizures	5	2
More Than One Illness	14	10
Smoking 5 Years or More	32	26
Parity ± 5	28	19
Gravidity ± 6	26	16

TABLE 16-XI

(WHITES)

PERCENT CASES AND CONTROLS WITH SELECTED
MATERNAL CHARACTERISTICS

Maternal Characteristics	Delayed Motor Development %	Normal %
Second Trimester Bleeding	10	4
Anemia	12	7
Smoking 5 Years or More	49	41
Cigarettes Smoked Per Day ± 11	34	29
Parity ± 5	18	11
Gravidity ± 6	16	10
Maternal Age ± 35	12	7

Febrile Seizures

Mothers of black children with febrile seizures had more frequent history of seizures, urinary tract infections, parity five or more, gravidity six or more, maternal age fifteen or younger, and maternal age thirty-five years or older than mothers of normal black children (Table 16-XII).

For white children, maternal histories of seizures, low parity, parity five or more, and low gravidity were increased (Table 16-XIII).

TABLE 16-XII

(BLACKS)

PERCENT OF CASES AND CONTROLS WITH SELECTED
MATERNAL CHARACTERISTICS

Maternal Characteristics	Febrile Seizures %	Normal %
History of Seizures	6	2
Kub Infections	17	11
Parity ± 5	29	19
Gravidity ± 6	26	16
Maternal Age — 15	8	5
Maternal Age ± 35	9	7

TABLE 16-XIII

(WHITES)

PERCENT OF CASES AND CONTROLS WITH SELECTED
MATERNAL CHARACTERISTICS

Maternal Characteristics	Febrile Seizures %	Normal %
History of Seizures	7	3
Parity — 1	45	40
Parity ± 5	15	11
Gravidity — 1	42	38

Abnormalities of Extraocular Movements

Among black children with abnormalities of extraocular movements there were increases observed of more than one maternal illness and of low parity (Table 16-XIV). Review of the data for white children with abnormalities of extraocular movements revealed higher rates of maternal anemia and of low gravidity (Table 16-XV).

Increases in abnormal characteristics of the mother among

TABLE 16-XIV

(BLACKS)

PERCENT OF CASES AND CONTROLS WITH SELECTED
MATERNAL CHARACTERISTICS

Maternal Characteristics	*Abnormalities of Extraocular Movements*	*Normal*
	%	%
More Than One Illness	14	10
Parity — 1	42	32

TABLE 16-XV

(WHITES)

PERCENT OF CASES AND CONTROLS WITH SELECTED
MATERNAL CHARACTERISTICS

Maternal Characteristics	*Abnormalities of Extraocular Movements*	*Normal*
	%	%
Anemia	9	7
Gravidity — 1	42	38

various groups of abnormals at one year were small and not
all were statistically significant. Aside from parity, gravidity,
maternal age, and bleeding during pregnancy, actual maternal
diseases which appear suspect are history of seizures, anemia,
urinary tract infection, and more than one illness during
pregnancy.

Among blacks, maternal seizures were associated with a small
increase in cerebral palsy, delayed motor development and
febrile seizures. Among whites, the history of maternal seizures
was followed by an increase in specific disease states among one
year olds, non-febrile seizures, hypotonia with deep tendon
reflexes, and febrile seizures.

Several reports[46, 52-55] suggest an increase in malformations
among the offspring of women with epilepsy, although the debate
is unresolved as to whether the increase is the result of the
disease, epilepsy, or therapy by various anticonvulsive medica-
tions, or other maternal characteristics which may be associated
with epilepsy.

Maternal anemia among blacks was associated with an increase in non-febrile seizures in one year old children. In whites,
too, an increase in non-febrile seizures was observed among the
children of women with anemia during pregnancy. Hypotonia

with deep tendon reflexes and delayed motor development were increased also.

Maternal urinary tract infections were associated with a slightly higher rate of non-febrile seizures and febrile seizures in blacks at one year. For whites, an increase in hypotonia with deep tendon reflexes, and specific disease states, were observed at one year of age.

The presence of more than one illness in black women was followed by an increase in cerebral palsy and in hypotonia with deep tendon reflexes at one year. For white women, increases in non-febrile seizures and in hypotonia with deep tendon reflexes were noted among their one year olds.

Obviously, the relationships which we need to examine are not quite as simple as this stage of the analysis makes it appear. There are undoubtedly important interactions between maternal age, parity or gravidity, and some maternal complications. Unfortunately, additional steps in this analysis have not been completed as yet, which is why a more definite statement regarding maternal health characteristics and neurological status of one years olds cannot be made. However, more complete analysis of pregnancy characteristics in relation to IQ in four year olds are available for further consideration.

Maternal Health and Intelligence at Age Four

A recent study will be published as a monograph in the near future and includes an analysis of variables reviewed in the tabulations of maternal characteristics and neurological abnormalities at one year.[57] Variables were identified for a detailed analysis based on significant simple correlation with intelligence at four years.

Simple correlations were thus identified between IQ at four years and maternal retardation, high parity, high gravidity, low height, low maternal weight, low hemoglobin, and anemia, urinary tract infection, number of hospitalizations since last menstrual period, low weight gain and maternal age. These variables were then entered into a multiple regression analysis of prenatal variables on four years IQ's separately for four subgroups. These groups included white males, white females, black males, and black females. Only a few variables were significant, and the variance contributed by maternal characteristics was small.

For white males the multiple regression analysis showed adverse effects from high gravidity, young maternal age, urinary tract infection, and anemia on four year IQ.

For white females, significant contributions came from low hemoglobin, high parity, and maternal age (−15 years and +35 years).

For black males the multiple regression analysis revealed small effects from maternal age (−15 years), number of hypertensive blood pressures during pregnancy and low hemoglobin.

Among black females, lowered four year IQ came from variables of maternal age (−15 years), parity, convulsions during pregnancy, and low hemoglobin.

Variables identified contributing to four year IQ were: maternal age in all four groups, anemia, low hemoglobin or low hematocrit in all groups, parity or gravidity in three out of four subgroups, and urinary tract infection, number of hypertensive blood pressure readings during pregnancy, and convulsions during pregnancy in one of each of the subgroups.

Borman, et al.,[57] carried forth a discriminate analysis between low and normal IQ groups by maternal characteristics of the four subgroups, white male, white female, black male, black female. In this analysis, significant contributions came from high parity among white boys. For white females, maternal hypertension was a discriminating variable. For black males, low parity and convulsions during pregnancy were significant variables, as were low maternal weight and convulsions in black females.

Summarizing this review of data on maternal health characteristics and developmental status at one year, and intelligence at four years of age, several maternal characteristics appear suspect. Aside from maternal age and parity, others include: bleeding during pregnancy, history of seizures and the related variable convulsions during pregnancy, anemia, low hemoglobin, low hematocrit, urinary tract infection, number of hypertensive blood pressure readings during pregnancy and possibly low maternal weight, and more than one disease during pregnancy.

Several in depth studies already in the literature from the Collaborative Perinatal Project which relate to maternal health characteristics and developmental measures in children should be briefly summarized.

The subject of maternal diabetes had been researched extensively with data from several investigators.[58-60] Comparisons between children of diabetic mothers and matched non-diabetic controls, reveals a small but significant difference in four year IQ. The children of diabetic women have a lower mean IQ than the controls. Churchill and Berendes[58] step-wise evaluation of these data clearly indicates that the association between 'maternal diabetes and four year IQ was limited to maternal diabetes associated with acetonuria on one or more occasions during pregnancy. Children of women with diabetes and acetonuria when compared to controls had a mean IQ which was 10 points lower at four years.

Increases in malformations have been reported among the offspring of diabetic women from the collaborative project. Mitchell and associates observed a higher rate of congenital heart disease among children of women with diabetes, with the risk being one in thirty-nine as compared to an expected one in 121, or a three-fold increase in risk. This increase in congenital malformations of the heart was due to a significant increase in congenital defects of the great vessels. An association was also made between maternal age and congenital heart disease of the offspring. Children of women thirty-eight years or older showed a two-fold increase in risk of congenital heart disease. Chung, *et al.*,[60] described an association between maternal diabetes and the congenital malformation hypospadias.

Because of associations between IQ in four year olds and maternal diabetes with acetonuria, the subject of acetonuria in pregnancy without diabetes was pursued.[61]

Comparison of the offspring of acetone positive women with matched children of non-acetonuric mothers showed a lower mean IQ among the offspring of acetonuric mothers, even when diabetes was not present. Whether this association is due to a direct toxic effect, or the disturbance of acid base balance, or is related to a possible deficiency in nutrient supply from the mother of the fetus, remains to be clarified. Since the association between maternal acetonuria and child IQ is limited largely to acetonuria during the third trimester of pregnancy the hypothesis of nutritional impoverishment was favored.

Associations have been observed and reported from the Perinatal Project regarding maternal hypertension and proteinuria during pregnancy and intelligence in the offspring. Holley[64] noted a decrease in mean IQ to 89.6 compared to 96.8 among controls. A puzzling observation concerned the fact that the IQ difference was not observed between children of primiparous hypertensive women and their controls.

Children of women who have proteinuria to a significant degree during pregnancy without hypertension when compared with certain characteristics to control children also showed an association with four year IQ.[63]

Children of women with proteinuria had a significantly lower mean IQ at four years than their matched controls. The differences could not be explained by gestational age or low birthweight.

Comparisons of four-year intelligence in children of women born within a year of birth of a prior child and who were of gestation thirty-six weeks or greater, with children born within two to five years of a previous gestation, equal to or greater than thirty-six weeks, revealed a depressed IQ among those children born after a short between-pregnancy interval. The IQ differences were relatively modest, around 4 to 5 IQ points.[64] The conclusion of this analysis advanced the probability that the IQ differences were due in part to an increase in low birth weight among gestationally mature children. The fact that offspring of the short interval group showed a considerably higher rate of suspicious or abnormal neurological findings than their controls was quite interesting. These differences consisted of delay or impaired motor development, small head size and hyperreflexia.

Discussion

The data reported from the collaborative project, and from other recent prospective investigations, have revealed associations between several maternal health characteristics and various neurological and developmental abnormalities of childhood. In general, the findings from these investigations of diverse populations have been consistent. They attribute to maternal complications a relatively small effect on the incidence of developmental abnormalties of childhood.

These findings do not permit the conclusion that obstetrical complications are the primary cause in cases of mental retardation.[46] There is agreement on important interactions between obstetrical complications and socioeconomic factors.[42] Investigators have observed significant differences in childhood performance caused by obstetrical-maternal factors in low socioeconomic groups. Developmental abnormalities were highest in low socioeconomic groups when maternal complications were present. On the other hand, these studies agree that among higher socioeconomic classes there were little consistent differences in developmental abnormalities caused by presence or absence of adverse maternal health characteristics.

Such observations can be attributed to possible compensatory effects of a favorable postnatal environment operating among higher socioeconomic groups, and which obliterate the adverse effects of prenatal influences. Conversely, findings show that in lower socioeconomic groups, a synergistic effect exists between an unfavorable prenatal and an equally unfavorable postnatal environment on developmental abnormalities.

Regarding neurological deficits at one year, the high prevalence of low birthweight children among the cerebral palsies, is also apparent in the material from the collaborative perinatal project. In pursuing these kinds of analysis, one constantly wrestles with an appropriate classification scheme. The one used here was based on prevailing symptomatology which may hinder rather than help in the search for etiologies. There really is no satisfactory compromise between what one may call the "lumpers" or "splitters." Lumpers face the problem of ending up with too few groups but somewhat larger numbers, of rather high etiological heterogeneity. The splitters define many groups, each may have too few cases for meaningful analysis.

The preliminary associations need to be pursued by sophisticated statistical techniques which make allowance for other differences which could account for the observed association. The observations agree in part with some findings of earlier retrospective studies of neurological and mental deficits.[2, 4, 6, 7] Aside from the systematic pursuit of data analyses based on the collaborative perinatal project and similar data bases available elsewhere, there is no substitute for intelligent, alert, pursuit of clinical observations which still produce important insights as attested to by recent publications on a particular syndrome of malformations and intrauterine growth retardation in children of women with alcoholism.

REFERENCES

1. National Action to Combat Mental Retardation. The President's Panel of Mental Retardation, October 1962. Washington, D.C., U.S. Government Printing Office, 1962.
2. Lilienfeld, A. M., and Parkhurst, E.: The study of the association of factors of pregnancy and parturition with the development of cerebral palsy; a preliminary report. *Am J Hygiene, 53*:262, 1951.
3. Lilienfeld, A. M., and Pasamanick, B.: Association of maternal and fetal factors with development of epilepsy. I Abnormalities in prenatal and paranatal periods. *JAMA, 155*:719, 1954.
4. Lilienfeld, A. M., and Pasamanick, B.: The association of maternal and fetal factors with the development of cerebral palsy and epilepsy. *Am J Obstet Gynecol, 70*:93, 1955.
5. Pasamanick, B., and Lilienfeld, A. M.: Maternal and fetal factors in development of epilepsy. *Neurology, 5*:77, 1955.
6. Pasamanick, B., and Lilienfeld, A. M.: Association of maternal fetal factors with development of mental deficiency. I. Abnormalities of prenatal and paranatal periods. *JAMA, 159.155, 1955.*
7. Lilienfeld, A. M., and Pasamanick, B.: Association of maternal and fetal factors with the development of mental deficiency. II. Relationship of maternal age, birth order, previous reproductive casualty, and degree of mental deficiency. *Am J Ment Defic, 60*:557, 1956.
8. Pederson, J.: Fetal mortality in diabetic pregnancy. *Diabetes, 3*:199, 1954.
9. Rubin, H., and Murphy, D. P.: Studies in human reproduction. III. The frequency of congenital malformations in the offspring of non-diabetic individuals and diabetic individuals. *J Pediatr, 53*:579, 1958.

10. Dekaban, A. S.: Occurrence of neurological abnormalities in infants of diabetic mothers. *Neurology,* 8:195, 1958.

11. Pederson, L. M.; Tygstrup, I., and Pedersen, J.: Congenital malformations in newborn infants of diabetic women: Correlation with maternal diabetic vascular complications. *Lancet,* 1:1123.

12. Gregg, N. McA.: Congenital cataract following german measles in mother. *Trans Ophthalmol Soc* (Australia), 3:35, 1941.

13. Swan, C.: Rubella in pregnancy as an etiological factor in congenital malformations, stillbirths, miscarriages and abortions. *J Obstet Gynaecol Br Commonw,* 56:341, 1949.

14. Dekaban, A. S.; O'Rourke, J., and Cornman, J.: Abnormalities in offspring related to maternal rubella during pregnancy. *Neurology,* 8:387, 1958.

15. Feldman, H. A.: Toxoplasmosis. *Pediatric Clinics of North America,* 1:169, 1955.

16. Sever, J. L.: Perinatal infections affecting the developing fetus and newborn. In The prevention of mental retardation through control of infectious diseases. Public Health Service Publication No. 1692, Washington, D.C., U.S. Government Printing Office, 1966, pp. 37-68.

17. Sever, J., and White, L. R.: Intrauterine viral infections. *Ann Rev Med,* 19:471, 1968.

18. MacMahon, B., and McKeown, T.: The incidence of harelip and cleft palate related to birth rank and maternal age. *Am J Hum Genet,* 5:176, 1953.

19. Stark, C. R., and Mantel, M.: Effects of maternal age and birth order on the risk of mongolism and leukemia. *J of the Natl Cancer Inst,* 37:687, 1966.

20. Penrose, L. S.: *The Biology of Mental Defects.* London, Sidgwick and Jackson, 1954.

21. Stein, F.; Susser, M., and Guterman, A. V.: Screening programme for prevention of Down's Syndrome. *Lancet,* 1:305, 1973.

22. Stevenson, R. E., and Juntley, C. C.: Congenital malformations in offspring of phenylketonuric mothers. *Pediatrics,* 40:33-45, 1967.

23. Frankenburg, W. K.; Duncan, B. R.; Coffelt, D. W.; Koch, R.; Coldwell. J. G., and Son, C. S.: Maternal phenylketonuria: Implications for growth and development. *J Pediatr,* 73:560, 1968.

24. Fisch, R. O.; Doeden, D.; Lansky, L. L., and Anderson, J. A.: Maternal phenylketonuria. *Am J Dis Child,* 118:847, 1969.

25. Man, E. B., and Jones, W. S.: Thyroid function in human pregnancy. I. Incidence of maternal serum low butanol extractable iodines and of normal gestational TBG and TBPA capacities; retardation of 8 month-old infants. *Am J Obstet Gynecol,* 104:898, 1969.

26. Man, E. B.; Holden, R. H., and Jones, W. S.: Thyroid functions in human pregnancy. VII. Development and retardation of 4 year-old progeny of euthyroid and of hypothyroxinemic women. *Am J Obstet Gynecol*, 109:12, 1971.

27. Man, E. B.; Jones, W. S.; Holden, R. H., and Mellits, E. D.: Thyroid function in human pregnancy. XIII. Retardation of progency aged 7 years; relationship to maternal age and maternal thyroid function. *Am J Obstet Gynecol*, 111:905, 1971.

28. Jones, K. L.; Smith, D. W.; Ulleland, C. N., and Streissguth, A. P.: Patterns of malformations in offspring of chronic alcoholic mothers. *Lancet*, 1:1267, 1973.

29. Jones, K. L., and Smith, D. W.: The recognition of the fetal alcohol syndrome in early infancy. *Lancet*, 2:999, 1973.

30. Baird, D.: The epidemiology of prematurity. *J Pediatr*, 65:909, 1964.

31. Donnelly, J. F.; Flowers, C. E.; Creodik, R. N.; Wells, H. B.; Greenberg, B. G., and Surles, K. B.: Maternal, fetal and environmental factors in prematurity. *Am J Obstet Gynecol*, 88:918, 1964.

32. Terris, M.: The epidemiology of prematurity: Studies of specific etiologic factors. In Chapman, S. S.; Lilienfeld, A. M.; Greenberg, B. G., and Connally, J. F. (Eds.): *Research Methodology and Needs in Perinatal Studies*. Springfield, Thomas, 1966.

33. Weiss, W., and Jackson, E. C.: Maternal factors affecting birth weight. In *Perinatal Factors Affecting Human Development*. Pan American Health Organization, *Scientific Publication No. 185*:54-59, 1969.

34. Lubchenco, L. S.; Horner, F. A.; Reed, L. H.; Hix, I. E.; Metcalf, D.; Cohig, R.; Elliott, H. L., and Bourg, M.: Sequelae of premature birth. *Am J Diseases of Children*, 106:101, 1963.

35. Bergner, L., and Susser, M. W.: Low birth weight and prenatal nutrition: An interpretative review. *Pediatrics*, 46:946, 1970.

36. Stein, Z.; Susser, M.; Saenger, G., and Marolla, F.: Nutrition and mental performance. *Science*, 178:708, 1972.

37. Pitkin, R. M.; Kaminetzky, H. A.; Newton, M., and Pritchard, J. A.: Maternal nutrition—A selective review of clinical topics. *J Obstet Gynecol*, 40:773, 1972.

38. Naeye, R. L.; Blance, W., and Paul, C. H.: Maternal nutrition and the fetus. *Pediatrics*, 52:494, 1973.

39. Berendes, H. W.: The structure and scope of the collaborative study of cerebral palsy, mental retardation and other neurological and sensory disorders of infancy and childhood. In Chipman, S.; Lilienfeld, A.; Greenberg, B.; Donnelly, Jr. (Eds.): *Research Methodology and Needs in Perinatal Studies*. Springfield, Thomas, 1966.

40. Buck, C.; Gregg, R.; Stravrsky, K.; Subrahmaniam, K., and Brown, J.: The effect of single prenatal and natal complications upon the

development of children of mature birthweight. *Pediatrics, 43*:942, 1969.

41. Werner, E.; Simonian, K.; Bierman, J. M., and French, F. E.: The cumulative effect of perinatal complications and deprived environment on physical, intellectual and social development of pre-school children. *Pediatrics, 39*:490, 1967.

42. Werner, E.; Bierman, J. M., and French, F. E.: *The Children of Kauai: A Longitudinal Study from the Prenatal Period to Age Ten.* Honolulu, University of Hawaii Press, 1971.

43. Pringle, M. L.; Kelmer; Butler, N. R., and Davie, R.: *11,000 Seven Year Olds.* London, Longman, 1966.

44. Davie, R.; Butler, N. A., and Goldstein, H.: *From Birth to Seven.* London, Longman, in association with the National Children's Bureau, 1972.

45. Hardy, J. B., and Mellits, E. D.: Does maternal smoking during pregnancy have a long-term effect on the child? *Lancet, 2*:1332, 1972.

46. Birch, H. G.; Richardson. S. A.; Baird, D.; Horobin, G., and Illsley, R.: *Mental Subnormality in the Community.* Baltimore, Williams and Wilkins, 1970.

47. Henderson, N. B.; Butler, B. V., and Clark, W. M.: Contributions of selected perinatal variables to seven year psychological and achievement test scores. Paper presented at the Western Psychological Association Meeting, April 1971.

48. Prechtl, H. F. R.: Neurological Sequelae of prenatal and perinatal complications. *Br Med J, 4*:763-767, 1967.

49. Lier, L., and Zachau, Christiansen, B.: Pre- and perinatal etiological factors in children with epilepsy and other convulsive disorders. A prospective study. *Acta Paediatrica Scandinavica*, Supplement 206:27, 1970.

50. Berendes, H. W., and Weiss, W.: The NIH collaborative study. A progress report. Proceedings of the Third International Conference on Congenital Malformations, The Hague, The Netherlands, 7-13 Sept. 1969. *Excerpta Medica*, International Congress Series No. 204:293, 1969.

51. Niswander, K. R., and Gordon, M.: *The Women and Their Pregnancies.* Philadelphia, W. B. Saunders Company, 1972.

52. South, J.: Teratogenic affect of anticonvulsants. *Lancet, 2*:1154, 1972.

53. *Are Anticonvulsants Teratogenic?* Editorial. *Lancet, 2*:863, 1972.

54. Lowe, C. R.: Congenital malformations among infants born to epileptic women. *Lancet, 1*:9, 1973.

55. Loughnan, P. M.; Gold, H., and Vance, J. C.: Phenytoin teratogenicity in man. *Lancet, 1*:70, 1973.

56. Niswander, J. D., and Wertelecki, W.: Congenital malformations among offspring of epileptic women. *Lancet, 1*:1062, 1973.

57. Broman, J. H.; Nichols, P. L., and Kennedy, W. A.: Prenatal and postnatal influences on I.Q. at age four. Monograph in preparation, 1973.

58. Churchill, J. A.; Berendes, H. W., and Nemore, J.: Neuropsychological deficits in children of diabetic mothers. *Am J Obstet Gynecol, 105*:257, 1969.

59. Mitchell, S. L.; Sellman, A. H.; Westphal, M. C., and Park, J.: Etiologic correlates in a study of congenital heart disease in 56,109 births. *Am J Cardiol, 28*:653, 1971.

60. Chung, C. S., and Myrianthopoulos, N. C.: Racial and prenatal factors in major congenital malformations. *Am J Hum Genet, 20*:44, 1968.

61. Churchill, J. A., and Berendes, H. W.: Intelligence of children whose mothers had acetonuria during pregnancy. In *Perinatal Factors Affecting Human Development.* Pan American Health Organization, Washington, D.C., *Scientific Publication No. 185,* 30-35, 1969.

62. Berendes, H. W., and Churchill, J. A.: Prenatal causes of mental retardation. A report of work in progress. Presented at XII International Congress on Pediatrics in Mexico City, Dec. 1968.

63. Rosenbaum, A. L.; Churchill, J. A.; Shakhashiri, Z. A., and Moody, R. L.: Neuropsychological outcome of children whose mothers had proteinuria during pregnancy. *Obstet Gynecol, 133*:118, 1969.

64. Holley, W. L.; Rosenbaum, A. L., and Churchill, J. A.: Effect of rapid succession of pregnancy in: Perinatal Factors Affecting Human Development. Pan American Health Organization, Washington, D.C. *Scientific Publication No. 185,* 41, 1969.

Chapter 17

RESPONSE OF THE PRIMATE
FETUS TO ASPHYXIA

R. E. MYERS

INTRODUCTION

THE PRINCIPAL THREAT to the health and well-being of the fetus is intrauterine asphyxia. Although precise knowledge is lacking, other disease processes including infection or intoxication likely account for a much smaller number of fetal deaths *in utero*. Likewise, the heaviest burden of brain pathology originating during early life is caused by asphyxia and its attendant circulatory disturbances.[5] Inborn errors of metabolism and the various storage diseases account for a minor proportion of cases. Hence, studies of the broad biologic and disease-producing consequences of fetal asphyxia are of major interest.

The brain abnormalities induced by intrauterine asphyxia or by disturbances of the cerebral blood supply vary according to the gestational age of the fetus at the time of stress. This variable brain pathologic response can be illustrated with respect to the experimental occlusion of the major blood vessels supplying the brain.[11] In early fetuses, this manipulation may cause no effect; it may produce focally destructive cerebral lesions; or it may induce specific brain malformations. When focal lesions occur, they vary from zones of lobar atrophy limited in distribution to hydranencephaly where much of the entire cerebrum undergoes liquifaction and disappearance. Cerebral malformations which may appear include disturbed overall cerebral structural

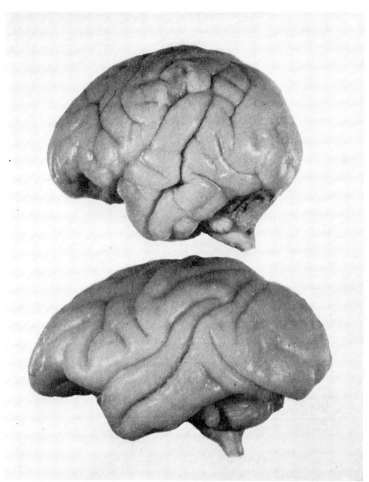

Figure 17-1. Gross cerebral malformation in the monkey caused by *in utero* ligation of both carotid arteries and jugular veins early during development. The malformation (above) consists of major alterations in the overall form of the brain and in the patterning of the cerebral convolutions. Compare to control (below).

development, altered patterning of the convolutions, and decreased cortical nerve cell populations (Fig. 17-1). Cerebral vascular occlusions or severe asphyxia during late fetal life or in the newborn, on the other hand, either cause no demonstrable changes or produce only focally destructive lesions. Distinct cerebral malformations in the sense of altered structural development without concomitant focal lesions fail to appear after injury at this stage since the cerebrum by this time has already attained its definitive form.

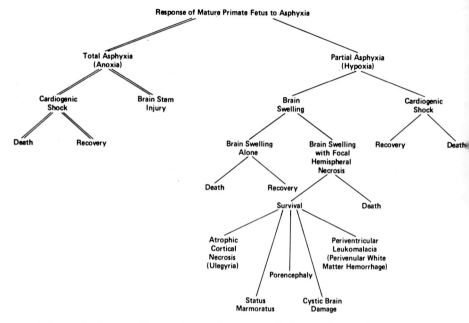

Figure 17-2. Cardiovascular and brain pathologic effects of severe fetal partial asphyxia.

Experience with human neuropathologic material also reveals distinct differences in the brain pathology of asphyxia according to whether it is sustained during earlier (22-35 weeks) or later (35-40 weeks) fetal life.[22, 23] Asphyxia of the early fetus or premature infant most commonly leads to infarction of the germinal matrix zones and intraventricular hemorrhage, while asphyxia of the mature fetus damages primarily the cerebral cortex, the hemispheral white matter, and the basal ganglia. The present discussion leaves aside the issue of cerebral malformations and their possible relation to early intrauterine asphyxia and focuses instead upon asphyxial brain injury as it affects the mature fetus. This decision is dictated by the paucity of experimental studies of asphyxially induced cerebral malformations in the primate and the fact that thus far most studies on perinatal asphyxia have been carried out on term fetuses.

The response of the mature primate fetus to asphyxia appears in Figure 17-2. As may be seen, two distinct categories of asphyxia are recognized, viz., *total* asphyxia where the interference with fetal respiratory gas exchange is complete and *partial* asphyxia where some gas exchange still remains though diminished in extent. These two types of asphyxia differ not only with respect to their circumstances of occurrence but also in their physiologic and pathologic consequences.

The response to total asphyxia was first investigated.[8, 13, 18] A term rhesus monkey fetus was delivered surgically and, prior to its first breath, a rubber sac was pulled over its head to prevent the initiation of lung breathing. The clamping of the umbilical cord then halted fetal umbilical circulation and marked the beginning of an episode of total asphyxia. Over the first 1½ minutes, the fetal arterial blood pO_2 decreased from its normal value of 28 to 35 to 4 to 6 mm Hg. This dramatic decrease in fetal oxygenation (anoxia) in turn brought about a severe respiratory and metabolic acidosis. In 10 to 15 minutes, the pH of the circulating blood decreased from its normal range of 7.28 to 7.34 to 6.70 to 6.80. The pCO_2 increased from its normal values of 38 to 45 to 120 mm Hg and higher. These marked changes in fetal blood composition were associated with dramatic alterations in the fetal blood pressure and heart rate (Fig. 17-3). The clamping of the umbilical cord by itself caused an abrupt increase in the peripheral vascular resistance and an instantaneous rise in the fetal blood pressure. After a short delay of about 20 to 30 seconds, the blood pressure begins a precipitous fall which, however, is interrupted at about sixty seconds by a second, more gradual blood pressure rise which peaks during the third minute. The early rapid blood pressure fall corresponds to the rapid fall in arterial blood oxygen partial pressure while the timing and characteristics of the subsequent gradual blood pressure rise relates it to the sympathetic nervous system stimulation and endogenous catecholamine release brought about by the asphyxia. Following this second catecholamine-stimulated peak, the blood pressure again gradually declines until it reaches tissue pressure levels. By the 10th to 12th minute, the fetal circulation ceases altogether. Thereafter, though the heart no longer accomplishes mechanical work output, it continues to generate pulses of electrical activity (ECG waveforms). The animal can be resuscitated after episodes of total asphyxia of as long as 25

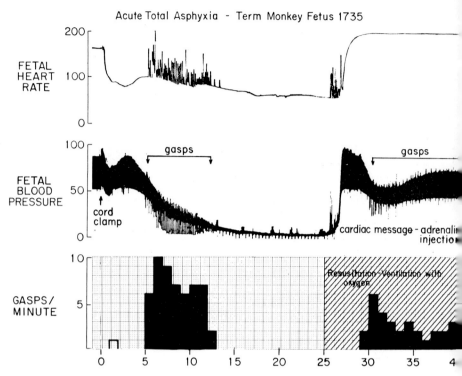

Figure 17-3. Cardiovascular changes in a term monkey fetus produced by a 25-minute episode of total asphyxia.

to 30 minutes with mechanical ventilation with oxygen, adrenalin injection and cardiac massage.

Anesthetized term monkey fetuses subjected to episodes of total asphyxia lasting less than 10 to 12 minutes fail to exhibit brain damage following resuscitation and long-term survival. Monkeys subjected to episodes of total asphyxia lasting longer than this, however, show injury to structures in the brain stem. The structure the earliest and the most severely affected is the central nucleus of the inferior colliculus (Fig. 17-4). Other structures injured somewhat later include the superior olives, the vestibular nuclei, the sensory and motor trigeminal nuclei, the posterior ventral and lateral nuclei of the thalamus, the intermediate grey matter of the spinal cord and the Purkinje cells of the cerebellum. The more prolonged the episodes of total asphyxia, the more extended the injury among these structures.

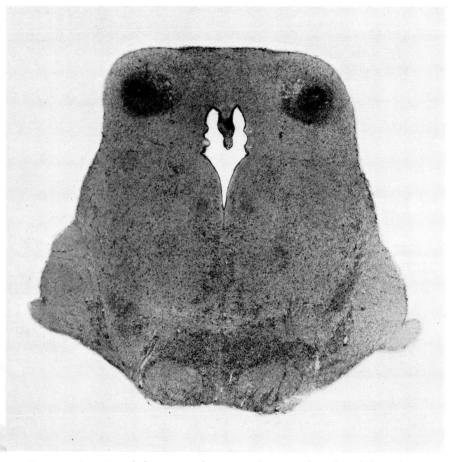

Figure 17-4. Focal destructive lesions in the central nuclei of the inferior colliculi of an immature monkey caused by a 12½-minute episode of total asphyxia at birth.

When the episodes of total asphyxia endure beyond twenty minutes, the animals uniformly exhibit cardiogenic shock following resusitation.[13] In most instances, the cardiogenic shock and its associated profound hypotension leads to death of the animal within 2 to 18 hours. Efforts at treatment, such as administration of cardioactive glycosides, the giving of plasma or whole blood transfusions, the infusion of pressor agents, are of no avail in more severe cases. In instances where the episode of total asphyxia was less prolonged and the induced cardiogenic shock less pronounced, the use of pressor agents may aid in bringing about an ultimate survival of the animal.

The predominantly brain stem pattern of injury caused by episodes of total asphyxia in the subhuman primate is commonly seen in the perinatally injured human. Rather, this pattern of injury seems more closely associated with infantile circulatory arrest in the human.[4] This paucity of human pathological material indicative of total asphyxia (anoxia) is explained by the fact that clinical circumstances which cause such rapidly developing total interruptions in respiratory gas exchange between the mother and the fetus occur only rarely in the human and, should such circumstances occur, the *in utero* status of the fetus would interfere with its recognition and relief in time to prevent fetal death in most instances.

In contrast to this, most circumstances which cause fetal asphyxia in the human are characterized by only partial impairments in respiratory gas exchange. Such obtains, for example, in most instances of abruptio placentae, placenta previa, umbilical cord wrapped around the neck, maternal circulatory or respiratory difficulties, or conditions leading to vasoconstriction in the uterine circulation of the mother. Further, the patterns of brain injury caused by subjecting term monkey fetuses to severe partial asphyxia closely resemble the patterns of injury which affect the brains of humans who survive perinatal asphyxia. Thus, the present paper assumes that human perinatal aspyhxial brain damage is caused in most instances by episodes of severe partial asphyxia (hypoxia). The remainder of the present paper will explore the response of the mature primate fetus to severe partial asphyxia.

Partial asphyxia implies some impairment in the respiratory gas exchange between the mother and the fetus. This impairment may be slight and cause only minimal alterations in the pO_2, pCO_2, and pH of the fetal arterial blood. Such a mild asphyxia causes no immediate or long-term effects even though it endures for hours. On the other hand, the partial asphyxia may be severe and approach the circumstance of total asphyxia. In this latter circumstance, the exchange of respiratory gases between the maternal and the fetal circulations may be largely halted. Between these two extremes there exists a continuum in the severity of the oxygen deprivation of the fetus.

In partial asphyxia, the impaired oxygen exchange is associated with a diminished carbon dioxide movement from the fetus to the mother so that fetal hypoxia tends to be associated with increases in the fetal CO_2 partial pressure. However, the development of hypercarbia and respiratory acidosis in the fetus may be delayed and of slight degree compared to the severity of the hypoxia. The frequent appearance of this dissociation in the behavior of the two respiratory gases during fetal asphyxia (depending upon its time course and the circumstances of its occurrence) relates to the higher diffusibility of carbon dioxide. Even so, as the severity of oxygen deprivation increases beyond certain limits (when the pO_2 of the fetal arterial blood falls below about 12 to 14 mm Hg), an acidosis of a metabolic type begins to develop and the pH of the fetal blood and tissue fluids decreases. This metabolic acidosis is caused by the impairments in fetal oxidative metabolism and the increased utilization of anaerobic pathways which give rise to significant quantities of fixed organic (lactic and pyruvic) acids. It is at this time that the pCO_2 of the fetal arterial blood shows its greatest increase when it reflects the decrease in pH of the fetal blood caused by the metabolic acidosis. Thus, the presence of a partial asphyxia of a significant degree ultimately implies, as evidence of its occurrence, diminished partial pressures of oxygen, elevated partial pressures of carbon dioxide, and increased concentrations of hydrogen ion in the fetal circulating blood.

The response of the term primate fetus to partial asphyxia of varying degrees of severity is depicted in Figure 17-5. As may be seen, the primate fetus may sustain a partial asphyxia of a considerable severity before it exhibits any alterations in vital functions or the brain shows signs of injury.[14] The fetal vital functions show their first alteration as the pO_2 of the fetal arterial blood decreases from its normal level (under anesthesia) of 28 to 30 mm Hg to 15 to 17 mm Hg (when the hemoglobin saturation with oxygen decreases from 60 to 70 percent to 25 to 35 percent or the oxygen content falls from 10 to 12 volumes percent to

NORMAL

pO₂ = 28+30mm Hg; Hgb Sat = 60-70%; O₂ content = 10-12 vol %

MILD ASPHYXIA   *(No change in vital signs)*

pO₂ = 15-16mm Hg; Hgb Sat = 25-30% O₂ = 3-4 vol %

MODERATE ASPHYXIA   *(Progressive change in vital signs)*

pO₂ = 11-12mm Hg; Hgb Sat = 12-14%; O₂ content = 0.8-1.5 vol %

SEVERE ASPHYXIA   *(Brain Damage)*

pO₂ < 6mm Hg; Hgb Sat < 10%; O₂ content < 0.5%

(Death)

TOTAL ASPHYXIA

Figure 17-5.   Cardiovascular and brain pathologic changes produced by partial asphyxia of increasing severity.

3 to 4 volumes percent). Even with beginning vital signs change, the fetus can withstand such oxygen deprivation for prolonged periods without showing signs of brain injury. As the severity of asphyxia increases still further, the fetal vital signs which have begun to change, progressively alter as the fetus shows ever greater bradycardia and hypotension.[16] Figure 17-6 depicts the relatively fixed relation between the value of the oxygen content of the fetal arterial blood (as sampled from the descending aorta) and the fetal heart rate during maternal exposure to carbon monoxide.[6] Again, severities of asphyxia sufficient to cause considerable vital signs changes can be tolerated without evidence of brain injury. Only as the asphyxial severity increases so the

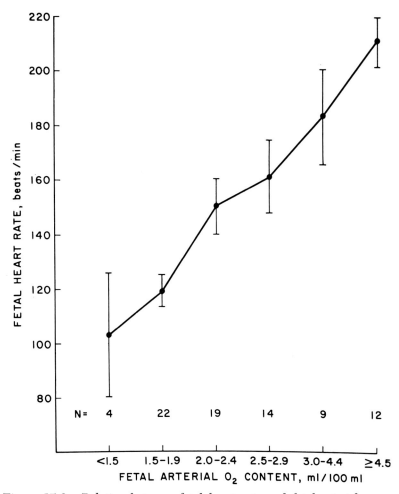

Figure 17-6.   Relation between fetal heart rate and fetal arterial oxygen content below 4.5 volumes percent during carbon monoxide exposure of the mother (after Ginsberg and Myers, 1974).

arterial pO_2 approaches 11 to 12 mm Hg (when the hemoglobin saturation with oxygen is 12 to 14 percent and the oxygen content is 0.8 to 1.5 volumes percent) does the fetus exhibit brain injury (providing the asphyxia endures for a miniumum of a half hour). Under these circumstances, the fetal heart rate decreases to 90 to 110 (normal = 200 to 240) and the mean arterial blood pressure

falls to twenty-five (normal $= 45$ to 55 mm Hg). The fetal state
with this severe an asphyxia is precarious and any further diminution in oxygen availability even of slight degree can precipitate
the rapid death of the fetus. One consequence of the slightness
of the difference in the severity of asphyxia required to produce
brain injury, on the one hand, and to produce rapid fetal death,
on the other, is that most fetuses subjected to asphyxia either
survive without evidence of brain injury or die *in utero*.

Thus, the response of the fetus to asphyxia depends on its
severity. The fetus normally tolerates asphyxia of moderate
severity even for prolonged periods. Only when the asphyxia
becomes severe do the first vital signs changes appear. An
asphyxia of still greater severity is then required to produce
brain injury.

There is both morphologic[15] and chemical[20] evidence that
severe partial asphyxia leads to brain swelling in the mature
primate fetus. Figure 17-7 depicts the brain of a term monkey
fetus subjected to three hours of severe partial asphyxia. As
may be seen, the cerebellar tonsils and vermis exhibit signs of
herniation through the foramen magnum. Small-vessel hemorrhages suffuse the zones of compressed and herniated cerebellar
tissue. Swelling of the fetal brain may also cause convolutional
flattening. Swollen brains appear pale and perfuse poorly when
saline or formalin solutions are infused under pressure into the
arterial tree at animal sacrifice. Electron microscopic studies of
the cortex of term fetuses subjected to severe partial asphyxia
show a major shift of fluid from the extracellular to the intracellular compartment resulting in a major ballooning of the
intracellular spaces.[2] When the asphyxial assault is less severe
and the swelling of the brain does not cause its softening, the
cerebral tissues show a gain in water and a loss in sodium and
potassium. The decrease in potassium reflects the migration of
potassium from the potassium-rich internal environment of the
cell to the potassium-poor fluid compartment outside the cell
under conditions of decreased oxygen availability.[1, 7] The decrease
in tissue sodium content likely is caused by the dramatic decrease
in the volume of the sodium-rich extracellular space due to water

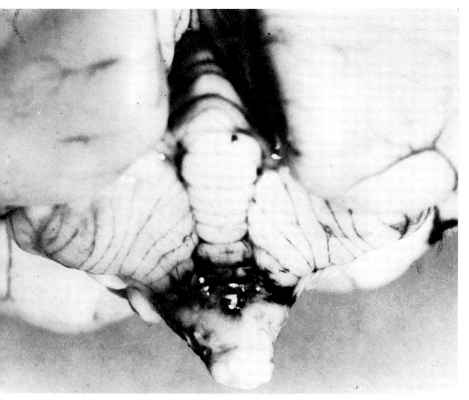

Figure 17-7. Cerebellar tonsillar and vermal herniation in a rhesus monkey newborn whose mother received excessive oxytocin infusions. Note hemorrhage into tissues which underwent compression-herniation.

movement from the extracellular to the intracellular spaces. Additionally, the decrease in cerebral blood content as it is expressed from the smaller cerebral vessels by the tissue swelling would account for some part of the total sodium loss. When the asphyxia is more extended and produces widespread cerebral necrosis or when tissue zones which show signs of necrosis are chosen for analysis, the brain swelling may lead to increases in tissue water and sodium and decreases in tissue potassium.[21] The tissue necrosis and softening causes a loss of integrity of the cell membrane and, for the first time, sodium may enter the intracellular compartment in high concentrations. Under these circumstances, the cerebral tissues show dramatic increases in their sodium contents while they continue to lose potassium.

Thus, the behavior of sodium, which may either decrease or increase during brain swelling, serves as a measure of cell membrane integrity and of tissue necrosis.

The swelling of the brain in relation to severe partial asphyxia is a primary process related directly to the diminished tissue oxygen availability. The hypoxia of the fetus is associated with a diminished energy availability to the cerebral cellular mechanisms including the sodium-potassium activated membrane ATPase. This leads to a disturbed regulation and control of ionic concentration differences between the inside and the outside of the cell. The depressed cellular energy state also in some manner leads to the release of potassium and/or sodium from their binding sites within the cell or at the cell membrane by the ammonium ion.[1] This release of the monovalent cation (or cations) from their binding sites within the cell leads to an increase in osmotic pressure, first expressed within the territory of the cell but early transmitted throughout the tissue mass and leading to an overall imbibition of fluid from the circulating blood and an increase in the mass of the cerebral tissue, i.e. to swelling of the brain.

The brain swelling may be slight or severe depending upon the asphyxial severity and duration. If the swelling is slight, an intact recovery is possible. If the swelling is of greater magnitude, it may lead to tissue necrosis. In some instances, the swelling and necrosis is focal and this generally affects specific predilection areas as, for example, the middle paracentral cortex, the posterior parietal-anterior occipital region, and the basal ganglia. In other instances, severe brain swelling causes a widespread necrosis of the entire cerebrum (see below).

The tissue necrosis with brain swelling whether focal or diffuse is due to the compression of the multitude of small vessels which permeate the tissue of the affected zones. Such small blood vessel compression by swollen tissue parenchyma leads to impairment of blood circulation through the small supplying vessels. In the final stages, blood flow stasis appears first focally and then diffusely throughout the cerebrum.[19] The stasis of flow is the final cause of parenchymal necrosis.

In those circumstances where the animals survive the asphyxial episode, the areas of tissue necrosis go on to tissue disintegration and removal with reaction of the still preserved surrounding brain tissue. The long term morphologic outcome depends upon lesion location and extent. If the tissue destruction is restricted in its distribution, the reparative processes may lead to zones of atrophic cortical sclerosis or ulegyria.[9] The affected areas (usually bilaterally and symmetrically but sometimes unilaterally) show loss of tissue mass with collapse of affected convolutions (Figs. 17-8 and 17-9). The surviving tissue in the lesion area becomes sclerotic with the development of astrocytic fibrosis.

In some instances, usually in association with atrophic cortical sclerosis, zones of destructive change and sclerosis also affect the neostriatum (the head of the caudate nucleus and the putamen). These nuclei then show reticulated zones of tissue destruction which, on long-term survival, exhibit glial sclerosis and nerve cell dropout.[9] Such damage to the basal ganglia occurs in specific types of cerebral palsy and the associated pathologic change is designated status marmoratus. An example of status marmoratus as it affects the rhesus monkey appears in Figure 17-10.

With more prolonged or severe episodes of asphyxia, the focal cortical necrosis produced may extend its boundaries beyond the restricted territories of the predilection zones to affect more widespread cerebral areas. Figure 17-11 illustrates such a circumstance as it affects both hemispheres of a Cynomolgous monkey.[17] The destruction and removal of such extended tissue areas, particularly in earlier fetuses, leads to large, punched-out defects which affect the entire thickness of the cerebral vesicular walls. These defects typically exhibit wide communications between the cavities of the ventricles and the subarachnoid spaces. This disease process, infrequent both in the human and in experimental animals, is called porencephaly.

In most instances, when the brain swelling is sufficiently severe that it causes brain injury, it leads to widespread necrosis of the cerebrum itself. Under these circumstances, the last

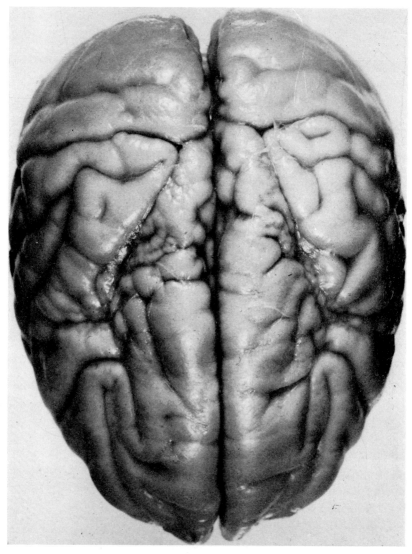

Figure 17-8. Bilateral symmetrical paracentral cortical sclerosis (ulegyria) caused by severe partial followed by total asphyxia. Note loss of tissue mass in affected areas.

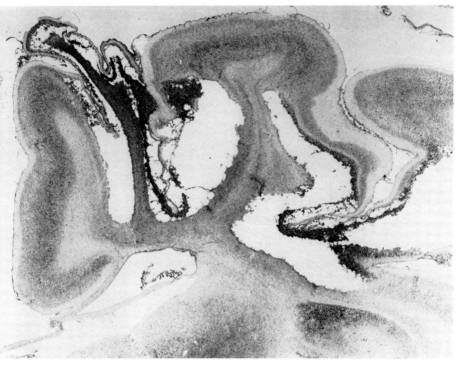

Figure 17-9. Brain appearance two weeks after severe birth asphyxia. Note the removal of necrotic grey matter tissue and the appearance of "mushroom" gyri.

structures to be affected are those located centrally and inferiorly within the hemispheres (Fig. 17-12). At the same time, the severity of asphyxia required to produce such extensive cerebral lesions also leads, in most cases, to the death of the fetus or the newborn. However, from time to time, animals sustaining such extensive cerebral injury may survive (usually when the disease process has occurred early enough during gestation that the fetus could still remain *in utero* for some days or weeks afterwards). Under these circumstances the cerebrum, which has undergone near-total necrosis, has had the opportunity to react to or to repair in varying degrees the zones of damage. With such prolonged survival, the reparative process has converted the widespread zones of cerebral infarction into areas of severe cystic degeneration.[10] Such cases are not infrequent both in

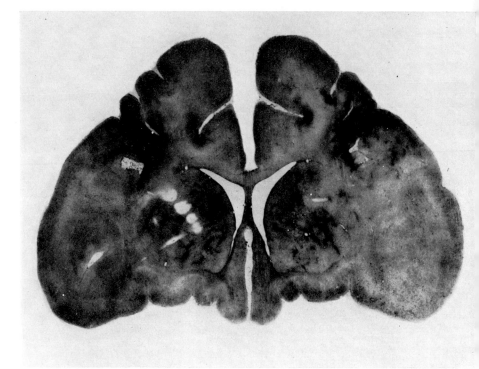

Figure 17-10. Status marmoratus of the basal ganglia associated with atrophic cortical and white matter sclerosis (Holzer stain).

monkey and human material. Two examples of severe cystic brain disease as produced by spontaneous abruptio placentae and by hypoxia of the mother appear in Figures 17-13 and 17-14 respectively.

A final type of brain injury occurs in relation to severe fetal partial asphyxia. Perivenular hemispheral white matter hemorrhage may appear in the monkey fetus or newborn in association with other types of hemispheral brain injury (brain swelling and/or focal cortical necrosis). This pathologic process preferentially affects the white matter of the prefrontal lobe and of the posterior parietal-anterior occipital region. Some cases have occurred in relation to experimentally produced severe partial asphyxia, but most have appeared in the brains of monkey fetuses dying during their gestational period of unknown causes.

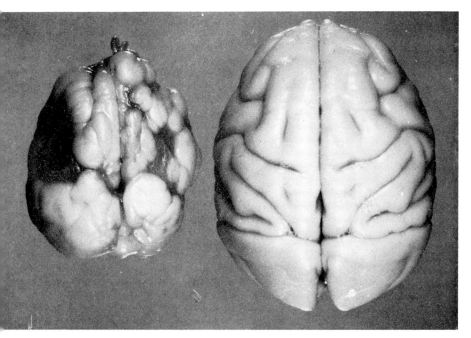

Figure 17-11. Porencephaly in a year-old monkey. The affected brain, much reduced in size compared to the control, shows bilateral symmetrical defects which consist of wide communications between the ventricles and the cortical subarachnoid spaces. The centers of these porencephalic defects correspond in their locations to the predilection areas for injury following severe partial asphyxia.

Figures 17-15 and 17-16 show two instances of hemispheral perivenular white matter hemorrhage, the first, as it affected a monkey fetus subjected to severe asphyxia by inducing fluorothane hypotension in the mother, and, the other, as it appeared in the brain of a fetus associated with an experimental abruptio placentae. Thus, perivenular white matter hemorrhage occurs naturally in the rhesus monkey and can be produced experimentally by subjecting term monkey fetuses to severe partial asphyxia. In many respects (including particularly its localization), this hemispheral white matter disease of the monkey fetus resembles periventricular leukomalacia as described in human newborns who have suffered perinatal brain damage.

The present survey has demonstrated that the patterns of

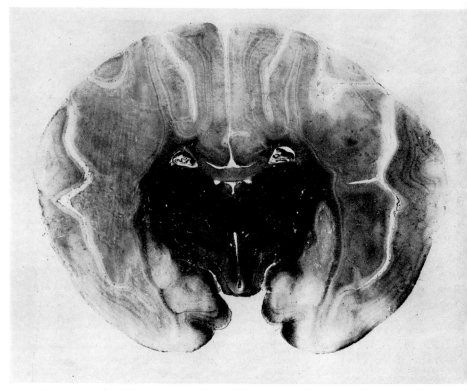

Figure 17-12.   Acute cerebral necrosis with softening affecting widespread areas of the cerebrum and causing a loss of tissue staining affinity. Note the perservation of centrally placed tissue zones which include the thalamus and portions of the hemispherical white matter. The medial aspects of the anterior temporal lobes frequently escape injury.

brain pathology produced in mature rhesus monkey fetuses by episodes of severe partial asphyxia are closely similar to the patterns of cerebral injury associated with perinatal brain damage in the human. This similarity of the experimentally produced and the naturally occurring pathologic changes associated with perinatal asphyxia makes clear that it is a severe partial asphyxia which leads to human brain injury in the vast majority of cases. Also, the circumstances used experimentally to produce partial asphyxia of the monkey fetus closely resemble the conditions which are well known as leading to perinatal brain damage in

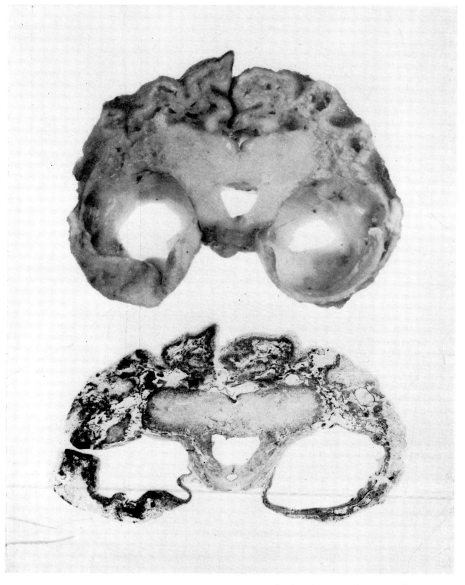

Figure 17-13. Severe cystic degeneration of the brain of a newborn caused by an abruptio placentae several weeks prior to delivery. The thalamus and basal ganglia show a coagulatory necrosis while the cortex and white matter exhibit a tissue dissolution and prominent macrophage response. Nissl-strained section (below).

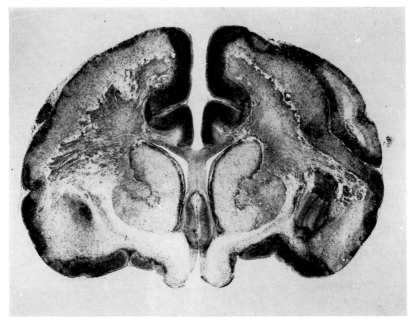

Figure 17-14. Early cystic degeneration of the brain in a six-day-old monkey which sustained severe birth asphyxia due to an experimental hypoxia of the mother.

the human. Thus, the rhesus monkey model of perinatal brain damage using partial asphyxia fits well into both the clinical circumstances which lead to its occurrence in the human and the patterns of brain pathology produced.

Severe partial asphyxia, like total asphyxia, also may cause cardiogenic shock (Fig. 17-2). Significant numbers of animals subjected to severe partial asphyxia, in addition to exhibiting brain swelling and cerebral necrosis, die in the early hours with intractible hypotension despite fully adequate support with mechanical ventilation and oxygen supplementation. Though some infants ultimately survive the shock and recover a normal blood pressure, most show an inexorable progression of the hypotension and expire within hours. This progressive hypotension is caused by an impaired heart action (a reduced myocardial contractility) rather than to decreased blood vessel tonus or to diminished peripheral vascular resistance as has been clearly

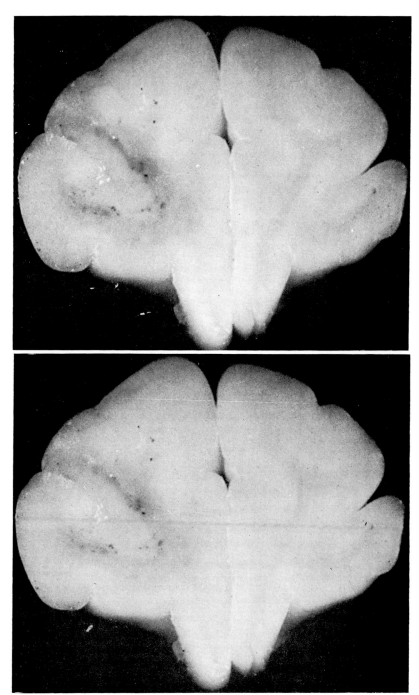

Figure 17-15. Perivenular hemorrhage in prefrontal white matter of a term monkey fetus subjected to severe partial asphyxia (maternal fluorothane hypotension—see Brann and Myers, 1974).

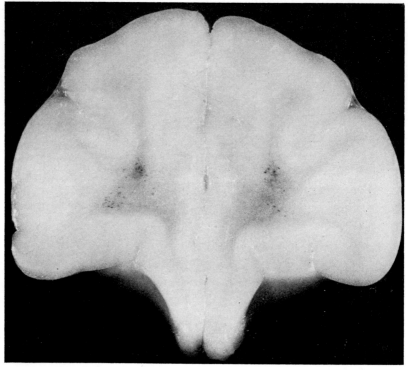

Figure 17-16. Perivenular hemorrhage in prefrontal white matter of a·
fetus subjected to an experimental abruptio placentae.

demonstrated by studies with juvenile rhesus monkeys (Kopf,
Mirvis and Myers, unpublished studies).

SUMMARY

Episodes of total asphyxia when sufficiently prolonged cause
both brain injury and death due to cardiogenic shock. The injury
to the brain with prolonged survival affects brain stem structures.
This circumstance of asphyxia is largely irrelevant to human
brain damage because of the rarity of clinical circumstances
which may cause total asphyxia but which are compatible with
fetal survival. The brain stem pattern of injury which results
from total asphyxia is almost never seen in the human except
following circulatory arrest in the infant. In contrast, to this,

severe partial asphyxia of the fetus causes primarily brain swelling and, when more severe, cardiogenic shock. As brain swelling develops, it produces a progressive narrowing of the lumina of small blood vesselsw hich permeate the affected tissue zones. The encroachment on small vessel lumina by tissue parenchymal swelling leads to progressive decreases in tissue perfusion, stasis of blood flow, and, ultimately, tissue necrosis. The tissue swelling and necrosis may be focal in distribution affecting certain predilection areas or it may become disseminated affecting the entire cerebrum. With survival, a variety of patterns of residual brain injury are described all of which have their close counterparts in the neuropathology of perinatal asphyxia in the human. These patterns of pathology produced by severe partial asphyxia include atrophic cortical sclerosis (ulegyria), status marmoratus of the basal ganglia, porencephaly, severe cystic brain degeneration, and perivenular white matter hemorrhage (periventricular leukomalacia). The occurrence of cardiogenic shock after resuscitation both with partial and total asphyxia is of major clinical significance and alone can terminate the life of the newborn subjected to asphyxia of sufficient severity or duration.

REFERENCES

1. Bito, L. Z., and Myers, R. E.: On the physiological response of the cerebral cortex to acute stress. *J Physiol, 221*:349, 1972.
2. Bondareff, W.; Myers, R. E., and Brann, A. W.: Brain extracellular space in monkey fetuses subjected to prolonged partial asphyxia. *Exp Neurol, 28*:167, 1970.
3. Brann, A. W., Jr., and Myers, R. E.: Central nervous system findings in the newborn monkey following severe *in utero* partial asphyxia. Neurology (in press).
4. Brierley, J. B.: In Proceedings of Fifth International Congress of Neuropathology, Amsterdam, Excerpta Medica International Congress Series No. 100, 1966, p. 21.
5. Freytag, E., and Lindenberg, R.: Neuropathologic findings in patients of a hospital for the mentally deficient: A study of 359 cases. *Johns Hopkins Med J, 121*:379, 1967.
6. Ginsberg, M. D., and Myers, R. E.: Fetal brain damage following maternal carbon monoxide intoxication: An experimental study. *Acta Obstet Gynec Scand,* (In press)

7. Meyer, J. S.; Kanda, T.; Shinohara, Y., and Furuuchi, Y.: Effects of anoxia on CSF/[Na] + [K] +. *Neurology, 21*:889, 1971.

8. Myers, R. E.: The clinical and pathological effects of asphyxiation in fetal rhesus monkey. In Adamsons, K. (Ed.): *Diagnosis and Treatment of Fetal Disorders*. New York, Springer-Verlag, 1969, pp. 226-249.

9. Myers, R. E.: Atrophic cortical sclerosis associated with status marmoratus in a perinatally damaged monkey. *Neurology, 19*:1177, 1969.

10. Myers, R. E.: Cystic brain alteration after incomplete placental abruption in monkey. *Arch Neurol, 21*:133, 1969.

11. Myers, R. E.: Brain pathology following fetal vascular occlusion: An experimental study. *Invest Ophthalmol, 8*:41, 1969.

12. Myers, R. E.: Conditions leading to perinatal brain damage in the non-human primate. In Crosignani, P. G., and Pardi, G. (Eds.): *Fetal Evaluation During Pregnancy and Labor: Experimental and Clinical Aspects*. New York, Academic Press, 1971, pp. 175-195.

13. Myers. R. E.: Two patterns of perinatal brain damage and their conditions of occurrence. *Am J Obstet Gynecol, 112*:246, 1972.

14. Myers, R. E.: Threshold values of oxygen deficiency leading to cardiovascular and brain pathological changes in term rhesus monkeys. In *International Symposium on Oxygen Transport to Tissue*. New York, Plenum Publishing Corp., pp. 1047-1053.

15. Myers, R. E.; Beard, R., and Adamsons, K.: Brain swelling in the newborn rhesus monkey following prolonged partial asphyxia. *Neurology, 19*:1012, 1969.

16. Myers, R. E.; Mueller-Heubach, E., and Adamsons, K.: Predictability of the state of fetal oxygenation from quantitative analysis of components of late deceleration. *Am J Obstet Gynecol, 115*:1083, 1973.

17. Myers, R. E.; Valerio, M. G.; Martin, D. P., and Nelson, K.: Perinatal brain damage: Porencephaly in a Cynomolgous monkey. *Biol Neonate, 22*:253, 1973.

18. Ranck, J. B., and Windle, W. F.: Brain damage in the monkey Macaca mulatta, by asphyxia neonatorum. *Exp Neurol, 1*:130, 1959.

19. Reivich, M.; Brann, Jr., A. W.; Shapiro, H., and Myers, R. E.: Regional cerebral blood flow during prolonged partial asphyxia. In Meyer, J. S.; Reivich, M.; Lechner, H., and Eichorn, O. (Eds.): *Research on the Cerebral Circulation, Fifth International Salzburg Conference*. Springfield, Thomas, 1972, pp. 216-227.

20. Selzer, M. E.; Myers, R. E., and Holstein, S. B.: Prolonged partial asphyxia: Effects on fetal brain water and electrolytes. *Neurology, 22*:732, 1972.

21. Selzer, M. E.; Myers, R. E., and Holstein, S. B.: Unilateral asphyxial brain damage produced by venous perfusion of one carotid artery. *Neurology*, 23:150, 1973.
22. Towbin, A.: Cerebral intraventricular hemorrhage and subependymal matrix infarction in the fetus and premature newborn. *Am J Pathol*, 52:121, 1968.
23. Towbin, A.: Central nervous sytem damage in the human fetus and newborn infant. *Dis Child*, 119:529, 1970.

INDEX

347